T. EDWARD COLLINS, D.O.

a clinician's view
of neuromuscular diseases
SECOND EDITION

a clinician's view of neuromuscular diseases

SECOND EDITION

Michael H. Brooke, M.D.

Professor of Neurology and Director,
Jerry Lewis Neuromuscular Research Center
Washington University
School of Medicine
St. Louis, Missouri

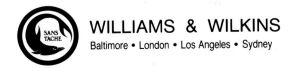

WILLIAMS & WILKINS
Baltimore • London • Los Angeles • Sydney

Editor: Nancy McSherry-Collins
Associate Editor: Victoria M. Vaughn
Copy Editor: William Vinck
Design: Bert Smith
Illustration Planning: Reginald R. Stanley
Production: Raymond E. Reter

Copyright ©, 1986
Williams & Wilkins
428 East Preston Street
Baltimore, MD 21202, U.S.A.

Accurate indications, adverse reactions, and dosage schedules for drugs are provided in this book, but it is possible that they may change. The reader is urged to review the package information data of the manufacturers of the medications mentioned.

Made in the United States of America

First Edition 1977

Library of Congress Cataloging in Publication Data

Main entry under title:

Brooke, Michael H., 1934-
   A clinician's view of neuromuscular diseases.

   Includes bibliographies and index.
   1. Neuromuscular diseases.   I. Title. [DNLM:
1. Neuromuscular Diseases. WE 550 B872c]
RC925.B76 1986   616.7′4   85-12452
ISBN 0-683-01064-6

Composed and printed at the
Waverly Press, Inc.

86 87 88 89 90
10 9 8 7 6 5 4 3 2 1

preface to the second edition

Almost a decade has passed since the publication of the first edition of this book. Age leaves its mark on books as it does on us all. This one has become a little stouter and has taken up exercise, albeit as a topic. I would like to believe that age has improved it. Those truths which have endured over the last ten years are reaffirmed in the present book in the confidence that they will probably endure for the next ten. Other paragraphs whose absurdities have become all too evident have been omitted. Ideas are a little like friends, some prove to be constant, unchanging and always helpful; others prove to be as embarrassing as an aquaintance who inhales soup or is revealed as an axe murderer. Only the reader can judge an author's ability to tell the two apart.

The first edition provoked some interesting correspondence. I received many letters from clinicians who extolled the book, not because they learned anything new, but because in the reading of it they found a kinship with their own experience. "You have put into words what happens in every Tuesday clinic," wrote one. Others were less enthusiastic and suspected that I had plumbed their minds and stolen their ideas. "I have always taught that to the residents and you gave me no credit," complained another about some clinical sign. I was equally flattered by both comments. What the book tried to express was the commonality of all our experiences in the treatment of neuromuscular diseases. Both writers recognize that we shared those experiences. The common chord was struck.

I hope to have retained this flavor in the present edition but it is the more difficult because the descriptive era in neuromuscular diseases has passed. The tide of basic science which is washing across our specialty is uncovering new and more fascinating entities. The present edition reflects this change. I know people with Duchenne muscular dystrophy and I can write about them with affection. It is hard to strike up a conversation with ATP or feel anything but threatened by HLA antigens. Nevertheless, the new entities which I have tried to describe in this book are not solely anomalies in biochemistry or immunology. They are people. Unless the clinician trains himself to remember that, medicine will be the poorer, and science barren. Mutatis, mutandur.

M.H.B.

v

preface to the first edition

This book will be prefaced by an apology, although probably not that which many will demand. It is a short work and will disappoint those who expect an encyclopedic compendium. Such tomes are often accompanied by so large a price that they are a luxury not to be afforded by the average physician with a peripheral interest in the subject. This book is aimed at the neurologist, pediatrician, orthopedist, and general practitioner who are aware that a bewildering array of neuromuscular diseases has surfaced in the last few decades unaccompanied by a simple text to describe them.

My own prejudices, carefully nurtured over a period of years, are here displayed for all to see. I have tried to identify such idiosyncrasies when appropriate but I do not apologize for them. They have been garnered during the time spent caring for patients with muscle diseases and I am reluctant to abandon them. A book is after all a personal thing. It is also delicate and the impassive citation of contradictory articles or the recitation of 200 rare but possible complications of a given disease can wilt it. I have chosen to emphasize some aspects of the illnesses and to ignore others. Such selectivity is not without purpose, reflecting the amount of time spent discussing the various topics in my own clinic and the frequency with which certain questions are asked.

My approach to the bibliography may appear capricious. I have often not quoted the original article, and those whose pioneer work is recognized in dozens of other texts may not necessarily find themselves in this one. Whenever possible I have tried to list the most recent references in the hope that interested readers will consult their bibliographies and begin that backward chase in the literature which will culminate in the discovery of the original sources. In areas which have been subject to much recent research or change I have tried to include a complete list of references. In other areas, where knowledge has progressed not in leaps but in a shuffle, the bibliography is less complete.

Of all these shortcomings I am unrepentant. The substance of my apology is of an entirely different matter. I was raised in a country where style was thought more important than substance; even, harsher critics may say, to the point of supplanting it on occasions. I was determined to write a literate book. Regrettably I failed. I found myself tainted by jargon, cliche, and tautology in a most inexcusable fashion. Inappropriate gerunds jostled with split infinitives. Weakness existed, not in isolation, but had to be "significant" or, even worse, "motor." Tenses mixed more readily than tonic water and the proper use of the comma eluded me, totally. The sentences which failed to contain the word "however" were all prefaced by "although." In short, it had all the characteristics of a standard medical text. Thanks to the unflagging efforts of the copy editor, the damage done to the English language has been healed but my literary style remains moribund.

And so, to our predecessors who felt that men of science were necessarily men of letters, to those whose clinical descriptions sparkled from the early texts so that in the reading of them one glimpsed the patient himself, to those whose letters to the editor made medical journals prior to 1920 so much less dusty than their recent counterparts—my apologies.

M.H.B.

acknowledgments

I would like to acknowledge the support of the Muscular Dystrophy Association. Those of us who work in their clinics or attend their summer camps have found that the MDA is more than just a source of research funds. I would also like to thank Kathy Brenner and Charlie Harper for their secretarial help. Like the good secretaries that they are, they took the blame for disasters that were entirely my fault and never once reminded me of it. I would also like to thank Dennis Duck whose helping hand was invaluable.

contents

1 the symptoms and signs of neuromuscular diseases

*Please listen to the patient, he's trying
to tell you what disease he has*

THE SYMPTOMS

If often seems that the urgency with which physicians rush their patients off for laboratory studies has its historical equal only in the migration of lemmings or the precipitous rush of the Gadarene swine. I sometimes suspect that students entering medical school are issued with a pamphlet entitled "How to Employ Your Time Usefully While the Patient Is Giving His History." It unnerves me when a physician misses the classical history of myasthenia because he is busy filling out requests for laboratory tests which will cost the patient a month's wages. Perhaps these feelings are unwarranted, but the exercise of diagnosing a patient's illness from his own words is a rewarding one and worth a few comments.

The way in which the history is obtained from a patient with neuromuscular disease is no whit different from the method used in any other illness. The symptoms may be different but the principles are identical. As each symptom is given, it should be pursued with a dogged tenacity until all the details are known. Thus, inquiry is made into the duration of the symptom, whether it is constant or intermittent, exacerbating or relieving factors, whether or not there are associated symptoms (such as pain), the effect of medications, and whether the symptom is progressing or diminishing.

In general, the symptoms of neuromuscular illnesses are those of weakness. However, the English language is on occasion an inexact form of communication. The statement that certain muscles are "weak" should not be accepted at face value. Indeed, patients often use the words "weak," "numb," and "tired" interchangeably. Some patients with a dense sensory loss complain that their legs are "weak." Equally, people with a marked motor disturbance may use the word "numb" for this loss of power. Any patient who complains of weakness must be pressed to describe the fashion in which the weakness affects him and what tasks he finds difficult.

It should be possible after obtaining the history of a patient with neuromuscular disease to predict with some accuracy which muscle groups are weak. When muscle strength is lost, the resulting symptoms depend more upon the muscle groups involved than upon the type of disease that causes the weakness. A patient who has a peripheral neuropathy may have the same

1

difficulty with hand movement as one whose weakness is due to a distal myopathy. Thus, from the patient's own description of his disease one will be able to say where the weakness is, but perhaps not what the disease is.

Much of what follows is self-evident, but the frequency with which these complaints occur in patients with neuromuscular disease and the infrequency with which hysterical patients manifest these symptoms make it worthwhile to catalog them.

Head and Neck

When the muscles of the head and neck are weak, clear-cut difficulties occur. Weakness of the upper eyelids may be noticed by the patient who may complain that they are drooping. On the other hand, this is not always the case and one patient with a moderate degree of ptosis presented with the complaint that her head was falling backwards. In an attempt to peer from under her ptotic lids she would hold her chin tilted upwards, the very image of the proverbial haughty dowager.

Weakness of the extraocular muscles is noted initially as blurring of vision and ultimately as diplopia. Since diplopia is not infrequently seen as a hysterical complaint, it is wise to ask whether the patient has discovered any maneuvers which improve the double vision. Those with diplopia due to extraocular weakness will usually state that if they cover one eye the diplopia disappears. By and large, this fact is unknown to the hysteric and although there are many causes of monocular diplopia, from lesions of the occipital lobe to abnormalities of the retina and cornea, the history of monocular diplopia must be regarded with some suspicion.

Weakness of the masseter and temporalis muscles is noted as a difficulty in chewing. Although the chewing of any food may be impaired, it is usually steak or other meat which causes the first symptoms. Occasionally the jaw weakness may be so severe as to give rise to the complaint that the jaw sags and the mouth opens uncontrollably.

Weakness of the facial muscles produces several characteristic difficulties. When severe, the face is expressionless, the mouth is unsmiling, and, when the patient sleeps, his eyes are open, only the whites showing between the unclosed lids. In a moderate degree of facial weakness the smile may have the appearance of a rather unpleasant snarl which is embarrassing to the patient. Ordinarily in smiling and laughing the orbicularis oris keeps the lips inverted in the nature of a purse string. In facial weakness the lips are allowed to evert. This snarling appearance may be so distrubing that the mouth is reflexly hidden behind the hand whenever the patient laughs. Other tasks that are impeded by facial weakness are whistling, drinking through a straw, and blowing up a balloon. All of these functions may be impaired in patients who have no idea that their face is at all weak. Patients presenting in middle age with facioscapulohumeral dystrophy who state that their disease began 2 or 3 years ago often admit on direct questioning that they have never been able to whistle with the lips pursed. This is not regarded by the patient as an abnormality, but as more of an idiosyncrasy.

It is not easy to get a clear history of speech abnormality from most patients. The abnormalities of speech are quite characteristic when one hears the patient talk, but it is often difficult to distinguish a spastic dysarthria from that due to palatal weakness on the basis of the history. Difficulty with swallowing, however, is usually well described. Patients with palatal weakness and weakness of the pharynx due to lower motor neuron disease or to a myopathy frequently complain of choking. They have more difficult swallowing liquids than solids, although both may present a problem, and they may suffer the regurgitation of fluids through the nose; the last symptom is less likely to occur with bilateral upper motor neuron disease (pseudobulbar palsy). With upper motor neuron lesions, there is a difficulty with the initiation of swallowing and often liquids will be aspirated into the trachea producing a coughing and choking spell.

Dysphagia is frequent enough in the hysteric and the symptoms are so similar in different patients that the term "globus hystericus" has been given to it. This symptom is usually associated with solid food; the patient has the sensation of a large ball of food which sticks in the back of the throat and will not go down or will descend part way to be lodged behind the larynx. This hysterical ball may last for hours and may be painful; nasal reflux and aspiration are not hallmarks of hysteria.

Other abnormalities of swallowing are produced by disturbance of esophageal function. The causes are varied and range from diseases of the esophagus such as scleroderma to compression by malignant lymph nodes. The patient often complains of a sensation of food sticking retrosternally. Unfortunately, the hysteric may complain of the same thing and it is difficult to distinguish this clinically.

Weakness of the neck muscles again produces difficulty in a characteristic situation. This is most striking when the patient is riding in a car or a bus. With sharp acceleration or braking, the strength of the neck muscles is not sufficient to counteract the inertia of the head and the head will snap uncontrollably backwards and forwards. This can be very disconcerting, and most patient with significant neck weakness give this history upon questioning. Neck weakness may give rise to problems in more bucolic situations, as illustrated by a man with weakness of the posterior muscles of the neck who was tending his rosebushes. As he bent forward from the waist to pluck one of the blossoms, his head fell onto his chest and he was unable to lift it again.

Limbs and Trunk

Weakness of the muscles of the limbs and trunk gives roughly four sets of symptoms: those associated with weakness of the shoulders, of the hands and forearms, of the hips and thighs, and of the lower legs.

Weakness of the shoulders is first noticed in performing tasks with the arms above the head: the housewife has difficulty lifting plates down from a high shelf; a carpenter complains that hammering nails into a beam which is over his head is becoming impossible. A more severe degree of difficulty may give problems with much simpler tasks. Thus, a man may have to use both hands to hold his razor while shaving or a patient may not be able to comb her hair without resting her elbows on a table and bringing her head down to a lower level. Patients may also complain that they have to "throw" their arms in order to get their hands onto a shelf at shoulder height. This throwing motion is a truncal movement which results in the arm being flung upwards; the hand then catches the desired spot and pulls the arm up onto the shelf. Another maneuver which patients often discover for themselves is to place the hand on the wall and, by using the fingers, to "creep" the hand up the wall, thus elevating the arm.

Weakness of the muscles of the hands and forearms gives rise to difficulty opening the screw cap tops on jars or opening door handles, particularly of the door knob type. Additionally, car door handles may present a problem. Occasionally very specific disabilities may occur with hand weakness. One lady's chief complaint was that she could not reach behind her back and undo her brassiere. Her abnormality was a median nerve palsy with weakness of the abductors of the thumb and of the opponens muscle.

Most are familiar with the symptoms associated with hip weakness. With mild hip weakness the patient runs poorly and in an ungainly fashion. He is unable to jump and, as the weakness becomes more severe, he cannot easily get up from a sitting position on the floor and may have difficulty climbing stairs or arising from a chair. In arising from the floor patients will mention that they have to pull themselves up on a nearby chair or use their hands to support their knees. They may suddenly grow to dislike a favorite arm chair because it is low enough to present difficulties in arising from it. In trying to stand they have to push themselves up with their hands on the arms of the chair. Often they will prefer to sit on a kitchen chair and then, eventually, a high stool to allow them to stand up using the minimum amount of muscle effort. Climbing stairs always presents a problem to the patient with hip and thigh weakness. Some will find it necessary to hang onto the banister to pull themselves up the stairs or to support the thigh with one hand while ascending. Others will turn sideways and, keeping the knees stiff, will climb the stairs crabwise, while supporting their weight with both hands on the rail. Interestingly, patients with thigh weakness have more difficulty coming down stairs than they do going up. As one foot descends to the lower step, the opposite quadriceps must take up the strain of the bent knee and support the entire body weight until the foot rests on the lower step. In those with quadriceps weakness there is a tendency for the knee to give way and collapse, causing the patient to fall the rest of the way down the stairs. This quadriceps weakness also may cause the patient to fall if he is jostled in a crowd. An unusual gait is that of children with severe hip abductor weakness whose quadriceps is relatively spared. They will walk with the knees locked together for support and slightly bent. Superficially this resembles the walk of a spastic child; closer inspection shows that the apposed knees are continuously braced against each other as the adductors of the opposite leg fill the role of the missing abductors.

It is important to distinguish the symptoms listed above from those which are seen in hysterical weakness. I try to avoid the use of leading questions while taking a history and, if a patient complains of weakness and does not spontaneously volunteer the information with regard to stairs and chairs, I will ask whether he has any difficulty with common objects around the house. If this does not elicit the history above, I will ask about difficulty with chairs or with stairs. The patient with real weakness immediately seizes upon this and provides the appropriate complaint. The patient with imagined weakness is still not clear as to the direction of the inquiry. Finally, when pressed to give specific details of their difficulty in getting out of a chair, patients with hysterical weakness will often say that they are just too tired and they cannot get out of the chair. When asked about climbing stairs they usually admit to climbing two or three, after which effort they must rest. Seldom do they experience the difficulties listed in the previous paragraphs.

Weakness of the calf muscles and the anterior tibial group of muscles leads to problems while walking. Weakness of the evertors and dorsiflexors of the foot causes the patient to lift his knee high in the air, and the gait may have a noticeable slapping quality. When the weakness is not so severe, the patient may complain only that he sprains his ankles very easily and that he finds it difficult to walk over a pebbled surface or a cobblestone street. This is due to the fact that, if he steps on a pebble with the medial side of the foot, the foot is inverted and the weight of the body acts to accentuate this inversion. The evertor muscles are too weak to correct the movement; the foot is twisted and the ankle sprained. One of my patients, when asked about walking over rough or uneven surfaces, told me that he thought he would trip over a cigarette paper were it in his path. Patients with such anterior tibial and peroneal weakness also catch their toes on curbs as they step over them. This may cause them to trip and fall. One interesting aspect of anterior tibial weakness is the problem which occurs in standing up from a sitting position. In order to stand up from a chair, the feet have to be dorsiflexed. If a patient is sitting in a chair with the knees at 90° and the feet firmly on the floor, the initial movement in getting out of the chair is a dorsiflexion of the feet. If you wish to prove this for yourself, sit in a chair with your hands over the anterior tibial muscles and feel them contract as you start to arise from the chair.

Weakness of the muscles of the calf will result in a loss of the "spring" to the step, which assumes a "flat footed" character, and, of course, the patient has difficulty standing on his toes.

THE SIGNS

The physical examination of patients with neuromuscular disease often perplexes those who are unfamiliar with these illnesses. Such perplexity is unnecessary since the examination is basically very simple. There are four aspects to it: inspection, palpation, examination of reflexes, and evaluation of muscle strength. It is also convenient to take the various parts of the body in sequence. The head and neck, the shoulders, the arms, the torso, the hips, and the legs are all examined separately. If one does this conscientiously, it is difficult to miss significant findings.

Inspection

Inspection of the muscles reveals the presence or absence of wasting as well as the occurrence of any spontaneous movements such as fasciculations or myokymia. Weakness of muscles also alters a patient's resting posture in some quite characteristic fashions. These postural alterations are often far more helpful in determining the extent of weakness than is the more formal evaluation of strength.

Examination of the muscles of the head and neck may reveal ptosis (Figs.

1.1 and 1.2). With ptosis of moderate degree the affected lid or lids will be obviously droopy and part of the iris will be covered. Ptosis may be so severe that the lid covers the pupil, making vision impossible in any direction other than downard. The patient must then retroflex the neck in order to see straight ahead. In a mild ptosis, the lower border of the affected eyelid may actually be at the same level with regard to the iris as the normal side. This is due to an elevation of the eyebrow, which hoists the ptotic lid upward. Such compensatory elevation of the eyebrow may be suspected when there is an increase in the number of forehead creases on the abnormal side. In such a case, when the forehead is smoothed out by the examiner's hand and the eyebrows are at the same level, the ptosis will become apparent. Hysterical ptosis is one of the easiest diagnoses to make from inspection. Because the upper lid cannot voluntarily be closed without the lower lid being raised at the same time, the patient with a hysterical ptosis always has a contraction of the lower lid. In other extraocular weaknesses the axes of the eyes may no longer be parallel and esotropia or exotropia may be noted.

Wasting of the temporalis muscles gives a hollowing of the temples and when it is associated with masseter atrophy imparts a cadaveric appearance. Severe weakness of the masseter muscles, such as is seen occasionally in myasthenia gravis, causes the jaw to open spontaneously. The patient counteracts this by supporting the jaw with one hand. The sight of a patient with his arm adducted and elbow flexed, propping the jaw on a table formed by the knuckles of his hand, is a characteristic and unmistakable one.

A large part of our communication with others is expedited by the play of emotion over our facial muscles. It is not surprising that weakness of these muscles is easily perceived. Although mild facial weakness may not be noticeable at rest, when the patient smiles or laughs the normally pleasant expression may be converted to a snarl. Spontaneous eye closure is frequently

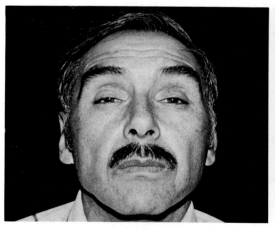 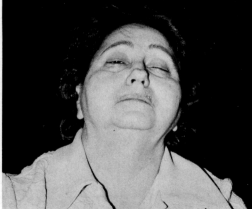

Figure 1.1 (*left*).   Ptosis. Notice the compensatory elevation of eyebrows with consequent wrinkling of the forehead. Oculopharyngeal dystrophy.

Figure 1.2 (*right*).   Ptosis. The head is retroflexed, allowing the patient to see from under her ptotic lids. This woman also has compensatory elevation of the eyebrows; she is keeping her left eye closed because of the diplopia from which she suffers. Myasthenia gravis.

incomplete and, when the patient blinks, the lids move slowly and without fully closing the eyes (Fig. 1.3). Sometimes facial weakness may be detected by having the patient open his mouth. During this maneuver the normal activity of the facial muscles causes an elevation of the upper lip. If there is facial weakness, particularly unilateral facial weakness, the elevation of the upper lip is lacking. This results in a flattening of the upper border of the "cupid's bow," that area of the upper lip to which lipstick is applied. Severe weakness wipes the face clean of all expression: the skin is smooth and unwrinkled, and the mouth with its downturned corners lends an unusually mournful cast to an immobile mask.

Although one of the characteristic signs of facial weakness is the "bouche de tapir"—the tapir's mouth—in which the lips are protruded in unconscious mimicry of the animal, my experience has been that facial weakness is more easily noticed when viewed full face, because the lips have a flat, two-dimensional appearance. Instead of showing the normal curve, they look like two opposed rectangles. There is a classical neurological dogma that, if the muscles of the forehead are spared the weakness affecting the rest of the face, the lesion is of the upper motor neuron. Oddly, in neuromuscular diseases, there are many exceptions to this rule.

Weakness of the palate may be difficult to see, although on occasion it hangs limp and unmoving. It is usually noted while listening to the patient talk. Although this section is devoted to inspection of the patient, it seems a convenient place to discuss abnormalities of speech. In lower motor neuron lesions involving the palate, the voice has an echoing, nasal quality, rather like that associated with a cleft palate. The vowels become hollow and the consonants, particularly such guttural sounds as the hard "G" and "C," are difficult to pronounce. Facial weakness will, of course, also give rise to speech

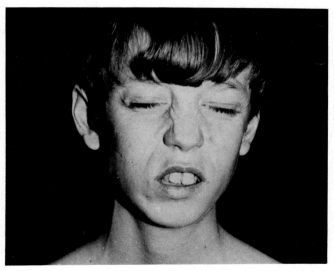

Figure 1.3. Facial weakness. Attempted eye closure does not result in complete occlusion of the palpebral fissure. The eyelashes are still visible and not buried within the tightly closed lids. Inflammatory myopathy with IgA deficiency.

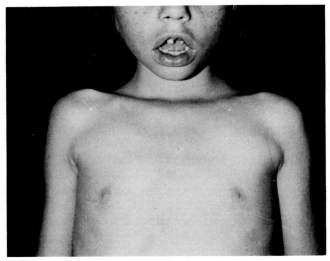

Figure 1.4. Neck and shoulder weakness. The clavicles form a "step" at the base of the neck. Infantile facioscapulohumeral dystrophy.

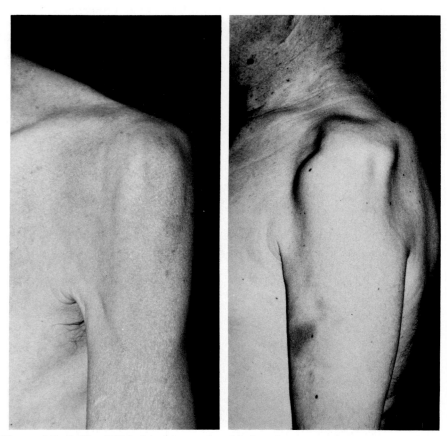

Figure 1.5 (*left*). Mild deltoid atrophy. Notice the stranded appearance of the underlying muscle, giving the appearance of ridges and hollows as one looks at the skin in oblique light. Motor neuron disease.
Figure 1.6 (*right*). Severe shoulder girdle atrophy. Motor neuron disease.

abnormalities, but in this case the difficulty lies in the plosive sounds such as "P" and "B." Two other abnormalities of speech, although not due to palatal weakness, should be easily recognized. Spastic speech, that associated with pseudobulbar palsy (bilateral upper neuron lesions), has a forced quality. The voice sounds strained and monotonous. One perceives a sense of great effort on the part of the patient as he attempts to force words out through a reluctant musculature. On the other hand, speech associated with cerebellar difficulties is quite different. Here the speech is broken up and disjointed, sometimes described as "scanning." When the patient is asked to say test phrases, such as "liquid electricity" or "methodist episcopal," not only are the syllables disjointed, but the emphasis occurs on the wrong ones. Indeed, the whole manner of speech is as irregular and ataxic as is the violent intention tremor associated with lesions of the cerebellum. Laryngeal weakness may be noticed as a hoarseness of the voice with a rasping, brassy quality. A useful test of laryngeal function is to listen for the glottal stop. Ordinarily, when one coughs there is a small click at the beginning. This click is the same sound that is produced when the phrase "sofa and chair" is pronounced correctly. It occurs between the word "sofa" and the word "and." It may disappear in those of us with slovenly speech habits, in which case an "R" is substituted, as in "sofa-r-and chair." In laryngeal weakness, when the patient is asked to cough, the initial glottal stop may be lost, the cough then resembling that of a dog in which the glottal stop is frequently not present.

Wasting of the sternocleidomastoids and of the trapezius is fairly easily noticed. When wasting of the sternocleidomastoids and the anterior neck muscles becomes marked, there is an odd appearance to the clavicles, which jut out in front of the wasted muscles (Fig. 1.4). Wasting of the tongue is

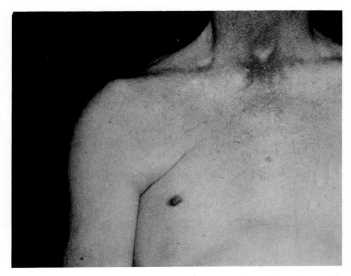

Figure 1.7. Shoulder weakness. The deep crease running from the axilla obliquely toward the neck is an indication of shoulder weakness with underlying pectoral atrophy. Limb girdle dystrophy.

often hard to see but when present the tongue may become characteristically wrinkled or scalloped, especially at the lateral border.

Wasting of the muscles around the shoulders is easily seen (Figs. 1.5 and 1.6). The bony prominences become more noticeable. Posteriorly, the spine of the scapula juts out, no longer hidden by the suprapinatus above and the infraspinatus below. The deltoid may be wasted, and a marked "step" is formed at the point of the shoulder. From the front, a characteristic sign may be present. As the shoulders become weak, the scapulae tend to slide laterally and upwards on the thorax as the muscle tone is no longer sufficient to brace them backwards. When this happens, the points of the shoulders tend to fold anteriorly, rather as if one were folding over the corner of a piece of paper in a dog-ear fashion. Since there is often associated pectoral muscle wasting, a crease is formed which runs diagonally from the axilla towards the neck (Fig. 1.7). Winging of the scapula, in which the lower medial corner or sometimes the entire medial border of the scapula juts backwards, may also be noticed

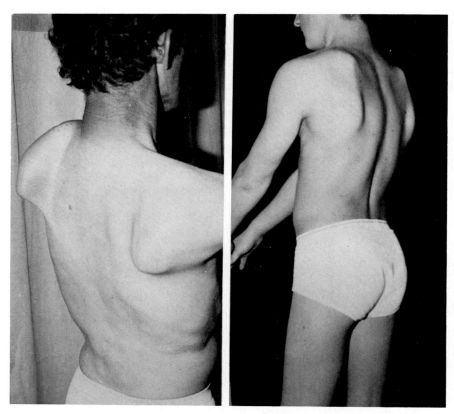

Figure 1.8 (*left*).   Scapular winging. The patient cannot hold his arms out in front of him, and an attempt to do this results in the scapulae riding upwards and laterally over the back of the thorax. Facioscapulohumeral dystrophy.
Figure 1.9 (*right*).   Mild scapular winging. When the patient is asked to hold his arms out in front of him and then to bring them slowly down again, as in this picture, the inferior medial corners of the scapulae pop back with a sudden movement. Limb girdle dystrophy.

(Fig. 1.8). In slender people it may be difficult to determine whether or not this winging is of pathological significance. Many physicians employ the technique of having the patient push against the wall in order to determine whether or not the winging is real. I have found the following maneuver more reliable: The patient is asked to raise his arms outstretched in front of him until they are horizontal. He is then told to bring the arms slowly down again until the hands are at his side. In patients with winging of the scapula, this downward movement always exacerbates the winging, and very often during the maneuver the medial inferior corner of the scapula pops backwards with a sudden rotary movement (Fig. 1.9). Another sign of shoulder weakness which is extremely useful is the "trapezius hump." This is a prominence in the mid portion of the belly of the trapezius which is easily seen from in front (Figs. 1.10 and 1.11). In patients with mild weakness, it is probably due to the activity of this muscle in trying to provide some support in fixation of the scapula. In more severe weakness, the scapula itself rides up over the shoulder and is visible from in front (Fig. 1.8). The trapezius hump is especially prominent during abduction of the arms, but may also be noticeable at rest. A secondary effect of shoulder weakness is on the position of the hands. In the normal standing posture the hands are held with the thumbs facing forwards. Weakness of the shoulder, with the attendant displacement of the scapula, causes the arm to turn so that the back of the hand now faces forward (Fig. 1.12).

Inspection of the arms and hands is relatively straightforward. One looks for wasting in the biceps, triceps, and forearm muscles. As a practical tip, it is easier to look for wasting of the forearm muscles when the patient holds the arms forward with the elbows flexed, putting the forearms in a vertical position, a posture similar to that used in boxing at the turn of the century. The bellies of the muscles on the medial and lateral side of the forearms may then be compared and any wasting detected.

In examining the muscles of the hands, the signs of flattening of the thenar

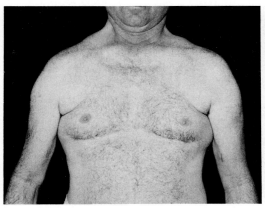 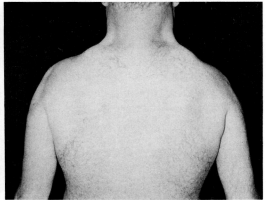

Figures 1.10 and 1.11. Shoulder weakness. Diagonal creases running from the axilla to the neck are visible. The clavicles slope downwards, and the "trapezius hump" is visible midway between the shoulder and the neck (Fig. 1.10, *left*). This is also seen from the back, and some webbing of the lateral aspects of the neck is noted (Fig. 1.11, *right*). Scapuloperoneal dystrophy.

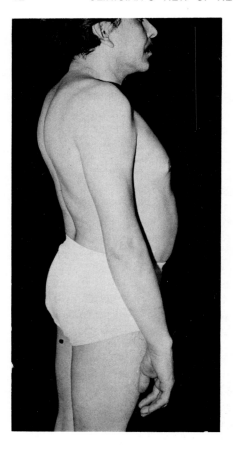

Figure 1.12. Shoulder weakness. Weakness of the shoulders allows the arms to rotate internally, and the backs of the hands and face forward. This is an abnormal posture. In addition, this patient has a slightly lumbar lordosis. Limb girdle dystropy.

and hypothenar eminence and of "guttering" of the interossei muscles are well known. One maneuver which is useful in patients who are suspected of having wasting of the first dorsal interosseous is to ask them to adduct the thumb to the first finger. Normally this results in a prominent belly of the first dorsal interosseous muscle. In patients with wasting, the belly does not develop and palpation of the muscle reveals it to be flabby (Fig. 1.13). Weakness of the muscles of the hand causes characteristic changes in the posture of the hand. Ordinarily the hand is held with the fingers semiflexed at all joints and the thumb held in a plane at right angles to the fingers (so that the thumbnail faces forwards when the hands are held by the side). In weakness of muscles of the thenar eminence, the thumb rotates so that it lies in the same plane as the fingers—the so-called simian or ape-like hand. An additional abnormality is associated with weakness of the other small muscles of the hand. The fingers are held loosely, neither adducted nor abducted, and the fingers, although remaining flexed at the interphalangeal joints, become extended at the metacarpophalangeal joints producing the "claw" hand (Fig. 1.14).

Inspection of the thorax and abdomen is less likely to be helpful in muscle illnesses. Wasting of the intercostal and paraspinal muscles accentuates the bony prominences of ribs and vertebrae. Laxity of the abdominal muscles

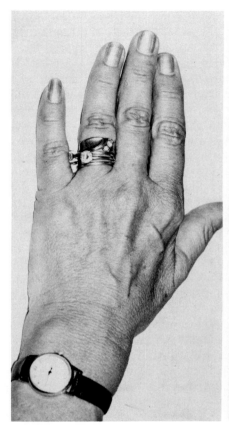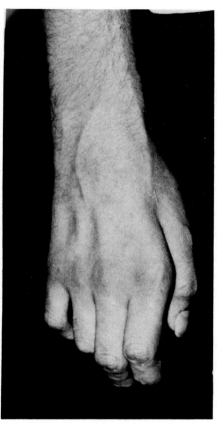

Figure 1.13 (*left*).   Wasting of the hand. Notice the hollowing between the first two fingers and between the first finger and the thumb. Even the apposition of the thumb to the next finger has failed to produce any palpable muscle mass. Motor neuron disease.

Figure 1.14 (*right*).   The posture of the paralyzed or claw hand. The fingers are held semiflexed, and there is some extension at the metacarpophalangeal joint. Motor neuron disease.

may cause sagging and folding of the skin when the patient stands, but, in general, these signs are more often associated with the chronically ill patient than one selectively affected by neuromuscular disease. About the most useful sign is the lumbar lordosis with its accompanying protruberant belly that is seen in cases with proximal hip and lumbar weakness. This is discussed in further detail below.

The quadriceps femoris, above all other muscles in the body, are most susceptible to wasting, and it is the vastus lateralis and medialis that bear the brunt of this wasting. The diagnosis of disuse atrophy should always be made with some reluctance, since focal atrophy of muscle groups is generally due to disease of the neuromuscular system rather than disuse, but it is remarkable how rapidly the quadriceps will waste following even a brief period of bed rest or as a result of pain in the hip or knee. Quadriceps wasting can be noticed more easily if the patient is asked to tense the thigh by making the knee stiff or fixing the kneecap. When this is done, the bellies of the normal medial and lateral vasti are prominent just above the knee. A wasted thigh is not only slender but also tapers perceptibly towards the knee.

When the muscles of the anterior tibial and peroneal groups are lost, the tibia assumes a "knife-edge" configuration owing to the prominence of its anterior border. A groove is seen immediately lateral to this knife-edge border. Sometimes a similar groove is seen in normal people of slight build, but if the patient is asked to dorsiflex the foot, a distinction between the normal and abnormal can be made. Normally during such dorsiflexion the bulge of the anterior tibial muscle obliterates this groove. In abnormal wasting the muscle belly is not prominent and the groove persists. Loss of the gastrocnemii causes the medial and lateral bellies of this muscle to change from their normally rounded configuration to a tapering and flabby appearance. It is also useful to inspect the size of the extensor digitorum brevis. Both myopathies and neuropathies may cause a foot drop, but if the cause is a disease of the peripheral nerve, the extensor digitorum brevis is usually reduced in size. In a foot drop caused by a myopathy, such as in the scapuloperoneal syndrome, the extensor digitorum brevis is often hypertrophied, perhaps because this small muscle is used in a futile attempt to dorsiflex the feet by pulling up on the toes.

Finally, all the muscle groups should be examined to look for the presence or absence of fasciculations or other involuntary movements. One of the many unanswered questions in neuromuscular disease is how to differentiate benign fasciculations from those of pathological significance. Some have maintained that the benign fasciculation is a brief, repetitive twitch of the same group of muscle fibers occurring over a period of 2–3 min, whereas pathological fasciculations appear in many muscle groups in a random fashion. Watching a patient with diffuse fasciculations is reminiscent of watching the surface of a pond in summer when the fish are rising: the ripples arise here and there with no seeming pattern. Unfortunately, there is no hard and fast differentiation of benign from pathological fasciculations. It has been our experience that perfectly normal people without any neuromuscular disease have periods of time when fasciculations may be quite intense and diffuse. Isolated fasciculations may last for many days in a patient who fails to develop any sign of neuromuscular disease when followed over many years. Fasciculations are exacerbated by many factors, such as fatigue, both physical and mental, cigarette smoking, and the consumption of coffee or other caffeine-containing drinks. There is perhaps one clue to the fact that a fasciculation is of pathological significance, and this is related to the size of the fasciculation. A fasciculation is an involuntary discharge of one motor unit resulting in the contraction of all the muscle fibers supplied by a single nerve cell. When denervation occurs, the several hundred muscle fibers supplied by a particular nerve may become devoid of their nerve supply. Ordinarily they atrophy, but reinnervation from a neighboring nerve cell may occur. This results in the accumulation of additional muscle fibers within the newly formed motor unit. By a constant process of denervation and reinnervation, motor units may come to contain several thousand muscle fibers rather than a few hundred. If such a large motor unit is the site of a fasciculation, a large part of the muscle may be involved in a single fasciculation so that the twitch extends across a good portion of the muscle belly. Thus, the presence of a sizable fasciculation may be some indication of pathology. Unfortunately, this is less useful in practice, since by the time denervation and reinnervation are extensive and the fasciculations are large, the disease is clinically apparent by other criteria. The origin of the fasciculation is not clear. It is a spontaneous discharge in some part of the motor nerve. Electrophysiological studies have suggested the distal part of the neuron is the culprit, but a contrary view has also been defined (1, 2).

A fasciculation is a brief twitch of a small portion of the muscle and should be distinguished from the phenomenon of myokymia. Some confusion has arisen in the literature, and on occasion the distinction is obscured. Myokymia is a repetitive train of action potentials causing a brief tetanic contraction of the muscle fibers of a motor unit. Because of the repetitive nature of the discharge, the visible contraction is longer in its time course. The twitch-like character of a fasciculation is different from the more sinuous movement of myokymia. Moreover, myokymia seldom involves one nerve fiber alone. The same abnormality affects many motor units, and their contraction and relaxation gives an undulating character to the whole muscle which resembles the movement seen in a field of wheat as the wind blows across it. Myokymia is also more apt to move the joint across which the muscle acts than are fasciculations. In spite of this, it may be necessary to obtain EMG studies before the two can be clearly differentiated.

Palpation

After the muscles have been examined, additional information may be obtained by palpating the muscle and by percussing it. There is really no way to describe the texture of normal muscle except to say that it has a certain resilience; it is equally difficult to describe the abnormal. However, the physician who learns to tell the difference between a flabby, atrophic, denervated muscle and the peculiar rubbery consistency of muscle in Duchenne dystrophy will find that palpation is a useful means of examination. One of the most characteristic signs is the feeling of the gastrocnemius muscle of a patient with the pseudohypertrophic form of muscular dystrophy (Duchenne). The children's stores often carry toys fashioned after spiders, snakes, or monsters of various kinds. They are made of a plastic which has a jelly-like consistency and shakes and trembles in an all too life-like fashion, and they are usually an iridescent green or other inexcusable color. The muscle of a patient with Duchenne dystrophy has almost exactly the same kind of feel as the substance out of which these toys are made.

A patient may experience pain while the muscle is being palpated, and this may also be helpful in the diagnosis. Sometimes fine nodules are felt beneath the skin or in the substance of the muscle in patients with inflammatory myopathies.

The evaluation of a patient's tone is more important in children than it is in adults. Even the concept of tone is a difficult one to explain. It means different things to physiologists, pediatricians, and neurologists. The word is used here to indicate the degree of resistance to movement that a limb has when the patient is relaxed. When the arm is picked up and the elbow flexed or the forearm gently shaken, the movements which occur at the elbow and the wrist are damped slightly by the normal tone in the muscles. The joints move freely and readily enough but a minimal amount of resistance can be perceived, even though it does not hamper the movement. In a patient who is hypotonic, the limb has all the resilience of overcooked spaghetti. It is impossible to describe this in words, and only the examiner's experience with patients with various degrees of tone will enable him to make an accurate assessment.

In children, the degree of head lag and the position of the body in ventral suspension are examined in addition to passive movement of the limbs. To evaluate head lag, the baby is placed on his back and his shoulders are raised by pulling his arms. Even the newborn child will make some attempt to flex his neck and bring the head up with the shoulders. Head lag is a phenomenon in which the head droops passively backwards and no attempt is made to raise it (Fig. 1.15). The degree of tone may also be evaluated by holding the child under the trunk and lifting him clear of the surface in the supine position. In hypotonic conditions the body will assume the posture of an inverted U, whereas in a normal child, shortly after birth, the back will be relatively straight and the arms and legs flexed.

Very often in hypotonic children the joints are hyperextensible; for example, the fingers may be bent backwards to touch the forearms or the feet dorsiflexed so that the toes can be made to touch the shins. Although the term hypotonic is sometimes used for such joints, it is better to name them hyperextensible or hypermobile.

Increased tone in neuromuscular disease is usually associated with contractures of the muscles. A contracture is a shortening which occurs in the muscle in the absence of any voluntary activity or any electrical signs of muscle activity. It is most often associated with a fibrotic shortened muscle. The muscles around any joint may be involved; they usually shorten into the

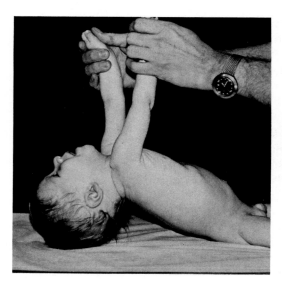

Figure 1.15. Abnormal "head lag." The baby is being pulled upwards by the arms, and the head lolls backwards without control. Infantile spinal muscular atrophy.

position which the patient adopts at rest. Thus, a patient confined to a wheelchair will have flexion contractures of the hips, knees, and elbows.

Percussion of the muscle may reveal the presence of myotonia, myoedema, or other abnormal direct percussion responses. Percussion myotonia is a sustained and uncontrollable contraction, associated with a delay in relaxation, produced by a sharp blow. It is characteristically sought in the thenar eminence, percussion of which causes an abrupt abduction of the thumb. The patient then struggles to get his hand back into the normal relaxed position. However, myotonia should also be looked for in muscles other than those of the hand. Percussion of the forearm over the extensor muscles of the fingers may result in the abrupt extension of the fingers followed by a slow downward drift as the myotonia relaxes. Another way of detecting myotonia is to slant a light obliquely across the belly of a muscle such as the deltoid. Percussion will then cause the contraction of a strip of the muscle, producing a depression which will be shadowed by the oblique light. This method is useful in eliciting myotonia of the tongue and muscles acting across large joints.

Myoedema is a phenomenon seen in hypothyroidism and in other metabolic abnormalities. Percussion of the muscle produces an initial depression which spreads outwards across the muscle rather like the ripples on a pond when a stone is thrown into the water. The initial depression then mounds upwards, giving the appearance of a small hillock where the muscle was percussed. The hillock may last for many seconds to minutes. Some have used the term myoedema for actual swelling of the muscle, as in a patient with a tender, painful muscle during an acute attack of polymyositis or of rhabdomyolysis. I think these two usages should be carefully differentiated and, at least in this book, myoedema will be used to indicate the percussion response.

Normal muscle will also contract upon percussion, particularly over the thenar eminence and the muscles of the forearm. However, the normal response is a brief contraction which immediately relaxes. It is usually not very marked, and the joint moves little if at all. Occasionally this percussion response may become quite brisk without having the characteristic delayed relaxation phase of myotonia. It is particularly seen in denervating illnesses and also in electrolyte imbalance in which the direct response to muscle percussion is augmented.

Reflexes

Examination of the deep tendon reflexes is an important part of the muscle examination. The reflexes which are evaluated are those of any standard neurological examination and include the biceps, triceps, supinator, knee, and ankle jerks together with the superficial reflexes of the abdomen and the plantar responses. With regard to the deep tendon reflexes, I have never really understood the system of grading which is used by many. I refer to the +, +⁻, +++, etc. system. I would like to believe that there are others equally baffled by this system, and I would, therefore, make a plea that reflexes be described as either absent, diminished, normal, or hyperactive. If it is necessary to add the comment that there is associated clonus, then so be it. At least this has the advantage of clarity when others subsequently read the patient's chart. In judging whether a reflex is hyperactive, attention is paid to the spread of the reflex to neighboring muscle groups and, most importantly, to the degree of "snap" in the muscle contraction. Ordinarily, when a tendon is tapped, the initial contraction of the muscle has a rather smooth quality before relaxing. If a tension recording were taken from the muscle, the familiar curve would be seen. In a hyperactive reflex, the initial upsweep of such a curve is very steep. This gives the appearance of a distinct snap to the muscle contraction. The tendon jerk becomes more jerky than usual, so to speak.

Muscle Strength

The evaluation of muscle strength is at the heart of the examination of the neuromuscular system. For the detailed evaluation of individual muscles, the classical monograph *Aids to the Examination of the Peripheral Nervous System* by the Medical Research Council (3) is enthusiastically recommended. The grading system therein is most useful. Strength is evaluated in the following categories: 0, no movement of the muscle; 1, flicker or trace of contraction; 2, active movement when gravity is eliminated; 3, active movement against gravity; 4, active movement against gravity and resistance; and 5, normal power. This elegant system of grading has been corrupted by at least a generation of neurologists. All of us insist on grading muscle as 4+, 3−, and so on. This disadvantage inherent in the system is that once a muscle becomes weak (grade 4) there is a wide variation in the degree of strength, until the muscle loses the ability to move the joint against any resistance and becomes grade 3. My own preferred version of the system includes the following grades: When it is difficult to decide when muscle strength is normal or not, I use a grade 5. This grade is meant to express uncertainty and should not be used for a muscle which is slightly weak. Grade 3− is used to indicate a muscle which can act against gravity, but not through the full range of motion for that joint. Thus, a hip flexor which can lift the leg so that it clears the examining table, but cannot move the leg through the full range, would be graded 3−. A quadriceps which can extend the knee against gravity, but short of its full range of movement, would receive a similar grade. Sometimes a muscle is able to move a limb its full range against gravity, but when resistance is placed on the limb, the muscle contracts feebly in response and then collapses. This brief contraction followed by collapse in a weak limb is then graded 3+. It should be noted that this is quite different from the hysterical phenomenon in which the muscle gives way suddenly after a relatively normal contraction. Attempts to quantitate muscle strength exactly, by the use of dynamometers and so forth, have not yet produced a more reliable method. This has led to the adoption of a system of functional muscle testing, a heresy which will be explained later.

It is time consuming to examine every muscle in the body, and most of us develop a shortened method. I think that an acceptable compromise is to examine the strength at each joint with all the movements possible at that joint. Thus, neck flexion, extension, and rotation are examined. Abduction, adduction, extension, and flexion of the shoulder, extension and flexion of the elbow are tested, and so on with all the joints of the body. This may not be pleasing to the purists, but it does have the advantage of enabling the examiner to see more than two patients in an afternoon.

It is important here to discuss another aspect of the evaluation of strength. It has been a frequent experience to see a patient whose weakness has been described as severe, only to find that his trouble is more psychological than muscular. Organic weakness gives very characteristic signs. The examiner can overcome the patient's best efforts to resist him, and the resistance which the muscle displays is uniform throughout the range of movement. If one is testing the abductors of the shoulders in a patient who is slightly weak, the patient is instructed to "make wings," the arms are held up horizontally, and pressure on the elbow allows the examiner to push the patient's arms downwards towards his side. The resistance that the examiner feels is the same at the beginning of this movement as it is when the patient's elbows have been forced down to 45°. This is quite different from hysterical weakness, in which there is a sudden "giving way" phenomenon. In the same situation of testing shoulder abduction, it may initially be quite difficult to depress the patient's elbow but then the muscle suddenly collapses and the arm falls down to the side. In fact a repetitive "catch and give" phenomenon may occur, resulting in a feeling rather like cogwheel rigidity in which small contractions are succeeded by periods of relaxation. This is never due to muscle weakness; however, if the patient has pain in the joint being tested, the same result may be obtained. Thus, when the phenomenon of "sudden give" is detected in examining a muscle, the patient should be asked whether the joint or the muscle hurts. If such pain is present, it is impossible to get an accurate assessment of muscular strength. This last point cannot be stressed too strongly.

If a patient is suspected of having hysterical weakness, he should be observed closely to see whether, when he is unaware of scrutiny, he makes movements with the limb, which he denies being able to perform upon command; a patient who is totally unable to step onto a small stool may do so readily when he uses the stool to climb onto the examining couch. Another sign of value in the testing of a patient with suspected hysteria is to palpate the antagonist muscles while testing muscle strength. If one feels contraction of the triceps while the biceps is being examined, one may surmise that all is not well. Since this paragraph is degenerating into the nature of random thoughts, I will add one further which is of value. The presence of biceps weakness carries with it a useful clinical sign. The biceps strength is obviously tested with the wrists supinated. Patients with biceps weakness invariably use one of two tricks to try and overcome the examiner. The first is to rotate the forearm midway between pronation and supination, in which position the added help of the brachioradialis comes into play. The other maneuver is to pull the elbow backwards. This is so like the movement used by a bartender in pulling up a glass of beer that it has been called "the bartender's sign."

A similar maneuver is noted in testing hip flexor muscles. When the patient is seated on the edge of the examining table and asked to raise the knee, the weak patient may accomplish this by leaning his entire body backwards, thus pulling the leg upwards. A proper test of hip flexor strength always includes the instruction to the patient to hold on to the edge of the table with both hands to prevent this movement.

If heresy is to be preached it might as well be florid heresy. That which follows will, I am sure, provoke disagreement. I have found that the formal examination of muscle strength in the fashion mentioned above has not been as useful as the functional evaluation of a patient's abilities. The whole concept of functional muscle testing is to determine in what way the patient's functional abilities such as stepping onto a stool, climbing, getting up from a chair, and so on are disturbed. It is remarkable how the way in which a patient walks and does certain tasks will allow a quite accurate deduction of the muscle groups that are weak. An evaluation of the functional disability of the patient also provides more accurate testing of the progression or improvement of an illness. A patient may be able to arise from the floor only with difficulty and with the support of both hands when first seen, but some months later may get up with transient hand support on one knee. Formal testing of muscle strength in both these situations may reveal only grade 4 muscles. Thus the improvement cannot really be gauged from formal strength testing. I think we all find it difficult to put down in words how strong a muscle is, and functional testing is an attempt to make the evaluation more accurate.

Gait

Functional evaluation begins with an examination of the gait. Consider what happens to the gait if the patient has progressive weakness of the hip muscles. In normal walking, as the heel hits the ground and the weight of the body is transferred to that leg, the strain is taken up by those muscles which abduct the leg on the hip. Obviously, this does not cause an abduction of the leg while walking but, rather, prevents the pelvis from tilting sharply so that the opposite hip is dropped. This function of the hip abductors is best thought of as a shock-absorbing mechanism which smooths out the shock transmitted from the leg to the pelvis. In minimal hip weakness, this action is lost. The patient's heel frequently hits the ground with a quite audible thud and the pelvis tilts abruptly to the opposite side. When the trouble is bilateral, as it usually is, this produces a heavy footed gait and a mild waddle. As the hip weakness becomes worse, other muscle groups are involved, particularly those of the hip and back extensors. This spreading weakness adds another characteristic to the walk. One normally stands with the back straight and the body's weight acts through the center of gravity in a line which lies anterior to the hip joints. Thus, without the help of any muscle tone, the body would jack-knife forward at the hips. The hip and back extensors prevent such a collapse. When these muscles become weak, the patient develops a compensatory posture. The shoulders are thrown backwards and a lumbar lordosis becomes apparent. This enables the body's weight to be thrown on a line behind the hip joints, further accentuating the backward lean. The body cannot collapse from this position, since it is supported as much by bony and ligamentous structures as it is by muscle. The walk in such circumstances has the previous waddling characteristic, superimposed on which is a lumbar lordosis and an associated protrusion of the abdomen. The attitude in which the patient waddles gently down the street, arms thrown back and belly thrust forward, has been termed the aldermanic posture, a term which will become obsolete as the literature of Dickens gives way to video tapes of Westerns.

Weakness of the quadriceps muscles gives rise to a phenomenon called "back-kneeing" (Figs. 1.16 and 1.17). During normal walking, the quadriceps act to stablize the knee joint. There used to be a schoolboy trick, and I doubt that the practice has disappeared, in which one approached the victim from behind and tapped sharply on the backs of the knees. In the unwary, this resulted in a sudden callapse of the knees causing the victim some momentary panic before the quadriceps took up the strain. It is exactly this collapse of the knee joint that the patient with quadriceps weakness fears most. To protect himself, he will lock the knee backwards in a position of hyperextension. He does this while standing and also with each step that he takes. As his heel hits the ground the knee is thrust backwards; the joint is stabilized mechanically by this thrust.

At first one might think that shoulder weakness would give little abnormality in the way a patient walks. However, abnormal posture of the shoulder is easily noticed during walking. The scapulae are allowed to slide forward and laterally when the muscle tone is no longer sufficient to keep them braced backwards. This causes the shoulders to hunch and allows the arms to rotate so that the backs of the hands are facing forward. As the patient walks, a curious floppiness of the arms is added to this hunched appearance. The floppiness is due to the lack of stabilization of the upper arm by normal

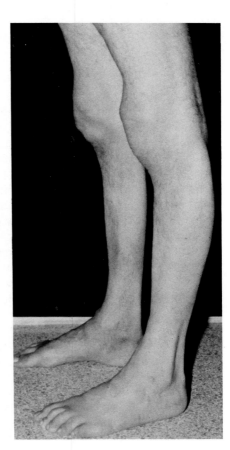

Figure 1.16. "Back-kneeing." In an attempt to stabilize the knee joint, it is thrust backwards and locked in a hyperextended position. Limb girdle dystrophy.

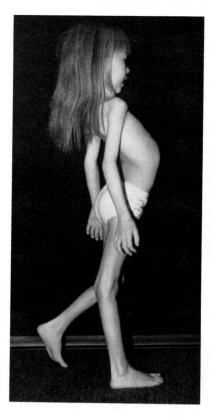

Figure 1.17. A more extreme example of "back-kneeing." The weakness of the quadriceps muscles in this young girl causes her to throw her knee backwards to stabilize it. In addition, there is some laxity of the joints resulting in pronounced hyperextension of the knee. Over the years this leads to joint pain and degenerative changes.

muscle tone. With each step the arm swings passively to and fro, a pendulum suspended from the shoulder.

Distal weakness of the legs causes another characteristic abnormality of gait. Weakness of the peroneal and anterior tibial groups hinders dorsiflexion of the foot. Walking is not easy for a patient with this problem; as the heel is lifted off the ground, the foot hangs limply from the ankle. The patient is in danger of tripping over any object which catches his toes, a danger which can be avoided only by lifting the knee high in the air. The patient is now faced with another problem. If he brings his foot downwards in a normal fashion, the toe will hit first and, because of weakness of eversion, he may well sprain his ankle as the foot collapses under him. Somehow or other he has to dorsiflex the foot, and since he cannot do this under muscular control he uses a short flinging movement of the lower leg in order to throw the toes upwards. He must get the foot quickly down on the ground following this, lest it passively falls back into plantar flexion. This quick throw and rapid descent produce the foot slapping gait. The sight of the high stepping walk with the foot being slapped onto the ground producing a noise like a clapperboard is almost unmistakable. Perhaps the word "almost" should be emphasized, because there is another gait that is superficially similar. Patients with loss of position sense in the feet also raise the legs high and stamp the feet on the ground, since they are not quite sure where the feet are nor yet where the ground is. They like to make firm contact with the foot, not only so that the forcible shock of the foot hitting the ground will force proprioceptive impulses through a somewhat jaded nervous system, but also so that they may hear the comforting sound of foot upon path. This results in a stamping gait as the patient goes on his uncertain way. The essential difference between these two kinds of walk is that, in the stamping gait of a patient with position sense loss, the foot is dorsiflexed when the knee is high, whereas in the steppage gait of a patient with anterior tibial or peroneal weakness, the foot dangles limply from the leg. In weakness of the muscles of the posterior aspect of the calf, the spring to the step is lost and the patient may walk with a shuffle. It should be stessed that a significant amount of gastrocnemius weakness may be present without any detectable abnormality of gait.

In patients with weakness of the muscles of both anterior and posterior compartments of the leg, the ankle joint is unstable in quiet standing and the patient may shift his weight uneasily from foot to foot.

Perhaps brief mention should be made of the hysterical abnormalities of gait. These are always difficult to evaluate and the patient's disturbance is usually a bizarre one. All varieties are seen, from the patient whose every step is a slow and cautious exploration into unknown territory to those whose wild and acrobatic movements seem to bring them to the brink of disaster. It is interesting that if the physician can forbear from holding out a helping hand when the patient seems imminently on the point of collapsing to the floor, the hysteric will miraculously regain his balance and proceed unsteadily to some new predicament.

There are, of course, other abnormalities which may be seen when a patient walks. It is beyond the scope of this book to describe the walk in upper motor neuron illnesses, the gait of a patient with Parkinsonism, or the gait of those with cerebellar disorders. Each has its own characteristics and these are well described in the standard neurological texts.

Observation of a patient while he is carrying out some simple tasks is an important part of the examination. The activities which are most useful to watch are arising from a sitting position on the floor, arising from a chair, stepping onto a chair, stepping onto a foot stool, walking on the heels, hopping on the toes, and raising the arms above the head. Weakness of muscles produces definite alterations in the way these tasks are carried out. The fact that it is easier to get the cooperation of young patients with this series of tests than in attempting a more formal evaluation of strength is an added advantage.

Arising from the Floor

Ordinarily, a patient can arise from a sitting position on the floor swiftly and easily. He flexes his legs, drawing the feet under him; one hand may be transiently placed on the floor to provide an added push; he then adopts a squatting position. From this position he stands, keeping the trunk erect, simply by straightening his legs. Children usually dispense with any hand support and bounce to their feet before one really has time to analyze the movement. With the development of hip weakness, there is a rather systematic deterioration in this performance (Figs. 1.18–1.28). Starting from the same position, sitting on the floor with legs outstretched, the patient with proximal hip weakness will start by making a quarter turn of the trunk, usually to the

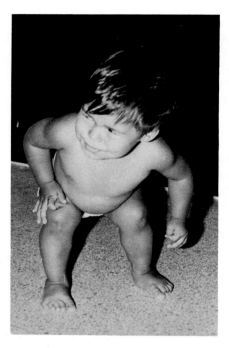

Figure 1.18. Mild hip weakness. In arising from the floor, this child placed his right hand transiently on his knee and required no other assistance. Duchenne dystrophy.

weaker side. The hand towards which he is turning is then placed on the floor, and simultaneously the knees are drawn up under the body. The whole weight is then shifted, so that the patient is resting either on hands and knees or on one hand and one knee. In the next movement the patient straightens his knees raising his hips in the air. Colloquially, I know this as the "butt first" maneuver; the patient forms an arch with the buttocks at the apex. It is much easier for a patient to stand upright by straightening at the hips from this position than to arise from a squatting position. When the weakness is mild, a patient may arise readily from the floor when asked to do so; only the fact that he hoists his hips in the air before the rest of his body reveals his loss of strength. When the weakness of the hips is severe, the patient adopts the butt first posture more laboriously and, indeed, the arch that the body forms is precariously balanced. The feet are wide spread and the hands firmly planted on the ground. One hand is then placed upon the thigh, leaving the body supported on both feet and one hand. This is the "tripod sign," so called because of the three-point base upon which the patient rests. A firm thrust of the hand on the thigh is sufficient to brace the trunk upwards and to allow some patients to stand. In others, both hands must be placed on the thighs to support the weight of the trunk. When viewed from the side, the body forms the shape of a capital A on its side with the apex being the hips and the cross bar the arms. The trunk is then inched laboriously upwards by the hands walking up the thighs. This entire maneuver is often known as Gowers' sign. Because the hand support on the thighs is crucial to the performance of this movement it should be noted that variations exist. Some patients, particularly children with mild weakness, bend the arm and rest the elbow on the thigh when assuming the upright position. In others with very mild weakness, the

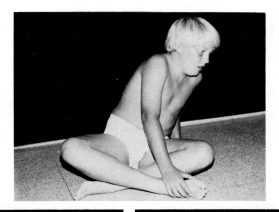

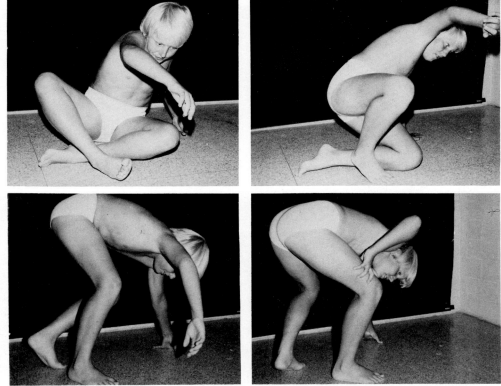

Figures 1.19 through 1.23. This series of photographs illustrates the various components which are analyzed in watching a patient rise from the floor. With a moderate degree of weakness such as this patient has, the first movement is a quarter turn of the body toward the weak side (Fig. 1.19, *top*). Supporting himself with one hand on the floor, he rolls over, bringing his knees and feet under him (Figs. 1.20 and 1.21, *center left and right*). The hips are then raised in the air while maintaining the support with one hand, the "butt first" maneuver (Fig. 1.22, *lower left*). Finally, one hand is placed on the thigh to provide the additional support needed in straightening the body from this position (Fig. 1.23, *lower right*). Nonprogressive congenital myopathy, undiagnosed.

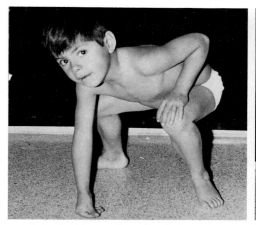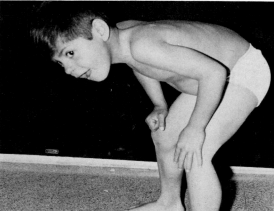

Figures 1.24 and 1.25.   This patient arises from the floor with unilateral hand support on the floor but then requires bilateral hand support on the thighs in order to attain the upright position. Duchenne muscular dystrophy.

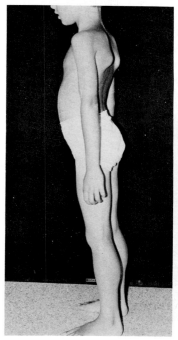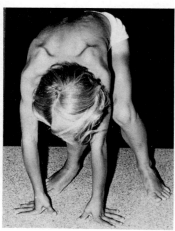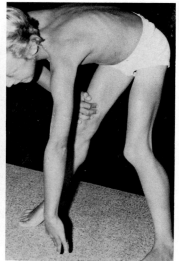

Figures 1.26 through 1.28.   In this child, the degree of weakness is sufficient to produce a moderate degree of lumbar lordosis. The shoulder weakness is also apparent in the way in which the scapulae jut backwards (Fig. 1.26, *left*). When he tries to arise from the floow (Fig. 1.27, *center*), he needs bilateral hand support on the floor in the "butt first" maneuver. He then transfers his hand to his thigh (Fig. 1.28, *right*), and stands by using bilateral hand support on the thighs. Duchenne muscular dystrophy.

hand may touch the thigh only transiently in a rather fluid movement as the patient stands. Some patients adopt a maneuver which is slightly different from the Gowers' maneuver. They find it easier to arise from a sitting position by first placing both hands slightly behind them flat upon the floor. This is termed "backhanding" (Figs. 1.29–1.31). The knees are then drawn up, and the initial few inches of movement are obtained by a push from both arms. The patient then arises from a squatting position in the usual fashion. This initial bilateral arm push is another indication of mild hip weakness.

In analyzing the various ways in which patients arise from the floor, each component movement should be noted. These are as follows: hand support on the floor, either unilateral or bilateral; the turning movement of the trunk; the butt first maneuver; and hand support on the thighs, either unilateral or bilateral, transient or labored. If all these aspects are observed during the course of an illness, there will be an easily noticed change in performance.

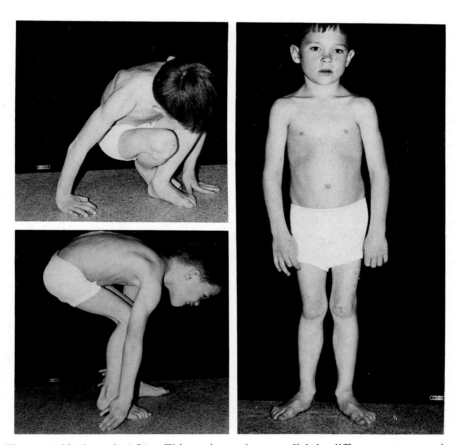

Figures 1.29 through 1.31. This patient adopts a slightly different maneuver in standing. He places his hands behind him on the floor (fig. 1.29, *upper left*), and then pushes upwards to assume the upright position (Fig. 1.30, *lower left*). This is colloquially known as the "back-hand" maneuver. This child also had some distal weakness, and in quiet standing (Fig. 1.31, *right*) it is seen that he has bilateral flat feet. In Figure 1.29, the scapular winging should be noted as he thrusts upwards off the floor. Juvenile spinal muscular atrophy.

This change may well occur at a time when formal testing of muscle strength does not show any difference.

Arising from a Chair

The patient is asked to sit in a chair and then to stand up. Most standard kitchen chairs are about 18 inches high. Ordinarily, this movement is performed without any assistance from the hands. Various changes are produced by different degrees of hip weakness. In early hip weakness the patient may lean his body forwards and place both hands on the chair seat to push himself up. He may need to put one hand on his knee or on the side of the chair and push briefly with this hand during the movement. As the weakness becomes more severe, it may be necessary to use both hands for support. Finally, not only must both hands be placed on the chair for support, but the patient then uses both hands to "climb up his thighs" in the typical fashion described above (Gowers' maneuver). The patient may also begin the task by rocking the trunk backwards and forwards in order to gain the momentum to enable him to stand.

Stepping onto a Chair

Stepping up onto a chair between 18 and 20 inches high is a difficult task and, unless the patient feels secure in doing it, the examiner should not insist. Anyone who can do this movement quickly, without hand support and without pulling himself up on neighboring objects, has fairly good muscle strength. Early weakness of the hips results in a slight "pause" during the step. The patient places one foot on the chair and seems to gather himself for the effort. This hesitation is one of the earliest signs of hip weakness. The patient bends the knee of the leg which is still standing on the ground and then thrusts himself upwards. He now has to transfer his weight to the foot which is on the chair; in patients with some hip weakness, this is very often a moment of difficulty. Patients who are unable to do the task will fall back to stand on the other leg. Other patients may start to fall backwards momentarily but then catch themselves and are able to pull themselves up onto the chair. This results in a sag of the hip in mid movement, known as the "hip dip." Both the hesitation and the hip dip are indications of proximal weakness.

Stepping onto a Stool

I use a stool about 8 inches high for evaluating the stepping power of patients who are unble to step up onto a chair. This movement is usually an easy one and should be within the capabilities of even the elderly or the debilitated patient. Abnormalities in this movement associated with mild hip weakness are very similar to those described when the patient steps onto a chair. There may be a slight hesitation at the beginning of the movement. The hip dip presents often as a wobble in mid movement, almost as if the leg is about to give way. In addition, patients who have hip weakness may attempt to "throw" themselves up onto the foot stool. It is as if the whole body takes part in the movement upwards in a "throwing" motion, in which the shoulders seem to take as great a part as the hips. When the weakness becomes more severe, the patient may place one hand upon his knee in order to straighten the knee out and brace the trunk upwards, rather in the fashion that he does when arising from the floor (Fig. 1.32). As the loss of strength progresses, the patient may have to use both hands, one on the knee and one on a nearby support, to pull himself up onto the stool. The movement is evaluated for both legs individually and is graded as to whether there is hesitation, a hip dip, an upward throw, and unilateral or bilateral hand support.

Walking on the Heels

Normally one can walk on the heel of either foot with the foot dorsiflexed, with no alteration in the posture of the trunk. Weakness of the anterior tibial muscles impedes this movement. It may be severe enough that the toes cannot be lifted from the ground at all. But in mild weakness the patient uses an alteration in his posture to enable him to do this. The knees are held stiffly and the hips are thrust backwards while slightly flexed, so that the trunk counterbalances the change in the weight distribution. This new posture results in the legs' slanting backwards when viewed from the side and gives the weakened anterior tibial muscles additional help in pulling the toes off the ground. Persons with normal strength never need to use this additional backward thrust of the hips to dorsiflex the feet.

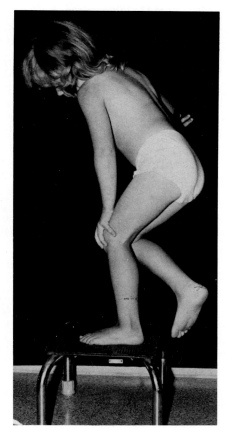

Figure 1.32. In stepping onto a stool a patient with a moderate degree of hip weakness uses the support of the hand on the knee to complete the task. Dermatomyositis.

Hopping on the Toes

The patient is asked to hop on the toes of one foot and then the other. Some patients whose walk is almost normal are not able to do this at all. This is one of the few sensitive tests to bring out weakness of the plantar flexors of the feet. The test should be interpreted with caution in those with severe thigh and hip weakness, since the performance may be hampered by the patient's real fear of the leg collapsing at the knee. In such cases the patient can be asked simply to walk on his toes.

Raising the Arms Above the Head

Ordinarily there is no difficulty in holding the arms straight and abducting them from the sides to bring them up above the head until the hands touch. When viewed from in front, the hands follow the circumference of a circle from the sides of the body to the mid line above the head. Patients with shoulder weakness adopt several tricks to try and overcome their difficulty. One of the earliest is a tendency to flex the elbows during the maneuver. A moment's reflection on the nature of levers and fulcrums will reveal that if the elbow is flexed the shoulder muscles have less work to do in supporting an arm abducted to 90°. The second abnormality that may occur is the use of the trapezius and other accessory muscles during the movement. This results in a shoulder shrug as the movement is attempted. The last abnormality, which is seen in severe weakness, is found when a patient is unable to get the arms above the head unless he clasps his hands in front of him and pulls. I am not sure what the mechanism is, but this makes it easier for the patient to get his hands above his head.

The preceding series of tests can be done quite quickly and will give much useful information with regard to proximal weakness of the hips and shoulders and distal weakness of the legs. It is also obvious that these maneuvers will not give information with regard to the strength in the hands, forearms, and upper arms. This means that formal examination of the biceps and triceps, of the forearm extensors and flexors, and of the small muscles of the hands must be carried out.

CLINICAL DIFFERENCES BETWEEN MYOPATHIES AND DENERVATION

One of the most hallowed tenets of physicians interested in neuromusclar disease has been that disease caused by denervation is quite different from that caused by primary illnesses of the muscles. What was at one time a clear-cut difference is now becoming a little blurred. Many times the distinction will be irrelevant because the actual diagnosis will be so apparent; a patient may be said to have facioscapulohumeral dystrophy or myasthenia gravis without even considering whether the disease is myopathic or neurogenic. At other times the cause of the weakness may be puzzling and it may then be useful to attempt the diagnosis of myopathy or neuropathy. The presence or absence of weakness is of no help, since both the denervating diseases and myopathies cause weakness. It has been said that wasting is more associated with the denervating conditions than with myopathies. This is by no means always true, particularly in the chronic dystrophies. However, if the degree of weakness is out of proportion of the severity of the wasting, the disease is more likely to be due to a myopathic process. An illustration of this is seen in Duchenne dystrophy, in which the muscles are bulky although the weakness may be quite pronounced. If, on the other hand, the wasting is severe and particularly if the muscle has a rather stranded appearance, as though it were broken up into individual bundles which can be seen through the skin, the disease is more likely to be a denervating one. Changes in the deep tendon reflexes tend to occur earlier in the myopathic conditions than they do in denervation. Again, the bulky muscle which is weak and in which the deep tendon reflex is absent is more likely to reflect a myopathy. Many neurology texts emphasize the loss of reflexes early in a denervating illness, a finding at variance with the previous statement. The explanation may lie in the type of patients seen in the muscle clinic. Such patients, if their muscles are denervated, often suffer from anterior horn cell involvement or other neuropathies in which the sensory changes are relatively minor. In this type of illness, the reflexes fade as the weakness worsens, but not before. In the patients with marked sensory signs, who are more likely to frequent the neurology clinic, the reflexes are indeed absent early in the process.

The presence of fasciculations, particularly when numerous, may indicate a denervating disease. Fasciculations occurring in the absence of weakness do not mean denervating disease, but if there is obvious weakness and wasting and fasciculations are pronounced, it is more certain that denervation underlies the process. In addition, the more pronounced the fasciculation the more likely it is that the disease is of the anterior horn cell or of the proximal part of the nerve. Contractures may occur in either process but are more likely to occur early in the myopathies. This is particularly true of young children.

However, when all is said and done, there are so many exceptions to the rules given above that one can make only a cautious interpretation. It is, indeed, much easier to arrive directly at the diagnosis after the physical examination and history than to become embroiled in the argument as to whether a disease is myopathic or neurogenic.

Most of the diseases in which weakness occurs are due to abnormalities of the anterior horn cell, peripheral nerve, neuromuscular junction, or the muscle itself. Upper motor neuron lesions will also cause paralysis, but the physical findings in this situation are so different that it rarely gives rise to confusion. It is true that, in cerebral hypotonia in young children, diffuse diseases of the central nervous system may present with floppiness, but weakness is generally not a prominent part of this picture. At any rate, it is useful in considering the differential diagnosis of muscle diseases to consider the neuromuscular unit in this sequential fashion. The diseases to be described will also be listed in this order and will commence with illnesses which are known to involve the anterior horn cell.

REFERENCES

1. Roth, G. The origin of fasciculations. Ann. Neurol. *12:* 542–547, 1982.
2. Wettstein A. The origin of fasciculations in motorneuron disease. Ann. Neurol. *5:* 295–300, 1979.
3. Medical Research Council. *Aids to the Examination of the Peripheral Nervous System,* Memorandum 45. Pendragon House, London, 1976.

Chart 1.1.   Functional Evaluation—Muscle Patients

Date _____

Name _____

Diagnosis _____

Gait
  1. Normal
  2. Not possible
  3. Loss of "shock absorbers"   Mild   Moderate   Severe
  4. Compensatory lordosis   Mild   Moderate   Severe
  5. "Back knee"   Mild   Moderate   Severe
  6. Foot drop   Mild   Moderate   Severe

Stepping onto a footstool

  Right foot   Left foot

  _____   Normal   _____
  _____   Not possible   _____
  _____   Hesitation   _____
  _____   "Hip dip"   _____
  _____   Throw   _____

                  Hand support
  _____   Unilateral   _____
  _____   Bilateral   _____
  _____   Transient   _____
  _____   Sustained   _____

Arising from floor
  1. Normal
  2. Not possible
  3. Initial turn   0°   90°   180°
  4. "Butt first" maneuver   Yes   No
  5. Hand support
      1. Floor   Left   Right   Both
      2. Thigh
          A.   Left   Right   Both
          B.   Transient   Sustained   Repetitive
      3. "Back hand" support

Arising from chair
  1. Normal
  2. Not possible
  3. Forward lean
  4. Hand support
      1. Chair   Left   Right   Both
      2. Thigh
          A.   Left   Right   Both
          B.   Transient   Sustained   Repetitive

Chart 1.1.—*Continued*

Stepping onto a chair
 Right foot   Left foot

Right foot		Left foot
_____	Normal	_____
_____	Not possible	_____
_____	Hesitation	_____
_____	"Hip dip"	_____
_____	Throw	_____
	Hand support	
_____	Unilateral	_____
_____	Bilateral	_____
_____	Transient	_____
_____	Sustained	_____

Time to walk/run 30 ft	__ sec
Time to climb 4 standard stairs	__ sec
Time to arise from floor	__ sec
Time to stand from chair	__ sec

FUNCTIONAL EVALUATION AND GRADING SYSTEM FOR NEUROMUSCULAR PATIENTS

Forms may be used in evaluating patients with neuromuscular disease. In Chart 1.1, a detailed analysis is made of the way in which patients perform certain tasks, such as walking or stepping onto a footstool. This analysis is derived from descriptions given above.

In Chart 1.2, an attempt is made to grade the severity of the patient's illness. The grading basically follows the outline suggested by Vignos et al. (1), but has been modified and expanded. The method which these authors proposed was of particular use in Duchenne's muscular dystrophy and focused mainly on hip weakness. In any neuromuscular disease it is the hip weakness that produces the maximum disability; therefore, this emphasis has been retained. In order to give some weight to disability of the arms and of the bulbar musculature, we adopted a modification. Patients are rated using a three-digit number. The first digit is determined by hip and leg function. The second digit refers to the shoulder and arm function, and the third to bulbar function. This makes the method applicable to other diseases although the first digit still gives the most useful evaluation of the overall severity of the disease. Thus a patient with Duchenne's dystrophy who is confined to a wheelchair, can feed himself, cannot raise his hands fully above his head, but has no difficulty swallowing or talking would be graded 941. A patient with motor neuron disease, on the other hand, who is able to walk relatively normally but cannot use his arms and has severe difficulty with bulbar musculature might be graded 164.

Pulmonary evaluation is also carried out, as illustrated in Chart 1.3.

Chart 1.2.   Grading System—Muscle Patients

Date_____

Name_____

Diagnosis_____

Hips and Legs

1   Walks and climbs stairs without assistance
2   Walks and climbs stairs with aid of railing
3   Walks and climbs stairs slowly with aid of railing (over 25 sec for 8 standard steps or over 3 sec for a single step)
4   Walks unassisted and rises from chair but cannot climb stairs
5   Walks unassisted but cannot rise from a chair or climb stairs
6   Walks only with assistance or walks independently with long leg braces
7   Walks in long leg braces but requires assistance for balance
8   Stands in long leg braces but unable to walk even with assistance
9   Is in wheelchair
10 Confined to bed

Arms and Shoulders

1   Starting with the arms at the sides, the patient can abduct the arms in full circle until they touch above the head. Can place a weight of 2-kg or more on a shelf above eye level with one hand
2   Can raise arms above head as previously but cannot place a 2-kg weight on a shelf
3   Can raise arms above head only by flexing the elbow (i.e. shortening the circumference of the movement) or using accessory muscles
4   Cannot raise hands above head but can raise 8 oz glass of water to mouth
5   Can raise hands to mouth but cannot raise 8 oz glass of water to mouth
6   Cannot raise hands to mouth but can use hands to pick up pennies from table
7   Cannot raise hands to mouth and has no useful function of hands

Bulbar Function

1   Normal speech and swallowing
2   Speech and/or swallowing is abnormal but presents no practical difficulty
3   Speech is occasionally difficult to understand and/or the swallowing difficulty causes occasional choking (on a daily basis)
4   Speech can be understood by close friends or relatives but it is difficult for casual acquaintances to understand and/or swallowing difficulty is always present and prolongs mealtimes
5   Speech is impossible to understand even by close friends or swallowing is impossible

Composite Grade — — —

Chart 1.3. Pulmonary Evaluation—Muscle Patients

Date _____
Name _____
Diagnosis _____

Forced vital capacity (L)	_____
% predicted vital capacity	_____
Peak flow (L/sec)	_____
% FEV[a] 0.5 sec	_____
% FEV 1 sec	_____
% FEV 3 sec	_____
Resting ventilation (L/min)	_____
Maximum voluntary ventilation (L/min)	_____
Maximum expiratory pressure (mm Hg)	_____

[a] FEV = forced expiratory volume

REFERENCE

1. Vignos, P. J., Spencer, G. E., and Archibald, K. C. Management of progressive muscular dystrophy in childhood. J.A.M.A. *184:* 89–96, 1963.

2

diseases of the motor neurons

INTRODUCTION

There is a group of diseases in which the most evident change is a selective deterioration of the motor neurons. There is particular involvement of the anterior horn cell, the cell body of the lower motor neuron, although in some of the illnesses, the upper motor neuron is similarly involved. These diseases have been grouped together under the rubric of motor neuron diseases, a term which is considerably more precise than the boundaries which separate these illnesses from others.

There is a famous *New Yorker* magazine cartoon, which purports to be a map of the United States. Upon it the island of Manhatttan is carefully drawn with recognizable detail as far west as 10th Avenue. Even the Hudson River and New Jersey are sketched in the appropriate places. Behind them an amorphous country stretches into the distance. A few features are noted, bearing uncertain names such as "Phoenix" or "California"; features which may have been read about or even seen on occasion, but which are placed on the map without the conviction that they really exist. In describing motor neuron diseases, there are some similarities. Ask any neurologist to give a talk on the subject, and he will immediately reach for his slides of amyotrophic lateral sclerosis, followed by others illustrating the various aspects of spinal muscular atrophy, both infantile and juvenile. This is territory made familiar by the large numbers of patients in any clinic. Beyond this are less certain areas. Poliomyelitis is certainly well characterized, but when encountered, often comes as a surprise. Infantile bulbar palsy and other spinal muscular atrophies with unusual inheritance or with a distribution of weakness peculiar to a particular family occupy an intermediate place. There is then an array of motor neuron disorders said to be associated with varied causes from electrocution to immunological abnormalities. In a book of this scope, which is devoted to the foreground of neuromuscular practice, they will be sketched with brief and often uncertain strokes of the pen. For a proper map, the interested reader may be advised to seek elsewhere (1).

ACUTE INFANTILE SPINAL MUSCULAR ATROPHY (ACUTE WERDNIG-HOFFMANN'S DISEASE, SPINAL MUSCULAR ATROPHY TYPE 1)

Clinical Aspects

This illness is a degenerative disease of the anterior horn cells and of the motor nuclei of some cranial nerves, generally inherited as an autosomal recessive gene. The majority of patients with acute infantile spinal muscular atrophy present a rather stereotyped picture. The child's mother may notice during the last months of pregnancy that the normal abrupt kicking movements of the healthy fetus are enfeebled or disappear entirely. When questioned about this change in fetal movements, as many as a third of the mothers acknowledge the symptom (2), although it is seldom volunteered. In more than half of the patients, abnormality is noticed at birth or within the first few days. The baby may be extremely limp, and the infant's lusty cry is supplanted by a plaintive mewling. Respiratory distress is apparent early, and the generalized weakness is often severe enough to prevent the child from moving arms or legs. Weakness of bulbar muscles may make each feeding time an arduous procedure lasting an hour or more.

In other cases the infant is normal for the first few weeks of life and then a generalized weakness of limbs, trunk, and bulbar muscles ensues. The child's parents often have difficulty in deciding the exact time of the first symptoms and it is only when one of the motor milestones, such as lifting the head, is missed that the effects of the illness are noted. Rarely, the weakness seems to appear with surprising suddenness and may be thought by the parents to be related to an injury, infection, or immunization. Whatever the mode of onset, the symptoms of acute spinal muscular atrophy are manifest by the age of 3–6 months. Early in the disease the child's posture is typical: he lies spread-eagled with the thighs splayed apart, flat upon the surface of the examining table. The knees are flexed in the characteristic "frog leg" position (Fig. 2.1). The arms assume a similar posture of abduction with the elbow flexed. The child's arms are usually externally rotated so that the forearms rest on the examining table beside his head. On occasion the arms may be internally rotated, bringing the forearms down parallel to the trunk. There may be small flickering movements of the feet and hands at rest. The chest is thin, with the ribs easily visible, and is often flattened as if the thorax were unable to support its own weight. Paradoxical movement of the thorax occurs so that during inspiration the descent of the diaphragm causes further flattening of the thorax; the rise and fall of the abdominal muscles are the major movements to be seen (Fig. 2.2).

Almost uniformly, such children have an alert and lively expression. The eyes turn quickly to the examiner even though the head cannot. The muscles

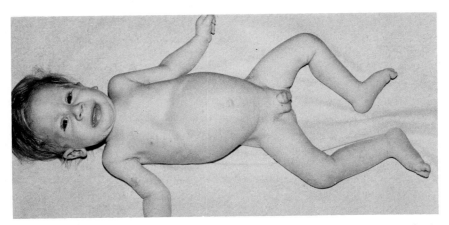

Figure 2.1. Infantile spinal muscular atrophy. This hypotonic child lies motionless with legs in the characteristic "frog leg" position.

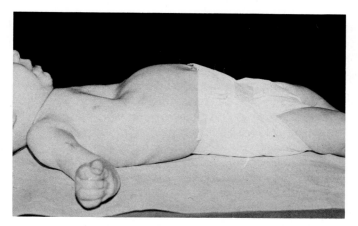

Figure 2.2. Infantile spinal muscular atrophy. The same child as shown in Figure 2.1. Pectus excavatum is to be noted. The protuberant abdomen is associated with respiratory movement; most of the respiratory effort is abdominal.

of facial expression are only mildly weak; one does not see in spinal muscular atrophy the paralysis of the face which is so common in infantile myotonic dystrophy and infantile facioscapulohumeral muscular dystrophy. The mild amount of facial weakness and wasting may give the expression an elfin look. The children are quick to smile and become the favorites of nurses and doctors alike. The extraocular muscles are not affected. Feeding difficulties are often an early complaint and severe weakness of the muscles of chewing or swallowing are early findings. Pooling of saliva in the nasopharynx together with the diminished respiratory movements results in a faint and continuous bubbling sound. Fasciculations of the tongue are seen in about half of the patients. They occur as discrete, tiny indentations which appear to be close to the surface of the tongue, and should not be confused with the slightly tremulous movement of the tongue at rest which is seen in a normal infant. Fasciculations of the limb muscles are seldom seen, perhaps because of the covering of subcutaneous fat. In those children who can move their limbs there may be an associated fine tremor, but it is not as marked in the acute form of spinal muscular atrophy as it is in some of the more chronic forms. A sensory examination, when it can be evaluated, is quite normal. Loss of the deep tendon reflexes is the rule.

It is sometimes said that the proximal muscles are more involved than the distal ones and that the legs are more involved than the arms. In evaluating the degree of weakness it should be realized that it takes less effort to move fingers and toes than to move arms or legs, and this may give the impression that the proximal muscles are more affected. In our clinic we have been struck by the rather generalized and symmetrical weakness in acute infantile spinal muscular atrophy. Children with the typical acute form of the illness are usually dead by 2 years of age and almost certainly are dead by 3 years of age. This should imply that the disease is progressive, but the progress of an illness in a patient who has lost almost all muscle function is difficult to evaluate. Respiratory difficulties do seem to be progressively worse, whether because of increasing weakness or because of the effects of repeated respiratory infections is difficult to say. The terminal event is usually a pneumonia with respiratory failure. In patients whose disease has lasted for some months, contractures may develop in the muscles; this sign is not often found early in the illness. Congenital deformities, such as a hip dislocation and contractures at birth, are uncommon and occur in less than 10% of patients (3). This may on occasion serve to distinguish acute spinal muscular atrophy from some of the other causes of severe hypotonia, such as congenital fiber type disproportion.

Of all cases of spinal muscular atrophy, 27% fall into the acute or Type 1 variety. The disease is almost always inherited as an autosomal recessive. Suggestions have been made that there are modifying factors to the expression of this autosomal gene (4, 5), but by and large, genetic counseling may be given on the basis of an autosomal recessive inheritance. The risk to any future children born to parents of a child with acute spinal muscular atrophy will stand at 1 in 4. The frequency of the carrier state in an English population is about 1 in 80 (4) and is probably of the same order in the American population. The risk of having an affected child will be about 1 in 400 for any unaffected sibling of a patient with spinal muscular atrophy if the carrier state of the sibling's spouse is not known. If either of an affected child's parents remarry, the risk of the half-siblings of the original case developing the illness will be 1 in 150. The incidence of the illness is about 1 in 15,000 to 1 in 25,000 live births (4, 6).

A complete discussion of genetic counseling must take into consideration the relationship of this illness to the chronic or arrested form of spinal muscular atrophy. It has been suggested that the various spinal muscular atrophies form a continuous spectrum from patients with severe infantile disease dying in the first year to those whose disease begins in late childhood and in whom survival until late adult life is commonplace (7–9). Families have been described in which some members have the acute variety, whereas others have more benign disease. Other investigators have put forward convincing arguments that these appearances are deceptive and that acute spinal muscular atrophy is genetically and clinically distinct from the more chronic forms (6, 10). They have suggested that the acute variety of spinal muscular atrophy has its onset usually before 3 months and certainly before 6 months. Death is considered inevitable by 3 years of age and usually occurs much earlier. About one quarter of all the cases of spinal muscular atrophy will be of the acute variety (11). If a child has this clinical course a similar prognosis may be given for any future siblings who are affected. Conversely, the chronic form usually commences at about 6 months of age and rarely before 3 months. These patients may live until early adult life or even later. There is a small area of overlap in the two groups. Some affected members of a family with the chronic variety may die before 3 years of age, but this is unusual enough to permit prognostic and genetic counseling on the basis of discrete forms of illness.

Pathology and Etiology

The disorder is genetically determined, but its cause is unknown. Examination of the spinal cord at autopsy shows marked abnormalities of the large anterior horn cells in the spinal cord. Overall, the number of these cells is reduced. Cells in all stages of abnormality can be seen from those showing changes of chromatolysis to others in which the empty space is the only indication of where the anterior horn cell was once located. Degeneration of large thalamic neurons, particularly in the nucleus ventralis posteriori, is also a feature of the disease (12). Large bundles of glial tissue have been found extending into the spinal nerve roots. These are up to 70 μm in diameter and are ensheathed by a basement membrane. They do not contain collagen, and it has been suggested that they represent a reaction to a mechanical force tugging on the nerve roots, compressing the axons and secondarily involving the anterior horn cell (13). Others have disputed this claim pointing out that similar, although not identical, glial bundles may be seen in poliomyelitis (14) and in amyotropic lateral sclerosis (15).

Laboratory Studies

The two most useful laboratory studies are electromyography and muscle biopsy. The serum "muscle" enzymes, such as aldolase and creatine kinase may be slightly increased but more often are normal. Electromyography often shows fibrillations at rest and either a decreased interference pattern or an absence of motor units if the limb is paralyzed. One does not usually see the bizarre giant polyphasic complexes characteristic of denervation and reinnervation, which are found in other illnesses.

Muscle biopsy may show changes which are diagnostic of the illness and different from those seen in other forms of denervation. There are often sheets of very atrophic fibers (Figs. 2.3–2.7). Almost all of these fibers are round. Only a few show the angulated appearance more characteristic of adult denervation. The large groups of atrophic fibers are intermingled with groups of markedly hypertrophic fibers. Nuclear changes are less frequently seen. There are often pyknotic nuclear clumps, particularly among the groups

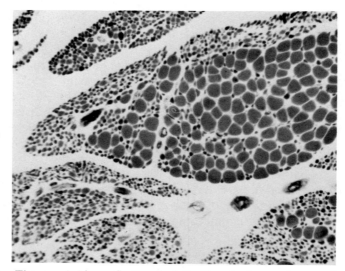

Figure 2.3.   The muscle biopsy findings in infantile spinal muscular atrophy are quite characteristic, with large numbers of round, atrophic fibers and clumps of hypertrophic fibers of uniform histochemical type (Type 1) (ATPase reaction, pH 9.4).

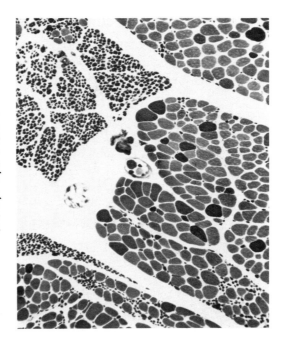

Figure 2.4. Infantile spinal muscular atrophy. The presence of occasional Type 2 fibers (dark fibers) among the population of hypertrophic fibers as illustrated here does not negate the diagnosis of infantile spinal muscular atrophy. Notice again the large sheets of extremely atrophic fibers next to the clumps of hypertrophic fibers (ATPase stain, pH 9.4).

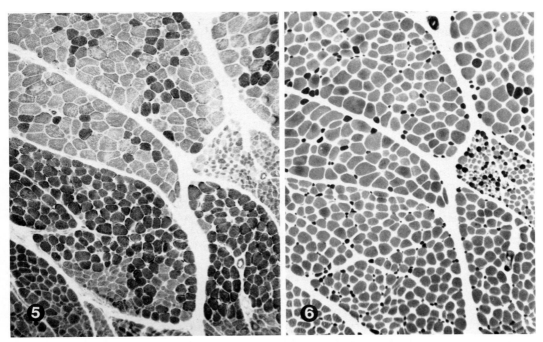

Figures 2.5 and 2.6. These two photographs, which are serial sections from the same muscle biopsy using different histochemical techniques, illustrate a problem which can occasionally confuse the pathologist. Figure 2.5 is an oxidative enzyme stain (NADH-tetrazolium reductase). This would appear to show two types of fiber which, by convention, are known as Type 1 (dark) and Type 2 (light). From the appearance of this stain it would seem that both fiber types are abundant among the hypertrophic fibers which would not be compatible with the diagnosis of infantile spinal muscular atrophy. When the ATPase reaction is examined (Fig. 2.6) all of the fibers are light or Type 1. This discrepancy is probably due to an anomaly in the NADH-tetrazolium reductase in this illness. It is for this reason that fiber typing for the purposes of pathological interpretation is always made with the ATPase stain. Again illustrated is a fascicle of tiny fibers.

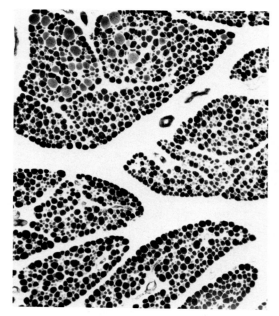

Figure 2.7. Sometimes the hypertrophic Type 1 fibers are lacking in the biopsy. This figure illustrates the biopsy from a patient with infantile spinal muscular atrophy who demonstrates the hypertrophic Type 1 fibers but only in one fascicle. If, by chance, the biopsy had not included this fascicle it might well have been read as a muscular dystrophy becasue of the variability in the size of fibers without any clear small group atrophy (ATPase stain, pH 9.4).

of atrophic fibers, but internalization of the muscle nuclei is not noted. Degeneration and necrosis are often not prominent even in severely atrophic areas. Although fibrosis may be seen in the atrophic fascicles, it differs from that noted in Duchenne dystrophy and is usually lacking around the hypertrophic fibers. The histochemical stains are helpful because the hypertrophic fibers are almost all Type 1 fibers when examined with the routine pH 9.4 ATPase stain (Figs. 2.5 and 2.6). A biopsy in which the hypertrophic fibers are absent may be quite difficult to interpret (Fig. 2.7). One then sees sheets of atrophic fibers of varying size and this biopsy may be mistaken for a myopathy or a dystrophy. Often in Werdnig-Hoffmann disease the PAS stain for glycogen shows large areas which are totally devoid of stain. This may be helpful in differentiating spinal muscular atrophy from other causes of severe weakness in the infantile period. The absence of hypertrophic fibers is a poor prognostic sign, but the presence of large numbers of hypertrophic fibers is less reliably associated with the milder form of the disease. As always, a sampling error may creep in when a biopsy is taken from any particular muscle and this complicates the direct correlation of biopsy with prognosis. The muscle spindles in Werdnig-Hoffmann disease seem to be unusually well preserved. Indeed, many of us have often wondered whether they might be more numerous than usual. The most sensible explanation is that the absolute number of spindles is unchanged but, because of the shrinkage of tissue and the atrophy of the extrafusal fibers, the spindles themselves become more concentrated and, therefore, in any given sample they are more numerous.

Many pathologists have puzzled over the reason for the large fibers being primarily Type 1, it would seem logical that these fibers have preserved their innervation. Why the Type 1 fibers are so favored is not clear. If both the spindles and some of the Type 1 fibers are spared, one might suspect that there is a reason common to both. There are nerve fibers which supply both intrafusal and extrafusal muscle fibers, the so-called beta (β) fibers, it is likely that in the muscle spindle these fibers supply some of the slow or bag fibers which are also Type 1. Since these nerves are not the usual alpha (α) motor neurons which supply the rest of the extrafusal fibers, there might be some biochemical difference which spares them from the effect of the disease.

Treatment

The typical patient with Type 1 or acute infantile spinal muscular atrophy usually dies within the first 2 years of life. In this sense, they differ from the children described in the next section with a milder form of the illness, in whom treatment has been quite successful. Since such treatment should be commenced at around 1 year of age, if there is any doubt at all as to whether a child belongs in the acute infantile form or in the more chronic variety, it is worthwhile being aggressive. The second year of life is critical for the success of any therapy designed to get the child in a standing position.

CHRONIC CHILDHOOD SPINAL MUSCULAR ATROPHY

In the middle 1950s, two reports (16, 17) focused attention on an illness beginning in childhood in which proximal weakness was due to denervation. Under the title juvenile muscular atrophy simulating muscular dystrophy, a clinical entity was outlined with a slow progression and the life of the patient measured in decades rather than years. Since then, there have been numerous case reports and several review articles (8, 18–20). It has been estimated that about 47% of all patients with spinal muscular atrophy are of the chronic variety.

As clinical experience grew, it became apparent that between the acute infantile spinal muscular atrophy and the juvenile form, often known as Kugelberg-Welander's disease, there were children with a wide spectrum of severity. Children who appeared to have the infantile variety and whose death was confidently predicted by 2 years of age would unexpectedly survive, albeit with severe disability, confounding the predictions of their physician and the expectation of their parents. Equally disconcerting was the appearance of patients with severe forms of Kugelberg-Welander disease or juvenile spinal muscular atrophy who would become rapidly wheelchair bound in teenage life. The idea that spinal muscular atrophy represented a clinical continuum between its most acute and its most chronic forms gained popularity. The patients who fell into the gap between the acute infantile type of spinal muscular atrophy and the juvenile form were characterized as having "intermediate" or "Type 2" spinal muscular atrophy.

Genetic analysis of large groups of these patients has been carried out in an attempt to determine whether this is one disease or many. Patients with the acute variety were excluded from the analysis since they appeared to be a genetic entity in their own right (21). Pearn et al. (22) analyzed the families of 124 index patients. They examined the age of onset of the illness together with the age at which the patients first consulted a physician. The technique they employed was to determine whether children in a given family demonstrated a similar clinical picture, which might be characteristic of that family and might differ from the clinical picture seen in another family. This would imply a different genetic origin. They thus compared the intrafamily variability of the illness with the interfamily variability between all the families in the study. There was basically no difference between the various families and it was concluded that 90% of the cases were due to a single autosomal recessive gene. The disease may be quite variable with relatively severe and milder forms occurring within the same family. The authors also suggested that all patients who experienced the onset of the illness after the age of 5 were isolated cases, possibly due to a new dominant mutant and that they were to be separated from the majority of the patients. Some have suggested that these conclusions should be modified. Hausmanowa et al. (23) pointed out that the majority of cases, which were analyzed by Pearn and coworkers, were derived from a children's hospital. This would account for a predominance of the more acute cases and a lack of those adults at the older end of the spectrum.

Whatever the resolution of this problem, from the standpoint of genetics, it is convenient to present the clinical picture of chronic childhood spinal muscular atrophy in two groups: the early onset and the late onset. This is done to emphasize that the clinical picture and treatment is different. They may still have the same genetic cause.

EARLY ONSET SPINAL MUSCULAR ATROPHY (CHRONIC WERDNIG-HOFFMANN DISEASE, SPINAL MUSCULAR ATROPHY TYPE 2, INTERMEDIATE SPINAL MUSCULAR ATROPHY)

Clinical Aspects

The illness usually begins in the middle of the first year but may occur earlier. It may begin so insidiously that it is difficult for parents to be precise as to the date of onset. As in the acute form, cases have been described which begin abruptly following immunizations, but this is the exception. A physician is often consulted when a major milestone, such as sitting unsupported or rolling over, is delayed or is not attained. Most of the children are able to move the arms and legs, and to lift the head from a prone position and about one-third of the patients are able to roll over at some stage in their life. The child may be able to sit independently for a brief period of time and may even learn to stand. Only the minority maintain sitting and standing for any substantial period, and most are confined to life in a wheelchair during the second and third years. Children who do manage to sit unsupported often do so by being placed in this position. They either sit with back straightened and chin tucked in, balancing so precariously that it seems as if the faintest breeze will cause them to tumble backwards, or they are hunched over with their spine forming an arc that owes it support more to the strength of ligaments than of muscle (Figs. 2.8–2.10). Some children with this illness may learn to walk with the aid of long leg braces for a few years. This may be expedited by physical therapy as discussed below.

The distribution of weakness in the chronic form is a little different from the acute illness. There may be mild facial weakness, but this is unusual. Fasciculations and wasting of the tongue are seen in at least one-half of the patients (2) (Fig. 2.11), but children with the chronic form of spinal muscular

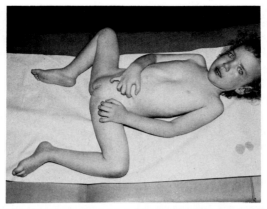

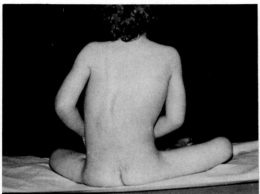 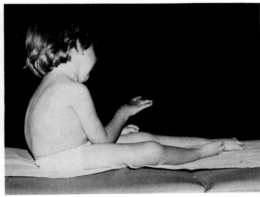

Figure 2.8 (*top*). Infantile spinal muscular atrophy, intermediate form. The child lies in the typical frog leg position. The posture of the weak hands should also be noted.

Figure 2.9 (*lower left*). Infantile spinal muscular atrophy, intermediate form. When this girl sits upright, which she can do unsupported, scoliosis is evident.

Figure 2.10 (*lower right*). Infantile spinal muscular atrophy, intermediate form. A characteristic posture of these patients during unsupported sitting is a rounded kyphosis, which this child exhibits. Notice, once again, the hand posture.

atrophy seldom have difficulty in chewing and swallowing. Truncal weakness and weakness of the limbs are marked, and the proximal muscles tend to be more severely involved than the distal muscles. In one report the arms were found to be weaker than the legs (24). But usually the reverse is true (7, 25). A fine tremor of the hands is so common that its presence can be regarded as substantiating the diagnosis (26). As the disease progresses, skeletal deformities are inevitably seen. The most common one is kyphoscoliosis. The kyphoscoliosis seen in chronic spinal muscular atrophy is more severe and, indeed, more frequent than that of Duchenne muscular dystrophy. This probably reflects the severity of the weakness in the early years rather than being a specific change due to the illness. Contractures of the joints at the hips and knees are often found and, less commonly, contractures of joints of the arm and hands are noted. Occasionally, dislocation of the hips occurs in the child confined to a wheelchair for many years. Deep tendon reflexes are usually decreased but may on occasion be abnormally brisk.

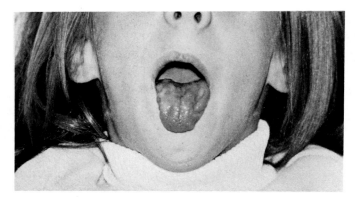

Figure 2.11. Infantile spinal muscular atrophy, intermediate form. The tongue is scalloped and atrophic.

The course of the illness is difficult to evaluate. After the initial progressive weakness the disease may remain static or brief periods of worsening may be interspersed with long periods of stability. The terminal event is respiratory insufficiency which may be provoked as much by the increasing chest deformity as by any progressive weakness of the respiratory muscles, and even the patients who are most severely involved may survive until adult life. Perhaps the wisest course is not to try and predict the time at which death may occur but to plan for possible survival into adult life.

Genetic counseling can be given on the assumption that the illness is inherited as an autosomal recessive. The majority of cases are so inherited, and those which conform to other patterns are rare enough (27) that the possibility can be ignored unless the family history clearly indicates otherwise.

Laboratory Studies

The laboratory studies of most help in the diagnosis are the same as those described under the acute form. The muscle biopsy will show the changes of denervation but may be slightly different from that seen in the acute disease. Although some patients with prolonged life span have biopsies which are identical to acute infantile spinal muscular atrophy (with rounded fibers and the majority of the hypertrophied fibers being Type 1), many of the biopsies show fiber type grouping and large Type 2 fibers. I have not seen the latter change in those children who die of the disease in the first 2 years, and it may be helpful in making the distinction. Again, it is possible that the changes on the biopsy merely represent the severity of the disease rather than reflecting a different etiology. The levels of the serum "muscle" enzymes, such as CK, may be either normal or elevated. The degree of elevation may be up to 5 times normal, but one does not see the astronomical levels of CK characteristic of Duchenne muscular dystrophy. There is also a difference in the progression of the serum CK values. In Duchenne dystrophy these are highest in the preclinical stage of the disease and drop progressively as the disease becomes more advanced. In spinal muscular atrophy, on the other hand, elevation of the CK usually occurs as the disease advances and is not noted early in the illness. EMG shows the pattern of denervation with occasional signs of reinnervation. Conduction velocities are usually normal. X-rays of the back and limbs are helpful in evaluating the progression of the kyphoscoliosis, the degree of osteoporosis, or the presence of hip dislocations but are not helpful in establishing the diagnosis.

Treatment

There is, as yet, no medication which will arrest or reverse the illness. On the other hand, there are often long periods during which it remains quiescent and the child can be trained to use what little muscle is available to the maximum advantage. It is possible that the muscle weakness due to the disease is compounded by a degree of disuse atrophy. Most of these children demonstrate severe weakness in the first year of their life. At a time when their normal siblings are beginning to take their first uncertain steps, these children are still relatively immobile. At best, they are placed on the floor and encouraged to crawl as best they can. Others are simply seated in a stroller. At worst, they remain in bed for much of the day. The use of devices, such as a scooter board or an A frame, at the appropriate time in the child's life, can be associated with some fairly dramatic gain in function.

During the first year, therapy should be directed at maintaining mobility of joints and avoiding contractures. At around the age of 12–16 months, it is often possible to place the child in an A frame. This device (Figs. 2.12 and 2.13) passively holds the child in a standing posture. Initially, it may be tolerated for only short periods, and lack of head control may prevent its use at all. It is often unpopular with the children as well as with the rest of the family in the beginning, and it is probably not realistic to expect the child to stand more than 15 or 20 minutes, until he becomes accustomed to it. The time can gradually be increased until, in many cases, the children can stand quite comfortably for an hour or so. When the child gains head control, the chest strap can be loosened for brief periods in an attempt to have the child gain trunk control. If this is successful over a period of months, the chest band can be removed entirely. The same procedure is then repeated with the pelvic band. When the child is able to stand in the A frame simply using the leg supports, he is ready to "graduate" to long leg braces and the use of a walker. Several of the patients may dispense with the walker and, on occasion, we have seen children able to walk independently without any further support. It is, of course, very difficult to prove that this type of treatment changes the spontaneous course of the illness. Common sense would seem to indicate it, but common sense is often betrayed by statistics. However, among the last 12 patients with early onset chronic spinal muscular atrophy, whom we have treated in this fashion, 10 were able eventually to walk with the aid of long leg braces and walker, although sometimes the walking was maintained only for a short period of time.

As the children grow older, the development of a kyphoscoliosis is to be expected, especially in children who are not walking. Whether this is due to the severity of the disease, or whether walking retards the development of the scoliosis is not certain. During early childhood, the scoliosis is best controlled by means of a back brace which provides passive support. Bear in mind, however, that the child who is walking with great difficulty may be quite

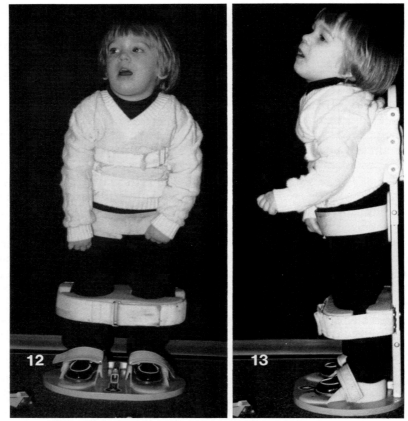

Figures 2.12 and 2.13.   An A frame. This device holds the child upright by supporting the thorax, pelvis, and knees. In this position many of the children gain adequate head control and then the upper straps can be loosened to encourage them to develop some trunk control. In some patients the pelvic straps may eventually be loosened and then the child is ready to "graduate" to long leg braces.

unable to do so when wearing a body jacket. As the children attain their teenage years, surgery is usually indicated. In the past, the prolonged postoperative period and the respiratory difficulties associated with extensive back surgery have dissuaded both patients and physicians from undertaking this procedure. With the advent of Luque instrumentation, which shortens the postoperative course, we may well see an increase in back surgery (28). The necessity of back surgery in scoliosis which is rapidly increasing or is greater than 30–40° is not simply due to cosmetics. The terminal event in the patient with spinal muscular atrophy is usually respiratory difficulty, which is compounded by the terrible spinal curvatures which used to be seen in this illness.

LATE ONSET JUVENILE SPINAL MUSCULAR ATROPHY (KUGELBERG-WELANDER DISEASE, SPINAL MUSCULAR ATROPHY TYPE 3)

Clinical Aspects

Typically, the disease is first noted between the ages of 5 and 15 years, although it may begin earlier. Cases have been described in which the illness begins in later adult life. Once again, it is difficult to decide whether this variability of the age of onset is due to the fact that this is not one disease but a collection of separate and unrecognized illnesses. Nevertheless, the great majority of cases seem to occur in childhood or early adolescence. There is some suggestion that the disease may be more severe and perhaps more frequent in the male than in the female, although this too has been disputed.

The disease begins gradually and, although there are sporadic reports of sudden exacerbations associated with acute illnesses, such as intercurrent infections, the weakness pursues a slowly progressive course. The muscles around the hips are among the first to be involved and cause difficulty in walking. As the weakness gets worse, the child's walk becomes a waddle and there is an increasing problem with climbing stairs. Later, the weakness is severe enough for the patient to use a Gowers' maneuver in arising from the floor. By this time, there is always some associated weakness of the shoulder muscles. This may not be noticed by the patient but is found on physical examination. The calf muscles have been described as pseudohypertrophic in about a fifth of the patients. Whether this really represents pseudohypertrophy or whether the atrophic thigh muscles make the normal gastrocnemius stand out in contrast is unresolved. I have seen several patients recently with quite massive hypertrophy in whom the muscle biopsy revealed groups of atrophic fibers scattered among muscle fibers which were much larger than usual with no fatty infiltration. Toe walking and early contractures of the gastrocnemii are unusual, which helps to differentiate the "pseudohypertrophy" from that seen in Duchenne muscular dystrophy.

Skeletal deformities are not common early in the disease, although the muscular weakness of the hips is associated with a compensatory lordotic posture. The progress of the disease may be slow enough to allow the patient to walk, although with difficulty, 10, 20, and even 30 years after the start of the illness. Most patients, however, will be using a wheelchair in their mid 30s and some will have a more rapid form of the disease which takes them off their feet by the time they are 20.

Shoulder and arm weakness becomes troublesome in the later stages of the illness. The muscles of the hands and forearms are among the last to be affected and there is sometimes a discrepancy between the flexors of the wrist, which may become quite weak, and the extensors, which retain a fair amount of strength. Although the weakness spreads in the late stages to involve almost all the muscles of the body, the general pattern, in which the legs are more involved than the arms and the proximal muscles are more involved than the distal muscles, holds true for most patients. Weakness of the neck flexors and extensors is also noted, and patients may find some difficulty in lifting the head off the pillow. Rarely, facial weakness, weakness of the tongue, and weakness of the palate are seen. It is seldom noticed by the patient, but friends may comment on the development of nasal speech. Cases have also been described in which ptosis has been found. However, the involvement of the cranial musculature is the exception rather than the rule. As with so many chronic neuromuscular diseases, skeletal deformities, kyphoscoliosis, and contractures of muscles around inactive joints occur in the later stages. There is no intellectual handicap in juvenile spinal muscular atrophy.

Fasciculations are found in about half of the patients at some stage.

Typically, these are seen around the shoulders and hips and are more noticeable in adolescence and early adult life than later on. Wasting of the involved muscles may be prominent. The deep tendon reflexes are often depressed, particularly at the knees and elbows, although some patients have normal or increased reflexes in spite of quite severe weakness. Extensor plantar responses have been noted in some patients but are extremely rare; no satisfactory explanation has been found for them.

Sporadic cases are common. When familial cases occur they often have an autosomal recessive inheritance. Other patterns such as autosomal dominant and X-linked recessive inheritance have been described, but they usually occur in cases which are otherwise atypical for juvenile spinal muscular atrophy and give rise to the suspicion that there may be forms of motor neuron disease which are as yet imperfectly characterized (29).

Laboratory Studies

The laboratory studies which are most useful are the serum "muscle" enzymes, the muscle biopsy, and the EMG. Indeed, without these studies, the diagnosis may be impossible. Elevation of the level of serum CK is reported in about half of the patients. In my own experience, abnormally high values were found in over three quarters of the patients. Usually, the values are about doubled, but they may be elevated up to 10 times the normal. One rarely sees in juvenile spinal muscular atrophy the very high elevation of CK which is so common in Duchenne dystrophy and, as with some of the other denervating diseases, the level of elevation remains steady or even increases with the progress of the disease rather than decreasing as it does in Duchenne muscular dystrophy. The EMG shows the changes of denervation and reinnervation. Fibrillations, fasciculations, positive denervation potentials, and giant polyphasic potentials may all be found. The muscle biopsy also shows the typical findings of denervation (Figs. 2.14–2.17), with a mixture of large and small groups of atrophic fibers and with some markedly hypertrophied fibers. Histochemical studies show type grouping and often a predominance of Type 2 fibers. This is a pattern which is quite different from that of the infantile form of the illness. Whether it is an expression of the age at which the disease begins or whether it is, in fact, a specific change associated with the illness is not known. Much has been written about the presence of "myopathic" changes in the muscles of patients with spinal muscular atrophy, some of which may cloud rather than clarify the issue. There is probably no immutable law which decrees that basophilia, fiber splitting, and internal nuclei must imply a primary disease of the muscle. Their presence in the spinal muscular atrophies merely reflects the variety of changes which muscle undergoes in a chronic disease.

The disease may be mistaken for other illnesses causing slowly progressive proximal weakness. There are, obviously, many of these but the classic confusion has arisen between limb-girdle dystrophy and juvenile spinal muscular atrophy. It is almost axiomatic that if you can make the clinical diagnosis of one, the other also remains a possibility. Even the serum CK cannot clearly separate the two entities, and EMG and muscle biopsy are necessary to allow an accurate differentiation. In the young patient with juvenile spinal muscular

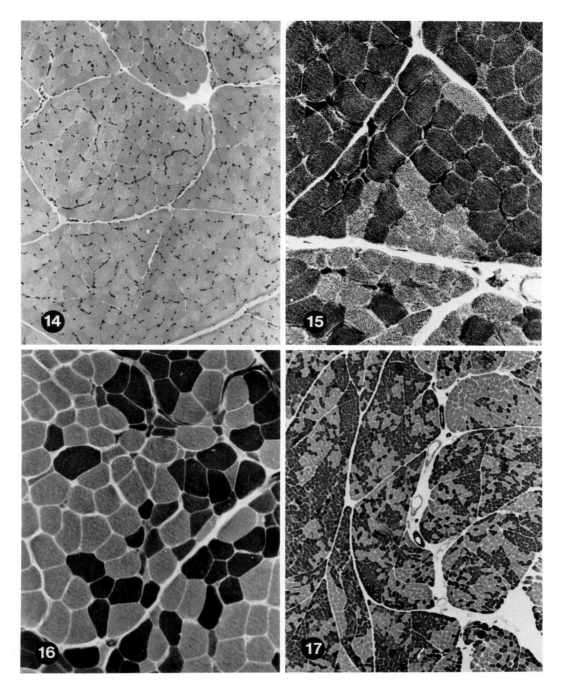

Figures 2.14 through 2.17. When denervation occurs at a later age the changes are somewhat different. The denervated fibers shrink and are compressed between the plumper normal fibers. This may be difficult to see with a routine hematoxylin and eosin stains (Fig. 2.14), but the fibers are often highlighted with the oxidative enzyme reaction, so-called "dark angulated fiber" (Fig. 2.15). These fibers often occur in small groups, the term "small group atrophy" denotes this change and suggests denervation. In order to interpret a biopsy as showing definite denervation, both Type 1 and Type 2 fibers must be affected. Fiber types are demonstrated in the routine ATPase reaction in Figure 2.16 where the atrophic fibers are both light (Type 1) and dark (Type 2). A further change which is noted with the ATPase reaction is "type grouping." In this change, the normal random mosaic pattern of Type 1 and Type 2 fibers is replaced by clumps of one fiber type next to clumps of the other (Fig. 2.17).

atrophy, the possibility of Duchenne muscular dystrophy must be considered, and evaluation of serum CK may be helpful as mentioned.

Treatment

Treatment of the disease is similar to that of the other forms of spinal muscular atrophy. Active assisted exercises should be carried out in order to strengthen the available muscles. Skeletal deformities should be prevented or corrected when they do occur. The use of a heavy back brace to prevent the kyphoscoliosis in patients with spinal muscular atrophy is not possible while the patient is still ambulatory. However, once the patient is confined to a wheelchair, either a back brace or, preferably, corrective surgery is eventually necessary. Very frequently, the patient with an increasing lumbar lordosis is troubled by low back pain. The possibility of degenerative disc disease should not be ignored in a patient complaining of pain and increased weakness. Unfortunately, these patients do poorly following surgery to relieve such symptoms, although they do well with surgery for the correction of scoliosis.

REFERENCES

1. Rowland, L. P. (ed.). *Human Motor Neuron Diseases.* Raven Press, New York, 1982.
2. Pearn, J. H. Fetal movements and Werdnig-Hoffman's disease. J. Neurol. Sci. *18:* 373–379, 1973.
3. Pearn, J. H., and Wilson, J. Acute Werdnig-Hoffman's disease: acute infantile spinal muscular atrophy. Arch. Dis. Child. *48:* 425–430, 1973.
4. Pearn, J. H. The gene frequency of acute Werdnig-Hoffman's disease (SMA type I): a total population survey in northeast England. J. Med. Genet. *10:* 260–265, 1973.
5. Zellweger, H., Hanhart, E., and Schneider, H. J. A new genetic variant of the spinal muscular atrophies in infancy. J. Med. Genet. *9:* 401–407. 1972.
6. Pearn, J. H., Carter, C. O., and Wilson, J. The genetic identity of acute spinal muscular atrophy. Brain *96:* 463–470, 1973.
7. Dubowitz, V. Infantile muscular atrophy: a prospective study with particular reference to a slowly progressive variety. Brain *87:* 707–718, 1964.
8. Gardner-Medwin, D., Hudgson, P., and Walton, J. N. Benign spinal muscular atrophy arising in childhood and adolescence. J. Neurol. Sci *5:* 121–158, 1967.
9. Byers, R. K., and Banker, B. Q. Infantile muscular atrophy. Arch. Neurol. *5:* 140–164, 1961.
10. Fried, K., and Emery, A. E. H. Spinal muscular atrophy, type II. Clin. Genet. *2:* 203–209, 1971.
11. Pearn, J. H. Classification of spinal muscular atrophies. Lancet *1:* 919–921, 1980.
12. Iwata, M. Neuropathology of Werdnig-Hoffmann disease. In: *Annual Report on ALS Research.* Ministry of Welfare, Tokyo, Japan, 1979, pp. 128–130. (Cited in Ann. Neurol. *8:* 81–82, 1980.)
13. Chou, S. M., and Nonaka, I. Werdnig-Hoffmann disease proposal of a pathogenetic mechanism. Neuropathologica *41:* 45–54, 1978.
14. Iwata, M., and Hirano, A. Glial bundles in the spinal cord late after paralytic anterior poliomyelitis. Ann. Neurol. *4:* 562–563, 1978.
15. Ghatak, N. R., and Nochlin, D. Glial outgrowths along spinal nerve roots in amyotrophic lateral sclerosis. Ann. Neurol. *11;* 203–206, 1982.
16. Kugelberg, E., and Welander, L. Heredofamilial juvenile muscular atrophy simulating muscular dystrophy. Arch. Neurol. Psychiatry *75:* 500–509, 1956.
17. Wohlfart, G., Fex, J., and Eliasson, S. Hereditary proximal spinal muscular atrophy: a clinical entity simulating progressive muscular dystrophy. Acta Psychiatr. Scand. *30:* 395–406, 1955.
18. Emery, A. E. H. The nosology of the spinal muscular atrophies. J Med. Genet. *8:* 481–495, 1971.
19. Namba, T., Aberfeld, D. C., and Grob, D. Chronic spinal muscular atrophy. J. Neurol. Sci. *11:* 401–423, 1970.
20. Hausmanowa-Petrusewicz, I., Askanas, W., Badurska, B., Emeryk, B., et al. Infantile and juvenile spinal muscular atrophy. J. Neurol. Sci. *6:* 269–287, 1968.
21. Pearn, J. H., Carter, C. O., and Wilson, J. The genetic identity of acute Werdnig-Hoffman disease. Brain *96:* 463–470, 1973.

22. Pearn J. H., Bundey, S., Carter, C. O., Wilson, J., Gardner-Medwin D., and Walton, J. N. Genetic study of subacute and chronic spinal muscular atrophy in childhood. J. Neurol. Sci. *37:* 227–248, 1978.
23. Hausmanowa-Petrusewicz, I., Zaremba, J., and Borkowska, J. Chronic form of childhood spinal muscular atrophy. J. Neurol. Sci. *43:* 313–327, 1979.
24. Munsat, T. L.,, Woods, R., Fowler, W., and Pearson, C. M. Neurogenic muscular atrophy of infancy with prolonged survival. Brain *92:* 9–24, 1969.
25. Van Wijngaarden, G. K., and Bethlem, J. Benign infantile spinal muscular atrophy: a prospective study. Brain *96:* 163–170, 1973.
26. Moosa, A., and Dubowitz, V. Spinal muscular atrophy in childhood: two clues to clinical diagnosis. Arch. Dis. Child. *48:* 386–388, 1973.
27. Zellweger, H., and Hanhart, E. The infantile proximal spinal muscular atrophies in Switzerland. Helv. Paediatr. Acta *27:* 355–360, 1972.
28. Luque, E. R. Segmental correction of scoliosis with rigid internal fixation in orthopedic transactions. J Bone Joint Surg. *1:* 136, 1977.
29. Emery, A. E. H., Davie, A. M., and Smith, C. Spinal muscular atrophy: resolution of heterogeneity. In: *Recent Advances in Myology*, edited by W. G. Bradley, D. Gardner-Medwin, and J. N. Walton. Excepta Medica, Amsterdam, 1975, pp. 557–565.

MOTOR NEURON DISEASE (AMYOTROPHIC LATERAL SCLEROSIS)

Clinical Aspects

The symptoms of this illness are associated with degeneration of the motor nerve cells throughout the nervous system. There is a progressive wasting and weakness of those muscles which lose their nerve supply, and signs of spasticity and hyperreflexia betoken the damage to the upper motor neurons. Various clinical varieties have been described, depending on the part of the nervous system which bears the brunt of the disease. There is probably no more terrifying disease in the medical textbooks than the acute form of motor neuron disease. The appalling plight of the patient, in whom a rapidly progressive weakness of the arms and legs is associated with an inability to speak or swallow but whose mind remains clear to the end, is obvious. One patient commented that having motor neuron disease was being given the privilege of a ringside seat at one's own dissolution. It is a disease that commands the respect of those who witness it, even if only briefly. Hence, more physicians and medical students have entertained the delusion that they are suffering from motor neuron disease than from any other neuromuscular disease. Most of us working in neuromuscular clinics have suspected occasionally that our common benign fasciculations represented the early ravages of this disease.

Because of the ominous prognosis which the disease usually carries, we have tended to ignore a significant percentage of patients with motor neuron disease who have a relatively benign course, with survival up to 20 or 30 years after the onset. In the following paragraphs a subdivision of motor neuron diseases into the more classical varieties of progressive spinal muscular atrophy, progressive bulbar palsy, and amyotrophic lateral sclerosis (ALS) will not be attempted. Instead, the typical severe form of the illness will be described, followed by an outline of the milder varieties.

Epidemiological studies of motor neuron disease are of great interest in trying to locate specific segments of the population which may be at risk, or to identify antecedent factors which may give clues as to the origin of the disease. The number of studies is small and they must be critically evaluated with regard to the accuracy of diagnosis and the completeness of the figures in any particular population (1–8). The incidence of the disease (number of new cases occurring each year) is between 1 and 2 per 100,000. The prevalence of the illness (the total number of cases seen in the population at any one time) is described in most series as between 2 and 7 per 100,000. The higher figure is probably more accurate. In the United States, it seems that whites suffer from the illness more frequently than blacks, and it is more common in men than in women (about 1.8 to 1). It is most often a disease occurring in the older person with the median age of onset at 66 years. In spite of this, it is well to remember that motor neuron disease is no respecter of age or gender, and may be found at almost any age. Approximately 5–10% of the patients may have a family history of the illness, although the mode of "inheritance" is not clear and the other cases may be quite remote from the patient's immediate family. Sometimes, an autosomal dominant pattern of inheritance is seen (7).

The early symptoms reflect a patchy distribution of weakness which is often distal. Frequently the hands become clumsy and there is difficulty in the performance of fine tasks, picking up pins while sewing, or threading a nut onto a bolt, for example. One patient noticed a sudden deterioration of his lifelong accuracy in casting with a fishing rod. Sometimes the weakness is in the legs, and the patient may trip over things easily because of a mild foot-drop. Bulbar symptoms are said to be the initial complaint in up to one-third of the patients (8, 9), but only a few of the patients presenting in our clinic experienced bulbar symptoms initially, although many said in retrospect that the bulbar symptoms were the first really troublesome complaints. Night cramps in the leg muscles are an early symptom. These pains, which are often in the calf or thigh muscles, may occur when the patient is resting in bed. There is a spasm and cramp of the muscles, often following a movement of the limb such as stretching.

Within weeks to months the disease spreads to involve almost all the muscles of the body. Distal involvement may be more severe than proximal, but this is not invariable. Fasciculations are often noticed early in the illness, may be prominent at night, and may even disturb the patient's sleep. Occasionally the patient will complain of sleep starts or myoclonic jerks when resting. Norris (10) found that a relative absence of fasciculations is associated with slow progression of the illness. Such is not always the case, and diffuse and abundant fasciculations have been associated with a relatively slow progression as with the severe disease.

The patient may complain of stiffness or of a "heavy," clumsy feeling in the legs, heralding the onset of upper motor neuron signs. Hyperreflexia can be so severe that ankle clonus is noted by the patient as, for example, when he presses his foot firmly on the brake pedal of a car.

Weakness of the bulbar musculature causes the patient to have difficulty with both speaking and swallowing. The speech is often difficult to evaluate and shares characteristics of both upper and lower motor neuron damage. Usually the upper motor neuron changes predominate, giving the speech a forced, monotonous quality. This abnormality progresses until in the terminal stages the patient may be completely mute or, at best, able to utter a strained, moaning sound. Difficulty in swallowing is also usually due to upper motor neuron damage. The patient has difficulty in initiating swallowing and will complain that solid foods lodge at the back of the throat. Saliva accumulates in the pharynx and causes choking spells. Milk and ice cream are poorly tolerated, because they leave a thick film at the back of the throat.

Some patients are bothered by a hyperactive cough reflex which causes the patient to cough when trying to talk or when stepping outside into cold air. Pseudobulbar affect may also be noticed in patients with the severe form of motor neuron disease associated with forced laughter or inappropriate crying. It should be borne in mind before the diagnosis of pseudobulbar affect is made that this disease is a devastating one and that frequently the patient has every reason to burst into tears.

The facial muscles are sometimes weak, but it is exceptional to find extraocular palsies or ptosis. Indeed, the occurrence of weakness in these muscles should give rise to some doubt about the diagnosis of motor neuron disease in spite of occasional reports to the contrary.

Although weakness of the individual eye muscles is almost unheard of in ALS, patients who have other bulbar brainstem signs of the disease may have an abnormality of pursuit movements (11, 12). The smooth pursuit movements, which the eyes make as they follow a moving target, are replaced by a series of step-like saccades. This phenomenon, which is exacerbated as the speed of the moving target increases, is similar to that seen in Parkinson's disease. It is also noted in the normal elderly patient and is one of the changes of aging. In the ALS patient, it is far more marked when compared with age-matched controls. It may be due to involvement of the extrapyramidal or corticobulbar tracts. All of the subjects described had other signs of brainstem disorder, although it was not stated whether they were of the upper or lower motor neuron variety. In my own experience, these movements are prominent in patients with the upper motor neuron changes of the bulbar muscles. In the few patients I have seen in whom the bulbar findings were limited to lower motor neuron changes, eye movements were normal.

Bladder and bowel problems are seldom noted. Urinary incontinence is rarely seen in patients with motor neuron disease and its basis is not clear.

With time, the patient becomes increasingly helpless. Confinement to a wheelchair often occurs within a matter of 12–18 months and finally the patient is bedridden, unable to move, talk or swallow. Death occurs from respiratory failure, which may be ushered in by symptoms of anoxia such as nightmares and confusion. Survival from the onset of symptoms to death is under 3 years in most cases.

The signs of damage to the lower motor neurons include wasting and weakness associated with fasciculations (Fig. 2.18). Even when the patient's symptoms are localized to one area, the findings of fasciculations and weakness in more than one limb may indicate diffuse disease. Motor neuron disease is one of the rare situations in which wasted, weak muscles are associated with increased reflexes. Other upper motor neuron signs are often surprisingly slight, and the plantar responses may be flexor even when the reflexes are abnormally brisk. The superficial abdominal reflexes may similarly be preserved.

Examination of the bulbar muscles may reveal some facial weakness

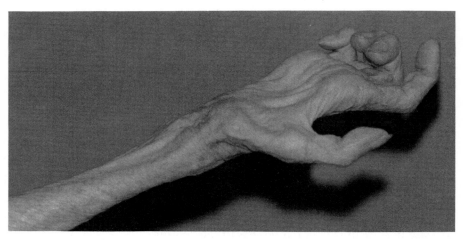

Figure 2.18.   Amyotrophic lateral sclerosis leads to severe wasting of muscles as in of the hand of this patient in the terminal stage of the disease.

although, as was mentioned, the extraocular muscles are not involved. There may be atrophy of the tongue, which looks "scalloped," with prominent indentations along its edge caused by the teeth. Fasciculations of the tongue may also be seen. They should be sought with the tongue resting quietly in the floor of the mouth, since the protruded tongue can be the site of quivering movements difficult to differentiate from fasciculations. Palatal weakness and poor movement of the posterior pharyngeal wall may also be noted. The upper motor neuron component of this weakness becomes obvious when the patient is asked to move his tongue rapidly from side to side; the movement is slow and stiff, and is often associated with a synkinetic movement of the lower jaw. Both neck extensors and flexors may be weak.

The diagnosis of motor neuron disease is made with some assurance if weakness, wasting, and fasciculations are found in three or more limbs, associated with hyperreflexia. If bulbar difficulties are also seen, the diagnosis is even more likely. Sensory abnormalities are not a major part of the disease, although careful quantitative sensory testing and pathological examination of the peripheral nerves show abnormalities more frequently than was thought previously (13).

Damage to other areas of the nervous system may be seen but is not typical of the disease. Some patients have a clear-cut dementia, and extrapyramidal tremor and rigidity have been noted on occasions. These patients' disease differs from the form of motor neuron disease found on Guam which is related to the parkinsonism-dementia syndrome (see below). Perhaps sometimes the non-Guamanian ALS-parkinsonism-dementia syndrome represents the chance association of two or three processes, particularly in the elderly patient with motor neuron disease. There seems to be no difference in the clinical course of this form of motor neuron disease from the classical variety.

The autonomic nervous system is spared; trophic changes in the limbs and pressure sores are not found. Sexual function is preserved.

Physicians in their hunt for eponymous fame have often collected patients with constellations of clinical findings, creating subclassifications within major disease groups. Motor neuron disease has not been exempt from this, and although such divisions are artificial they are hallowed by time and usage. When motor neuron disease involves the lower motor neurons of the spinal cord without upper motor neuron involvement, it is called progressive spinal muscular atrophy of Aran-Duchenne. Such patients have wasting and weakness of the arms, legs, and trunk with little hyperreflexia. Some patients with this form of the illness have a better prognosis than do patients with the other varieties. When the illness primarily causes difficulty with chewing and swallowing and other "bulbar" functions, it has been termed progressive bulbar palsy of Duchenne. The survival of these patients is expected to be shorter than that of the preceding group. The name amyotrophic lateral sclerosis was coined by Charcot in 1875. The term was used to denote the variety of illness which involved both upper and lower motor neurons supplying the trunk, extremities, and bulbar muscles. Because this is the most common and most diffuse form, the name is synonymous with motor neuron disease.

It was at one time thought that the differentiation into various syndromes had some prognostic significance. Such attempts at forecasting the outcome of the disease may equally well be based on common sense. Patients who have more severe disease are likely to die earlier than those with less severe disease, and those with involvement of the vital functions such as swallowing and breathing are inclined to have more trouble than those whose only difficulty is weakness of the arms and legs.

Pathology

At postmortem, the changes are limited to loss and degeneration of large motor neurons. The earliest changes are difficult to ascertain for obvious reasons, although in the rapidly progressive illness, with patients dying relatively soon after the onset of the disease, argentophilic spheroids are found in the proximal portion of the axons of anterior horn cells. These consist of rather irregular bundles of neurofilaments (14, 15). Another type of cytoplasmic inclusion, the Bunina body, is found in the anterior horn cell. These inclusions are eosinophilic. Their structure is uncertain, but they seem to consist of dense granular material, sometimes around a core containing filaments. Chromatolytic changes of the neurons are also noted, although they differ from the typical change of central chromatolysis, which is a secondary change more indicative of axonal damage to the nerve. Gliosis of the anterior horns is also found.

Laboratory Studies

Laboratory studies are helpful in the diagnosis of this illness and should be aimed at demonstrating denervation in widely separated areas of the musculature. EMG, shows widespread fibrillations associated with giant polyphasic potentials and fasciculations. There may be slight slowing of motor nerve conduction velocities, although they are typically normal. The use of muscle biopsy in the evaluation of a patient with ALS is not governed by the usual criteria. Only the patients with early and predominantly lower motor neuron involvement give rise to much difficulty in diagnosis. The patient who presents with a weak hand or forearm may as easily have a local lesion of the brachial plexus as motor neuron disease. It is useful in such patients to biopsy the quadriceps muscle, even in the absence of clinical involvement. In motor neuron disease there is almost always pathological abnormality of all muscles whether or not clinical weakness is apparent (Figs. 2.19–2.21).

Evaluation of serum CK and other "muscle" enzymes is of less help in making the diagnosis, since although typically the levels are normal in denervating illness, in almost half of the patients with motor neuron disease the serum CK may be increased to 2–3 times normal (16, 17). Spinal fluid protein is usually normal but mild elevation (less than 100 mg/100 ml) may be seen (18).

Some biochemical abnormalities have been noted in motor neuron disease associated with muscle breakdown. There is an increase in the ratio of 3-methylhistidine (3-MeH) to creatinine in the urine (19). This amino acid is present in the contractile protein of muscle and muscle wasting leads to an increase in its excretion in the urine. The amount of creatinine in a 24-hour urine sample reflects the muscle mass fairly accurately. Since the muscle mass is also dramatically reduced, the abnormality in 3-MeH excretion is best appreciated when expressed in terms of creatinine excretion (i.e., mg 3-MeH per mg creatinine). Concomitant with the increasing breakdown of muscle is an increase in hydrolytic enzymes, such as acid protease in the muscle and collagenase in the skin (20). Plasma and erythrocyte cholinesterase and acetylcholinesterase activity was found to be no different in patients with ALS than in the normal population (21).

Although motor neuron disease is often easy to recognize, certain other illnesses may mimic some of the changes and should always be considered in the differential diagnosis. Thus, cervical spine disease with cord compression and root compression may give signs of widespread denervation in the arms together with upper motor neuron changes in the legs. In rare patients, widespread fasciculations are associated with cervical cord disease. A popular aphorism is that patients with motor neuron disease are not allowed to die before a myelogram is carried out. Although this may be an extreme statement, the possibility of a cervical lesion should always be considered. When myelography shows definite evidence of cervical spine disease, it is difficult to decide whether this alone is responsible for the symptoms or whether it is merely an incidental finding in a patient with real motor neuron disease. I have usually erred on the side of enthusiasm and have recommended surgical exploration in such cases. Unhappily, my experience has not beeen reassuring. Some patients may improve temporarily after operation only later to resume their downhill course.

There is also the occasional patient who appears at first sight to have motor neuron disease, without any of the upper motor neuron bulbar signs, who is found to have slow conduction velocities and a raised cerebral spinal fluid protein. It is worthwhile instituting a therapeutic trial of steroids in suppressive doses in these patients. Occasionally, they have a dramatic response. Obviously in retrospect, the diagnosis is more likely to be a motor neuropathy than motor neuron disease, but unless this possibility is borne in mind, it will be missed. A patient with a clinical picture identical to motor neuron disease who demonstrated macroglobulinemia as well as slow conduction velocities

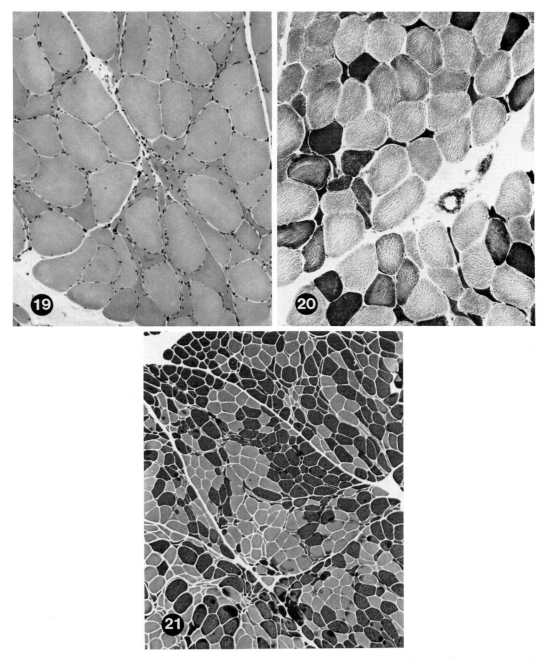

Figure 2.19. A biopsy from a patient with amyotrophic lateral sclerosis. The routine hematoxylin and eosin stains demonstrate small angulated fibers and small groups of atrophic fibers. Internal nuclei are seen but are not profuse.

Figure 2.20. With the oxidative enzyme reaction the small dark angulated fibers are highlighted.

Figure 2.21. ATPase stains show that the atrophic fibers consist of both fiber types (light and dark). There is also a suggestion of type grouping with clumps of Type 2 (dark) fibers and clumps of Type 1 (light) fibers in contrast to the usual normal random mosaic pattern. Type grouping is not as pronounced in ALS as in most of the chronic denervating conditions. Furthermore, in the biopsy from a patient with ALS, the Type 2 fibers (dark fibers) tend to be the largest fibers in the biopsy, although precise measurement is necessary to be certain of this.

and raised cerebrospinal fluid protein was shown at postmortem to have chromatolysis of the anterior horn cells and evidence of a radiculoneuropathy not an anterior horn cell disease (22).

Heavy metal intoxication has been suggested as an occasional etiology for motor neuron disease (see below) (23). Lead intoxication may present as a motor neuropathy in the absence of any sensory signs. The weakness is most marked in the wrist extensors. There may also be hyperreflexia and fasciculations. Usually there are other signs of systemic lead poisoning, but these may be subtle enough to be overlooked. Organic mercurial compounds were reported as a cause of motor neuron disease in a report of 11 patients poisoned by a fungicide used in wheat (24). Although these patients had atrophy and fasciculations of the limbs, there were sufficient differences to make the diagnosis of motor neuron disease doubtful. More recent and extensive case reports of organic mercurial poisoning have not described conditions which might be confused with motor neuron disease (25).

The neuromuscular complications of hyperparathyroidism may sometimes include weakness, fatigability, and increased reflexes. Hyperthyroidism may also be associated with muscle weakness and, in some cases, with either myokymia or fasciculations. Some authors have suggested that underlying malignancy might be a cause for motor neuron disease (26), but recent experience has not confirmed this. There are patients with malignant tumors who do seem to have loss of anterior horn cells, but this does not present as the usual and classical motor neuron disease.

Etiology

We know neither the cause of, nor the cure for, motor neuron disease, a situation which has encouraged a good deal of inventive thinking. In many ways, motor neuron disease seems to be a disease of aging. The gradual deterioration of nerve and muscle is a normal phenomenon of advancing age, although obviously not to the same extent as occurs in ALS. The epidemiological studies in the Rochester, Minnesota, population would support this (2). The incidence of ALS in that population was found to increase steadily with increasing age. On the other hand, other studies have shown that there is a peak incidence in the 7th decade and the occurrence of the disease declines thereafter. This would imply that the disease has a different etiology since there would otherwise be no explanation for the declining incidence in the later years. The authors of the Rochester study, however, make a good case for the accuracy of their data and, at present, it seems that ALS is an illness associated with increasing age. Other epidemiological studies have examined the question as to whether any preexisting factors may influence the development of motor neuron disease. Kurtzke and Beebe (1) identified 504 men dying from ALS and matched these with normal controls. When the medical records were reviewed, the patients with ALS suffered more frequently from trauma, limb fractures, and surgery. Also, a significantly larger number of the ALS patients had been truck and tractor drivers. The increased incidence of trauma has been noted in previous studies and the series of Holloway and Emery (4) suggested that farmers were more susceptible to ALS. It has been a common assumption that motor neuron disease occurs in males who have been very active, participating in sports and organized exercise, but Kurtzke and Beebe's study gave no support to this belief. A previous retrospective study, less carefully controlled (27), had suggested that a history of exposure to mercury and lead, the consumption of large amounts of milk, and participation in athletics characterized patients with ALS.

An increased incidence of exposure of patients to small household dogs from birth to 10 years prior to the onset of the illness was reported (28). If this is borne out in larger studies, one might suppose that exposure to an infectious agent (with the dog as the animal resevoir) in early life is responsible.

In many studies, an increased concentration of trace metals have been found in tissues of patients with ALS. The most popular one has been lead, but aluminum, calcium, selenium, and manganese have all been implicated. Unfortunately, because of technical difficulties, many of these findings could be due to chance contamination in the laboratory. In other patients with ALS there was a prior history of lead exposure, which may have resulted in a coincidental elevation of lead levels. The relationship between lead and ALS cannot be a simple one since treatment of ALS with chelating agents is not effective, and experimental lead toxicity does not really resemble ALS. The question as to whether trace metals play a significant role in the disease is unanswered, but they have been a recurrent theme in the discussion of etiology for many years (21, 29, 30).

The search for a circulating compound, either toxin or antibody, has been inconclusive. Schauf et al. (31) described that the serum of ALS patients had a mild effect in blocking the neuroelectric response in the ventral root, subsequent to a volley of discharges in the dorsal root in a frog spinal cord preparation. This effect was not as severe as that seen in multiple sclerosis and it was not altered by plasmapheresis of the patient (31). Wolfgram and Myers (32) found that serum from patients with ALS was toxic and selectively killed the neurons grown in tissue culture. They did not speculate on the nature of this toxic substances, and other workers could not confirm the findings (33). A more recent study pointed to a neuron-specific cytotoxic factor in the serum of patients with ALS and their relatives which destroyed anterior horn cells cultured from mouse spinal cord (34). A flaw in the study was the small number of normal controls. Playing a variation on this theme, Askanas et al. (35) measured neuron-specific enolase, an enzyme which is limited to the neurons, in tissue cultures which were treated with cerebrospinal fluid from ALS patients. There was no decrease in the amount of enzyme in the tissue culture, suggesting that the neurons were undamaged. In view of the technical difficulties in tissue culture, it is probably wise to interpret all of these results as showing no definite evidence of a toxic factor in the serum or cerebrospinal fluid of patients.

An autoimmune hypothesis is always popular in diseases which have no known cause and motor neuron disease is no exception. Most of the evidence so far is indirect. Immune complexes have been described in renal glomeruli, together with an increase in serum complement consumption (36). Antibodies directed against a constituent of the motor neurons have been detected in the majority of patients with ALS (37, 38). These findings were not absolutely specific for ALS but occurred more frequently in this group than in patients with other neurological illnesses or in normal controls.

The finding of autoantibodies in patients with ALS which block terminal nerve sprouting has sparked renewed interest in immune mechanisms (39, 40). Denervated rat muscle grown in tissue culture secretes a 56 kilodalton protein. Antisera prepared against this protein will decrease the terminal nerve sprouting ordinarily induced by botulinum toxin. This suggests that the protein is a "growth" factor secreted by denervated muscle which may play an important role in restoring the innervation. In about half of the patients with ALS the serum contained a factor, probably IgG, which was both an antibody against the 56 kd protein and suppressed nerve sprouting. Although ALS is not thought to be a deficit of the distal part of the neuron the same protein may be identical with a factor which promotes the survival of cultured spinal cord neurons (41). If this is substantiated it would represent a major step toward understanding the illness.

The histocompatibility antigens (HLA antigens) are of many different types and may serve as markers for the genes involved in the immune response. Thus, a particular pattern of HLA antigens recurring in a given disease might imply a similar genetic substrate in the immune system of susceptible patients. This would then suggest that the basis of the illness may be an abnormality of the immune response. An increased incidence of HLA-A3 antigen has been found in ALS patients, particularly those with the classic or severe variety (42, 43). Bartfeld et al. (44) found no increase in HLA-A3, but did note an increase in HLA-Bw35. Abnormalities have been sought in the immune proteins and, although a monoclonal elevation of IgG kappa (κ) has been noted in one patient (45), no consistent abnormality in IgG levels has been found.

From the time of a report that intracerebral inoculation of extracts of the central nervous system of patients with motor neuron disease into monkeys produced a similar disease, there has been a hunt for a culpable virus. Many different attempts have been made to trap this hypothetical elusive agent and all have failed (46, 47). Techniques have run the gamut from inoculation of neural extracts in animals to the propagation of neurons in tissue culture (48, 49).

An association between poliomyelitis and ALS has been noted. Not only do the two diseases show a predilection for the anterior horn cell, but some patients who have had poliomyelitis may develop a chronic progressive form of motor neuron disease after a period of many years (50, 51). The illness often begins in the limb affected by the poliomyelitis. There may, of course, be a commonsense explanation. Most muscles have so much reserve function that 25% may be lost without the patient being aware of any weakness. A muscle which has been previously affected by poliomyelitis has no such reserve. Thus, if ALS begins diffusely, the first weakness the patient will notice will be in the muscles already weakened by the poliomyelitis. Virus-like particles have been noticed in the muscle of patients with ALS, but it is impossible to say whether they represent merely an incidental finding (52). An attempt to unmask the poliovirus' role in ALS used a radioisotopically labeled DNA (produced by using a poliovirus RNA as a template) as a "probe" in the evaluation of tissue from patients with ALS. This failed to demonstrate any evidence of the poliovirus (53). Perhaps a more telling example was a patient with ALS who suffered from antecedent poliomyelitis and in whom no poliovirus was demonstrated at autopsy using the same probe (54). The viral etiology of motor neuron disease remains thus unproven, but not disproven.

The sparing of the extraocular muscles in ALS led to speculation that androgens may play a role in the disease. Androgen receptors are found in cranial nerve nuclei, with the exception of the 3rd, 4th, and 6th nerves and in spinal motor neurons. A defect in these receptors was postulated by Weiner (55) as a possible cause for the illness. There is, however, a normal suppression of luteinizing hormone and follicle-stimulating hormone by testosterone in patients with ALS, suggesting that at least the pituitary response to androgen was normal (56).

Thyrotropin-releasing hormone (TRH) is a tripeptide, pyroglutamyl-histi-dyl-prolineamide, originally recognized for its ability to promote the release of thyroid stimulating hormone. It is widely distributed in mammalian nervous system and is now regarded as a possible neurotransmitter. It is present in the nerve terminals in networks around the ventral horn cells and in nerve endings associated with cranial nerves V, VII, and XII. Engel et al. (57) have suggested that the substance is deficient in patients with ALS, because of the low values of TRH found in the spinal fluid of such patients. Conversely, others have found normal levels of TRH in the spinal cord accompanied by increased levels of one of its metabolites, cyclic histidyl-prolinediketopiperazine (58).

Defects of carbohydrate metabolism have been noted on several occasions. Abnormal glucose tolerance and tolbutamide tolerance and subnormal insulin excretion have been found (59). Impairment of pancreatic exocrine function has been reported with decreased neutral fat uptake, mild steatorrhea and an abnormal response to secretin stimulation. These findings have been disputed by others (60, 61), and it now seems likely that they represent a secondary alteration to the carbohydrate metabolism because of profound wasting of the muscles.

Appel (62), in an intriguing speculation, pointed out similarities between motor neuron disease and two other diseases often associated with increasing age, Parkinson's and Alzheimer's. In all three diseases, a particular group of nerves disappears and the target tissue which they supply deteriorates. In ALS the motor nerves disappear and the muscle atrophies; in Parkinson's disease dopaminergic neurons are lacking and the striatal nuclei do not function; and in Alzheimer's disease the neurons from the septal area and the hippocampal region are involved. All three illnesses occur sporadically. All have a familial form in between 5% and 10% of the patients, and, in all, the neurons involved are those which may deteriorate in normal aging as well as in the accelerated degeneration seen in the illness. All may have unusual cytoplasmic features in the neurons (Lewy bodies, Bunina bodies, neurofibrillary tangles). If the disease is simply the acceleration of the normal process of aging, then some property intrinsic to the neurons may be at fault. Appel suggested that perhaps the target tissue is responsible for the deterioration. There is plentiful evidence that muscle contains factors which maintain the integrity of motor nerves or may promote neuron growth. Similarly, extracts of the striatum promote the survival of dopaminergic neurons from the substantia nigra and extracts of the hippocampus may have a beneficial effect on septal neurons. Thus Appel theorized that the defect in all of these illnesses may lie in a deficiency of the neurotrophic "hormones" released from the target organ. The theory would imply that replacement of the "hormone" could be an effective way of treating the illness.

Bradley and Krasin (63) also speculated on the similarity between the disease and accelerated aging. They wondered whether this might be due to an accumulation of abnormal DNA. Given the large number of different proposed etiologies, all might exert their effect through a final common pathway, such as a change in cellular DNA. DNA may be damaged by a large number of different agents, such as ultraviolet light, chemical agents, or radiation. The cell has several mechanisms to rescue such damaged DNA which might be defective in motor neuron disease. As support for their hypothesis they pointed out that the RNA content in the normal sized neurons of ALS patients is reduced by 30–40% and the base composition of the nucleic acid is altered with less adenine and more uracil than normal (64, 65). The decrease in RNA and the abnormal composition of RNA might be a consequence of the accumulation of abnormal DNA. Such a mechanism would also explain the increasing incidence of the disease with age, since there would be continuing failure to repair DNA and a progressive accumulation of abnormal nucleic acid eventually resulting in cell death.

Treatment

There is no medicine known which will cure or arrest the disease. As is so often the case in such situations, there have been many attempts at treatment, each of which has enjoyed popularity for a certain time. Therapeutic attempts with antiviral agents have not awaited proof of a viral etiology of motor neuron disease. Thus, amantadine, idoxuridine, cytosine, arabinoside, levamisole and isoprinosine have all been tried without success (66–74). Guanidine, a drug which may be an antiviral agent, but which also promotes the release of acetylcholine at the neuromuscular junction, has been employed. Initial encouraging results were not borne out on a long-term controlled trial (72, 75). Amantadine and guanidine were tried in 20 patients with ALS in a double-blind crossover trial; 10 patients being on guanidine and 10 on amantadine. The results were equally poor (75). Another precursor of acetylcholine, lecithin, has also been reported as ineffective (76). Some patients with motor neuron disease demonstrate fatigability and respond to the use of anticholinesterase such as pyridostigmine. Edrophonium can be used as diagnostic test to select those patients who might benefit from these drugs.

At the time of writing there is considerable interest in the use of TRH in motor neuron disease. Although best known for its role in stimulating the release of thyroid-stimulating hormone (TSH), TRH has other less well known properties as well as a rather wide distribution in the mammalian nervous system (77). In many ways TRH fulfills the criteria defining a neurotransmitter. It is localized within presynaptic nerve terminals, it is released upon stimulation of the nerve, there are high affinity receptors for TRH in the extrahypothalamic region of the brain, and direct iontophoresis can alter neuronal excitability. When applied to frog motor neurons the action of TRH was excitatory with a potency similar to that of glutamate (78). The neurons were seldom depolarized beyond the threshold necessary for a propagated potential but TRH might provide a facilitatory action changing the resting depolarization level and making the neuron more sensitive to subsequent depolarization past the threshold level. The fact that nerve terminals staining positively for TRH were present in networks around the anterior horn cells in the spinal cord as well as around those motor nuclei in the brainstem which are involved in ALS made it attractive to study the possible effect of TRH in the illness. The first study showed that high intravenous doses (2–19 mg/min) of TRH produced a moderate to marked improvement in the patient's strength (79). Subsequent studies using a subcutaneous route in an unblinded study have confirmed this impression (80). The drug is used in doses of about 150 mg in the average adult ranging from 25 to 200 mg daily. There are almost immediate side effects of shivering, slight hypertension, increase in the breathing rate, a peculiar sense of warmth or cold in the skin, and the feeling of bladder or rectal fullness and sometimes mild nausea. These side effects last for 15–30 minutes. The effect on the patient's function and strength lasts for up to 2 or 3 days and then disappears. An "autorefractory" period has been postulated to account for loss of therapeutic effect with continued drug usage. A drug-free interval of 1–3 days may reverse this.

There is some debate at the present time as to how much change in muscle function occurs, many investigators feel that the effect is not as dramatic as originally believed but, nevertheless, some muscles in some patients may show a definite increase in strength. Whether this effect is due to the release of inhibitory factors on the muscle activity or whether it is, in fact, a reversal of the lower motor neuron malfunction is not settled. TRH itself is rapidly destroyed in the blood and other tissues. In an attempt to deliver the TRH directly to the anterior horn cells, one group of investigators has used intrathecal infusion with results similar to the intravenous route (81).

An initial double blind placebo controlled trial of 150 mg TRH subcutaneously for 2 months in 30 patients showed improvement in the strength of scattered muscles but no change in the patient's function or in the course of the illness (82). Other studies, which have employed double blind control techniques, have failed to demonstrate the effectiveness of TRH, although in one the dose of the drug employed was different (83, 84). Investigations into the detailed physiological effect of TRH on muscle function have suggested improvement in such measurements following administration of the drug, although gains of clinical significance were more modest (85, 86). Last, the route of administration in most of the studies so far is either intravenous, subcutaneous, or intramuscular and there may be persuasive reasons to administer this drug more directly to the central nervous system using the intrathecal route (87). Where all of this is leading is not yet clear, the effect needs to be confirmed by using double blind techniques, particularly in view of some euphoria which seems to be associated with the administration of the TRH. It is also possible that the modification of the original TRH may lead to analogues which are more stable with a longer lasting effect.

The immune theory has received no support from treatment trials. Steroids are ineffective and plasmapheresis was without benefit (88). The use of interferon, in two patients with ALS who received subcutaneous injection of this substance, did not alter the illness (89). Penicillamine has been used in both short- and long-term treatment. It causes an increase in the excretion of lead, but has no clinical effect on the illness (21). Other drugs which have been used without benefit include vitamins E and B_{12}, phthalazinol (90), and amitryptiline. Snake venom enjoyed some notoriety but was discredited in two controlled studies (91, 92).

This gloomy litany of failed drugs should not be taken to indicate that there is no treatment in the disease. Perhaps the first point to emphasize is that a continuing dialogue between the patient and the physician is of great importance to the patient. Many physicians are uncomfortable in the presence of incurable disease and discourage frequent visits by the ALS patient. This act of banishment can cause a real sense of hopelessness and despair. I have often asked ALS patients, when I have been singularly unsuccessful in coping with their problems, why they returned to the clinic. The answer is usually the same. It begins with the statement, "I know you can't do anything for me, doctor, but just having someone who knows about the illness and will answer my questions helps." Patients, when told that they have a fatal disease, develop many fears which are irrational as well as others which are reasonable. They may believe that they will go blind or demented, or that death will come suddenly and unexpectedly, that they will lose bowel or bladder control, or that their friends may "catch" the illness. The proper medical management of ALS includes a quiet discussion period which may allay many of these fears. The practice of medicine has, after all, a major tenet that patients should feel better after visiting the physician. One does not always have to cure people.

In addition to the need for supportive devices, such as walkers, raised toilet seats, wheelchairs, and braces, the patient with motor neuron disease has, at some stage, three other problems. The first difficulty is with saliva pooling in the posterior pharynx. This produces choking spells and can be extemely disturbing. A portable suction device, properly used, can make an enormous difference to the patient's comfort. The second problem occurs at a stage when it is difficult to swallow solid foods. Many times patients struggle on, trying to swallow solids, not realizing the homogenized foods can be swallowed relatively easily. The use of a blender should be urged at the appropriate time. Sometimes the question arises as to whether a gastrostomy should be performed in order to circumvent the dysphagia. There is certainly much to be said for this procedure in patients whose mealtimes are spent in paroxysms of choking. From a practical point of view, we have found that the patient for whom a gastrostomy is being considered should be admitted to the hospital for a few days to evaluate the caloric intake with a properly balanced diet which is pureed or homogenized. In such a situation, the patient usually learns to take the semiliquid diet without too much problem. In one or two patients we have used feeding via nasogastric tube for brief periods of time.

Cricopharyngeal myotomy has been used in selected cases when dysfunction of this muscle can be demonstrated (93, 94). This simple procedure is far more acceptable to the patient than the unpleasantness of gastrostomy. In normal swallowing, the cricopharyngeal muscle plays an important part in initiating the movement of food down the esophagus. If its contraction is incoordinated, it may hamper swallowing, rather than help it. Surgical division of the muscle allows the food to enter the esophagus by gravity and may considerably improve swallowing. Such is the case in many patients with ALS. In one series, 15 patients with motor neuron disease underwent cricopharyngeal myotomy. Five died in the postoperative period. The other 10 all showed improvement of varying degrees. The deaths occurred because of respiratory failure. A mortality rate of 30% may seem excessive, but many patients with ALS, whose lives are made miserable by the severe bulbar symptoms, will gladly accept such a risk in the chance of deriving some benefit (95).

Another major source of discomfort in the ALS patient stems from the immobile shoulder. Patients who are developing shoulder weakness may very rapidly suffer from a "frozen" shoulder. The pain is associated with excursion of the arm through an ever decreasing range of motion, and finally, severe pain is present even with the arm immobile by the side. It is good practice to start shoulder mobilization exercises, in which the shoulder is put through the full mechanical range twice daily, as soon as the patient develops any signs of shoulder weakness.

Frequently a disturbance of sleep is noted by patients. Some may suffer from the terminal sleep disorder which accompanies their depression. There are two other symptoms, one of which occurs early and the other late. Night cramps are very troublesome and they are sometimes relieved by the use of quinine, diazepam, or, occasionally, calcium gluconate. Late in the disease, when the respiratory involvement produces mild anoxia, sleep is disturbed by frequent arousals and nightmares. Portable oxygen by the bedside can make the difference between a terrifying and restless night and a sound night's sleep. In the classical form of motor neuron disease, death is inevitable and heroic efforts to keep the patient alive at all costs are a disservice. It is equally obvious that the patient and his relatives should be consulted in any decision with regard to management.

In the last few years, there has been a major change in the management of some patients with motor neuron disease. The terminal event in all patients is respiratory failure of one kind or another. The ALS patient who is placed on a mechanical ventilator is seldom weaned from it. Most patients feel that survival in a hospital on a mechanical ventilator is unacceptable. The development of the portable ventilator has changed the situation for some patients. Life at home in a wheelchair is now possible. It is even possible for patients to be employed and lead a productive life. In my own opinion, it is the exceptional patient who can handle this type of independence. The patient will have to cope with everything from the curiosity of their friends in public, to their fear of a mechanical failure and sudden death. A necessary part of the management will be the presence of a spouse, close friend, or relative who is prepared to cope with the stress of looking after the patient's needs and who is willing to learn how to use the ventilator. The time to discuss this is before the need arises and the decision must not be taken lightly. The moment of crisis is not the time to be making such decisions. Those who volunteer most readily for this task are often the ones who have given it the least thought. A sensible discussion of the problems involved in this is the paper by Sivak et al. (96).

Slow Motor Neuron Disease

The existence of a form of motor neuron disease, which is only slowly progressive, has been known for some time. It is often not emphasized in medical texts because only a small minority of the patients were thought to be thus affected. It now seems that slow motor neuron disease may be more common than was previously thought. Obviously physicians who see a large number of patients with motor neuron disease will see a disproportionate number with the benign form; the mere fact of their survival ensures a steadily increasing population of such patients in the muscle clinic. This is in contrast to patients with the rapidly progressive illness, who die in a short time, and, therefore, disappear from the clinic population. Nevertheless, it seems that about 20% of the patients with motor neuron disease will conform to the "benign" variety with survival in excess of 5 years (97). There is no basic difference between the slow form and the more classical variety of motor neuron disease except that bulbar symptoms and upper motor signs are often absent in the early phase of the illness. Wasting, weakness, and fasciculations of the limbs are found, often in a patchy distribution and frequently more distal than proximal. Some signs of denervation may be noted in the tongue. It is only to be expected that those patients with the mildest form of the disease should have the longest survival. Whether slow neuron disease is a different illness characterized by absence of bulbar findings or whether the absence of bulbar paralysis permits the patient with motor neuron disease to survive longer is thus an unanswerable question. Slow motor neuron disease may be differentiated from the Kugelberg-Welander form of juvenile spinal muscular atrophy by the characteristic proximal distribution of the latter disease.

Focal Motor Neuron Disease

An interesting but only tentatively identified form of motor neuron disease is one in which only one area of the body is attacked. The disease begins insidiously with wasting and fasciculations involving one group of muscles. The shoulder girdle is particularly susceptible (Fig. 2.22), and I have also seen the small muscles of one hand and forearm and the thigh muscles involved. Typically, the disease is progressive for several months and may result in quite severe localized disability. The process then stops and the patient is left with a fixed deficit, from which he does not recover. I have seen some patients with atrophy of one shoulder girdle who have had an identical episode some years later involving the other shoulder girdle. Yet others with apparent focal motor neuron disease develop the slowly progressive variety after an interval of some years. No autopsy studies have been performed and, therefore, the diagnosis is still not proven pathologically. However, the muscle biopsy findings and EMG studies are characteristic of those seen in amyotrophic lateral sclerosis.

Over 100 patients have been described with focal atrophy of the small muscles of the hand and the forearm. Distribution of wasting is unusual

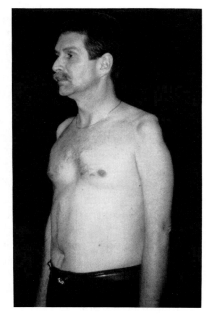

Figure 2.22. Focal motor neuron disease. This patient has been followed for 10 years and, although there is severe wasting of the shoulder, the disease has progressed hardly at all in the last 8 years.

because the brachioradialis muscle is spared. The disease is usually unilateral, at least initially, and may be associated with an exacerbation of the weakness with cold. EMG studies suggest a neurogenic disease. There may be preservation of the reflexes in spite of the wasting, a feature which it shares with motor neuron disease. The disease may be rapidly progressive initially, and then further progression appears to be slow or absent (98–100).

When there is such localized involvement, it is extremely important to rule out other possible diagnoses such as root compression, spinal cord tumors, or various forms of mononeuritis, diabetic and otherwise. Such lesions of the nerves or spinal cord are usually revealed by the presence of sensory abnormalities, although these may be slight. One patient, in whom the diagnosis of focal motor neuron disease was thought likely, developed some numbness of the lateral aspect of the shoulder 6 years after first noticing weakness of the shoulder. A benign tumor involving the C_5 root was found at exploratory surgery. When the shoulder girdle is involved, the possibility of brachial neuritis or neuralgic amyotrophy should be considered. This may be differentiated from focal motor neuron disease by the antecedent history of pain and by the tendency for recovery to occur following the episode of weakness. In summary, if focal motor neuron disease is to be considered as a diagnosis, great care should be taken to exclude other causes of focal atrophy. The final proof of its existence will depend upon autopsy studies.

OTHER MOTOR NEURON DISEASES

Since we neither know the cause of motor neuron disease nor have an absolute marker (such as a missing enzyme) with which to characterize the illness, it is difficult to decide whether the following diseases are merely variants of the classical form or whether they exist as clinical or pathological entities in their own right. At any rate, there are sometimes distinguishing characteristics which warrant inclusion in a separate category. Some of the syndromes occur recurrently in the literature and may have assumed an independent existence for that reason alone.

Geographic Pockets of Motor Neuron Disease

Guam

Motor neuron disease occurs among the Chamorro population on the islands of Guam, Rota and Tinian in the Western Pacific (5, 8, 101, 102). When originally described, the incidence of the disease was about 30 times higher than in the rest of the world, and was the cause of death in almost 10% of the adult population. The incidence is now declining in all age groups. Another major illness in the same population is the parkinsonism-dementia complex. These two syndromes are related, although the nature of their association is not clear. Guamanian patients who present with motor neuron disease rarely develop the parkinsonism-dementia complex, although patients with the latter illness may develop motor neuron disease terminally. The degree of involvement of the lower motor neurons in the parkinsonism-dementia syndrome is rather mild, and it has been suggested that this is merely the type of muscular atrophy associated with a very ill patient. Although clinically the two diseases are dissimilar, their appearance in the same populations on Guam and in other areas is more than coincidental. Pathologically, both illnesses show similar changes, changes which are different from those seen in classical motor neuron disease (103). Alzheimer's neurofibrillary degeneration has been described in various locations in the nervous system including the cerebral cortex, Ammon's horn, various basal ganglia, and some cranial nuclei of the brainstem. Granulovacuolar bodies were noted particularly in the pyramidal cells of Ammon's horn. Crystalloid inclusion bodies were also described. Guamanian ALS demonstrates a familial incidence of the disease in 14% of the patients. Further analysis of this does not reveal any particular form of inheritance and it is possible that the familial incidence represents an abnormal genetic stratum on which motor neuron disease develops from other causes. A declining incidence of Guamanian ALS has been associated with the increasing modernization of these previously isolated communities, suggesting some factor in the environment which predisposes the population to the disease. Should this be the case, studying segments of the population who have left Guam and emigrated to other countries or who have migrated into Guam from elsewhere would be of interest. The illness attacks Philippino migrants to Guam with a frequency about 6 times that of the continental United States, and yet not as frequently as Chamorros living on Guam (104). Migrations of Chamorros from Guam to other countries has also been studied (105). ALS developed in 28 of them, all of whom had spent their childhood and adolescence on Guam. Although the incidence of the illness in these patients was lower than that seen in the population from which they emigrated, it was nevertheless higher than in the country in which they settled. The disease appeared from 1 to 34 years after the patients left the island. This again suggests an environmental influence on the island of Guam which predisposes the patients to the development of ALS. Whatever factor this is, it seems to be associated with relatively primitive living conditions. The use of the cicad nut, a staple part of the diet, was investigated, but no definite evidence of its role in the disease was found. More recently, the soil and the drinking water in the areas in which the disease is endemic have been found to have a relatively high concentration of aluminum and manganese and a deficiency of calcium and magnesium (106). X-ray spectrometry has shown a high aluminum content in the neurofibrillary tangle bearing hipocampal neurons in Guamanian ALS (107). The decline in the incidence of ALS on Guam has reached the point where the population on Guam now has only a slightly higher risk of developing the illness than people elsewhere in the world (108), perhaps related to environmental factors such as changing dietary calcium and magnesium levels.

Kii Peninsula

A similar pocket of motor neuron disease has been found in the Kii Penisula in Japan (109–111). This is centered around the relatively isolated areas of Hobara and Kazagawa on the main island of Honshu. The clinical and pathological findings are very similar to those found in the Guamanian patients. Postmortem studies show neurofibrillary tangles. Another similarity is the low magnesium and calcium levels and increased amounts of aluminum and manganese in the soil and drinking water. The incidence is also declining in this area, again implying that modernization of the society is in some way associated with a decrease in the incidence of the disease.

West New Guinea

The highest incidence of ALS anywhere in the world is seen among the Auyu and Jakai people living under extremely primitive conditions in the southern coastal plain of West New Guinea (112). The prevalence in this rather small population of 7,000 people is over 1,300 cases per 100,000. This is over 100-fold the incidence in the rest of the world. As in the previous two examples, there is an association between ALS and the Parkinson dementia complex in the population. The clinical and pathological features are again similar, although the onset of the disease is earlier. This population is of particular interest because, although the same features of a deficiency in calcium and magnesium and an overabundance of aluminum and manganese is found in the drinking water, the population has no access to many factors which are abundant in developed countries. Domestic fowl and cattle, sheep and goats are not found in the area. Grain, such as rice, corn and wheat are absent from the diet, as are milk and dairy products. Manufactured goods of all kinds are missing, particularly petrochemicals, organic solvents, insecticides, fertilizers, medicines, and many other products. Since there are affected and unaffected villages in relative close proximity and since there seems to be no natural barrier to travel between these villages, either on the part of the people living in the region, or any possible vectors in the region, it seems unlikely that a communicable agent is responsible for the illness.

Ryukyuan Muscular Atrophy

In a fascinating report, Kondo et al. (113) outlined the historical, clinical, and pathological features of a neuromuscular disease with a high incidence in the Ryukyu Islands south of Japan. The disease clinically resembled juvenile spinal muscular atrophy with a slowly progressive, predominantly proximal weakness in which the legs were more involved than the arms. Some patients had fasciculations. Kyphoscoliosis and pes cavus were features of the disease. Although the results were not clear-cut, the authors felt that EMG and biopsy studies showed more evidence of neurogenic changes than of myopathic changes. The inheritance was through a recessive gene, attributed to a co-ancestor from northern Okinawa living in the 14th century.

Progressive Juvenile Bulbar Palsy (Fazio-Londe Disease)

A very rare disorder may be a variant of juvenile motor neuron disease. The disease is not present at birth which helps to differentiate if from other causes of facial diplegias such a myotonic dystrophy, infantile facioscapulohumeral dystrophy, and Möbius syndrome. A progressive weakness of the facial, ocular, and bulbar muscles occurs in the first decade. As the disease progresses, there is atrophy and weakness of the trunk and limb muscles; the prognosis is similar to that in the more common motor neuron diseases, with death occurring in months to years. Postmortem examination shows loss of motor nuclei throughout the brainstem and also loss of anterior horn cells in the spinal cord (114, 115). I have seen only three cases of this illness. The pathological findings on muscle biopsy from a clinically unaffected limb were those of denervation.

Scapuloperoneal and Facioscapulohumeral Syndromes

There are several entities which by implication are thought to represent anterior horn cell disease, but the literature seems to be in some disarray. Part of the problem reflects the changes which have occurred in the last decade in the criteria by which denervation or myopathic abnormalities are ascertained. Some years ago, the classification of muscle biopsies into the two categories of "neurogenic" and "myopathic" seemed to be clear-cut. EMG studies showed an equally clear-cut difference between the two groups. Recently this classical interpretation has been revised and the distinction blurred. Basophilia and phagocytosis may be seen in denervating diseases. Grouped fiber atrophy may, in fact, not be due to denervation but may reflect fiber type-specific atrophy or fiber splitting. Fibrillation potentials may be seen in the dystrophies and short, polyphasic potentials in neuropathies. About the only acceptable evidence that an illness is of the anterior horn cell is the autopsy demonstration of selective damage to these neurons. Such reports are conspicuously lacking from much of the literature.

A syndrome in which weakness of the anterior tibial and peroneal muscles is associated with weakness of the muscles around the shoulders has been termed the scapuloperoneal syndrome. This is a rather common combination in the muscle clinic, and about half of the patients seem to have an illness which is related to facioscapulohumeral dystrophy by its genetic, EMG, chemical, and pathological characteristics. The other patients may have any of a number of illnesses ranging from central core disease to nemaline myopathy. Many reports suggest the existence of a form of the illness caused by anterior horn cell disease. Close analysis of these reports reveals some discrepancies between the findings and the conclusions. In one family with a dominant inheritance, only 2 out of 12 members had definite shoulder weakness, and both EMG and muscle biopsy studies showed "myopathic" changes in some instances and "neuropathic" in others. A single autopsy report showed changes only in the cranial nerve nuclei (116). In another case, the published photograph of the muscle biopsy does not show convincing evidence of denervation, although the EMG revealed reduced motor unit activity with associated large potentials (117). The child described by Emery et al. (118) developed severe and generalized weakness after the initial symptoms of peroneal weakness, and the disease resembled a progressive motor neuron disease. This paper was criticized by Meadows and Marsden (119) who felt that the patient might have had Charcot-Marie-Tooth disease and cited one of their own patients with a similar clinical picture who later developed progressive slowing of the nerve conclusion velocities. Feigenbaum and Munsat (120) have pointed out in their paper on the subject the difficulties involved in determining the underlying pathology.

Motor neuron disease has also been implicated as a cause of facioscapulo-humeral syndrome clinically identical to the more familiar dystrophic form (121). Again, the evidence for this is disputable. The neuropathic etiology was based on the presence of small angulated fibers. Such fibers, however, have never been shown to be pathognomonic of denervation alone, and, in our experience, have been part of the picture of classical facioscapulohumeral dystrophy. The patient's EMG did not show any evidence of denervation. Although the girl's mother (who did not undergo a muscle biopsy) had an EMG which revealed fibrillations, this was only in the small hand muscles and not around the shoulders. I do not wish to imply that there are no scapuloperoneal syndromes caused by denervation. There may be such. It might be prudent, though, to await better definition of these cases before predicting their genetics and prognosis.

Distal Spinal Muscular Atrophy

The usual varieties of anterior horn cell diseases seldom spare the proximal muscles and the patient who presents with distal weakness and wasting should first be suspected of having a peripheral neuropathy. Nevertheless, there are patients who have distal wasting unaccompanied by such sensory symptoms as might incriminate the peripheral nerve with certainty. If, in addition, the conduction velocities are normal and the biopsy shows difinite evidence of denervation, the diagnosis of some form of spinal muscular atrophy seems likely. Some believe the illness represents a form of peroneal muscular atrophy differing in the lack of evidence of peripheral nerve pathology as well as in some of the clinical symptoms. For example, the arms are less involved than the legs, the incidence of foot deformity is higher, and the deep tendon reflexes are more commonly retained than in the usual forms of hereditary motor and sensory neuropathy. The symptoms usually begin in the first 20 years and the patterns of inheritance include autosomal dominant and autosomal recessive, as well as sporadic cases (122). Similar cases with an autosomal recessive inheritance were found during a survey of spinal muscular atrophy in the Northeast of England. Although a later onset was recognized in some patients, the illness usually begins in infancy or early childhood (123). Clinically, it again resembles the hereditary motor and sensory neuropathies of the Charcot-Marie-Tooth variety without the sensory component. The distal muscles of both the arms and legs are involved. The disease is progressive, although some patients still walk unaided in adult life. A third report details the clinical picture in six patients whose wasting and weakness is limited to the intrinsic muscles of the hands and is often asymmetric and accompanied by only the mildest involvement of any other muscle. The patients differ from those with focal motor neuron disease by the slow but steady progression of their illness (124).

Spinal Muscular Atrophy with Vocal Cord Paralysis

The same distal distribution of weakness and wasting resembling Charcot-Marie-Tooth disease but with normal nerve conduction velocities was seen in a family in which six members had an associated paralysis of the vocal cords. The EMG in two patients was said to show spontaneous fibrillations with a reduced interference pattern. No biopsy confirmation of denervation was available (125).

X-Linked Recessive Spinal Muscular Atrophy with Bulbar Involvement

This illness, inherited as an X-linked recessive, commonly begins in early or middle adult life with progressive weakness of the limbs which is usually more proximal than distal (126). There is also marked facial weakness often with fasciculations around the mouth and difficulty with swallowing. Gynecomastia is a curious and unexplained companion of the disease. Other occasional findings are elevated cerebrospinal fluid protein as well as mild elevation of CK.

Hexosaminidase Deficiency

Hexosaminidase is an enzyme which exist in three major forms in tissue. Its action is to cleave the N-acetylgalactosamine component from various naturally occurring glycolipids as well as some artificial substrates which are used in the determination of hexosaminidase levels. The compounds include gangliosides such as GM_2 gangliosides, globoside and asialogangliosides which are related to the gangliosides but do not contain neuraminic acid. Other substrates which occur naturally include oligosaccharides, glycoproteins and mucopolysaccharides (127).

There are three major isozymes, hexosaminidase A, B, and S. The first two of which are the most important in normal tissue. Hexosaminidase A is composed of both alpha (α) and beta (β) subunits. Hexosaminidase B consist entirely of β subunits. Hexosaminidase S comprises α subunits alone. The best known disorders of hexosaminidase deficiency are primarily disorders of the central nervous system, such as Tay-Sachs disease (hexosaminidase A deficiency), Sandhoff's disease (deficiency of both A and B isozyme due to an abnormality of the β subunit), as well as some ataxias of the spinocerebellar type which may be due to defects in the A or B isozyme or both. The correlation between the enzyme defect and the actual physiologic cause of the illness is, at present, unclear but an enzyme which has an effect on glycoproteins and mucopolysaccharides could well cause changes in the properties in the cell surface membrane.

It has become apparent recently that the clinical complexity of the hexosaminidase related diseases is greater than was originally thought and now includes some varieties of lower motor neuron disease (128–131). The patients described may not have identical disorders but the lower motor neurons were involved in all. It has been described both in an Ashkenazi Jewish man as well as in two non-Jewish patients. The clinical symptoms included proximal muscle wasting and weakness which was slowly progressive, fasciculations, cramps, hyperreflexia, stiffness, extensor plantar responses and, in general, a clinical picture which suggested motor neuron disease of either the ALS or the Kugelberg-Welander type. Spinocerebellar or cerebellar involvement has also been described. One family demonstrated mild mental retardation as part of the picture. Muscle biopsy shows chronic denervation and sural nerve biopsies have demonstrated loss of large myelinated fibers. Head scans revealed marked cerebellar atrophy. More cases will need to be studied before the "typical" clinical picture becomes apparent.

Triose Phosphate Isomerase Deficiency

A deficiency of the enzyme triose phosphate isomerase is associated with hemolytic anemia in infancy. Some of the patients express neurological abnormalities including ataxia, dystonic posturing, and pseudo rhythmic jerking of the extremities (132). Wasting and weakness of the limb muscles with an EMG which indicated denervation and with normal nerve conduction velocities pointed to an accompanying involvement of the motor neurons.

The enzyme, which is active in the glycolytic pathways interconverting glyceraldehyde phosphate and dihydroxyacetone, is absent in red and white blood cells, spinal fluid, skin fibroblast and muscle tissue.

"Incidental" Motor Neuron Disease

Degeneration of motor neurons undoubtedly occurs as part of several other diseases. In such illnesses the brunt of the pathology is borne by other areas of the nervous system and the presenting symptoms reflect this. The motor neuron disease is only an incidental finding, although it is no less real.

In Jakob-Creutzfeldt disease, a disorder due to a transmissible agent (66), there is a widespread neuronal degeneration. The disease begins with an increasing dementia, sometimes heralded by depression and behavioral disturbances. Early on, the patient may become fidgety and jumpy, later developing frank myoclonic movements and abnormal startle responses. As the disease progresses, difficulty with the bulbar musculature affects swallowing and talking. The rapidly progressive dementia may be associated with either spasticity or rigidity; other cases have been described with cerebellar ataxia. The wasting of the muscles, which is particularly seen around the shoulders, occurs late in the disease, but gives the typical appearance of motor neuron disease with fasciculations, wasting, and weakness. The disease runs a rapid course, and usually death occurs in less than a year. The terminal patient is often obtunded, blind, and mute, with a decorticate posture. If brain biopsy is performed in an attempt to confirm the diagnosis, care must be taken in the handling of the specimen, since this is a transmissible disease.

Muscular wasting and weakness associated with anterior horn cell degeneration has also been described in a number of other entities including high voltage electric shock, x-ray radiation, hyperparathyroidism, and asthma.

REFERENCES

1. Kurtzke, J. F., and Beebe, G. W. Epidemiology of amyotrophic lateral sclerosis: I. A case controlled comparison based on ALS deaths. Neurology *30:* 453–462, 1980.
2. Juergens, S. M., Kurland, L. T., Okazaki, H., Mulder, D. W., and Kurtzke, J. F. Epidemiology of amyotrophic lateral sclerosis. In: *Human Motor Neuron Diseases*, edited by L. P. Rowland. Raven Press, New York, 1982, pp. 281–302.
3. Jokelainen, M. Epidemiology of ALS in Finland. J. Neurol. Sci. *29:* 55–63, 1976.
4. Holloway, S. M., and Emery, A. E. H. The epidemiology of motor neuron disease in Scotland. Muscle Nerve *5:* 131–133, 1982.
5. Kurland, L. T., Choi, N. W., and Sayre, G. P. Implications of incidence and geographic patterns on the classification of amyotrophic lateral sclerosis. In: *Motor Neuron Diseases*, edited by F. H. Norris and L. T. Kurland. Grune & Stratton, New York, 1969. pp. 28–48.
6. Bobowick, A. R., and Brody, J. A. Epidemiology of motor neuron diseases. N. Engl. J. Med. *288:* 1047–1055. 1973.
7. Horton, W. A., Eldridge, R., and Brody, J. A. Familial motor neuron disease. Neurology *26:* 460–465. 1976.
8. Mulder, D. W., and Espinosa, R. E. Amyotrophic lateral sclerosis: comparison of the clinical syndrome in Guam and the United States. In: *Motor Neuron Diseases*, edited by F. H. Norris and L. T. Kurland. Grune & Stratton, New York, 1969, pp; 12–19.
9. Brain, W. R., Croft, P., and Wilkinson, M. The course and outcome of motor neuron disease. In: *Motor Neuron Diseases*, edited by F. H. Norris and L. T. Kurland. Grune & Stratton, New York, 1969, pp. 20–27.
10. Norris, F. H. Adult spinal motor neuron disease. In: *Handbook of Clinical Neurology*, Vol. 22, edited by P. J. Vinken and G. W. Bruyn. North Holland, Amsterdam, 1975, pp. 1–56.
11. Jacobs, L., Bozin, D., Heffner, R. R., and Barron, S. A. An eye movement disorder in amyotrophic lateral sclerosis. Neurology *31:* 1282–1287, 1981.
12. Leveille, A., Kiernan, J., Goodwin, J. A., and Antel, J. Eye movements in amyotrophic lateral sclerosis. Arch. Neurol. *39:* 679–686, 1982.
13. Dyck, P. J., Stevens, J. C., Mulder, D. W., and Espinosa, R. E. Frequency of nerve fiber degeneration of peripheral motor and sensory neurons in amyotrophic lateral sclerosis. Neurology *25:* 781–785, 1975.
14. Carpenter, S. Proximal axonal enlargement in motor neuron disease. Neurology *18:* 842–851, 1968.
15. Hirano, S. Aspects of the ultrastructure of amyotrophic lateral sclerosis. In: *Human Motor Neuron Disease*, edited by L. P. Rowland. Raven Press, New York, 1982, pp. 75–87.
16. Welch, K. M. A., and Goldberg, D. M. Serum creatine phosphokinase in motor neuron disease. Neurology *22:* 697–702, 1972.
17. Williams, E. R., and Bruford, A. Creatine phosphokinase in motor neuron disease. Clin. Chim. Acta *27:* 53, 1970.
18. Kjellin, K. G., and Stibler, H. Isoelectric focusing and electrophoresis of cerebrospinal fluid protein in muscular dystrophies and spinal muscular atrophies. J. Neurol. Sci. *27:* 45–57, 1976.
19. Corbett, A. J., Griggs, R. C., and Moxley, R. T. Skeletal muscle catabolism in amyotrophic lateral sclerosis and chronic spinal muscular atrophy. Neurology *32:* 550–552, 1982.
20. Antel, J. P., Chelmicka-Schorr, E., Sportiello, M., Stefansson, K., Wollmann, R. L., and Arnason, B. G. Muscle acid protease activity in amyotrophic lateral sclerosis: correlation with clinical and pathological features. Neurology *32:* 901–903, 1982.
21. Conradi, S., Ronnevi, L. O., Nise, G., and Vesterburg, O. Long term penicillamine treatment in amyotrophic lateral sclerosis with parallel determination of lead in blood plasma and urine. Acta Neurol. Scand. *65:* 203–211, 1982.
22. Rowland, L. P., Defendini, R., Sherman, W., Hirano, A., Olarte, M.R., Latov, N., Lovelace, R. E., Inocre, K., and Osserman, E. E. Macroglobulinemia with peripheral neuropathy simulating motor neuron disease. Ann. Neurol. *11:* 532–536, 1982.

23. Boothby, J. A., deJesus, P. V., and Rowland, L. P. Reversible forms of motor neuron disease: lead "neuritis." Arch. Neurol. *31:* 18–23, 1974.
24. Kantarjian, A. D. A syndrome clinically resembling amyotrophic lateral sclerosis following chronic mercurialism. Neurology *11:* 639–642, 1961.
25. Rustam, H., and Hamdi, T. Methyl mercury poisoning in Iraq. Brain *97:* 499–510, 1974.
26. Norris, F. H., and Engel, W. K. Carcinomatous amyotrophic lateral sclerosis. In: *The Remote Effects of Cancer on the Nervous System*, edited by W. R. Brain and F. H. Norris. Grune & Stratton, New York, 1965.
27. Felmus, M. T., Patten, B. M., and Swanke, L. Antecedent events in amyotrophic lateral sclerosis. Neurology *26:* 167–172, 1976.
28. Tarras, S., Schenkman, B. A., Boesch, R., Mulvihill, M., and Caroscio, J. T. ALS and pet exposure. Neurology *35:* 717–720, 1985.
29. Pierce-Ruhland, R., and Patten, B. M. Trace metals in motor neuron disease. Ann. Neurol. *8:* 193–195, 1980.
30. Mizumoto, Y., Iwata, S., Sasajima, K., Yase, Y. and Yoshida, S. Alpha particle excited x-ray fluorescence analysis for trace elements in cervical spinal cords of amyotrophic lateral sclerosis. Radioisotopes *29:* 385–389, 1980.
31. Schauf, C. L., Antel, J. P., Arnason, B. C., Davis, F. A., and Rooney, M. W. Neuroelectric blocking activity and plasmapheresis in amyotrophic lateral sclerosis. Neurology *30:* 1011–1013, 1980.
32. Wolfgram, F., and Myers, L., Amyotrophic lateral sclerosis: Effect of serum on anterior horn cells in tissue culture. Science *179:* 579–580, 1973.
33. Horwich, J. S., Engel, W. K., and Chauvin, P. B. Amyotrophic lateral sclerosis sera applied to cultured motor neurons. Arch. Neurol. *30:* 332–333, 1974.
34. Roisen, F. J., Bartfeld, H., Donnenfeld, H., and Baxter, J. Circulating neurotoxins in amyotrophic lateral sclerosis. Adv. Neurol. *36:* 403–417, 1982.
35. Askanas, V., Marangos, P. J., and Engel, W. K. CSF from ALS patients applied to motor neurons in culture fails to alter neuron specific enolase. Neurology *31:* 1196–1197, 1981.
36. Oldstone, M. G. A., Wilson, C. B., Perrin, L. H., et al.: Evidence of Immune complex formation in patients with amyotrophic lateral sclerosis. Lancet *2:* 169–172, 1976.
37. Kletti, N. B., Marton, L. S., Antel, J. P., and Stefansson, K. Antibodies against neuroantigens in the serum of patients with amyotrophic lateral sclerosis. Neurology, *34* (Suppl. 1): 238, 1984.
38. Brown, R. H., Ogonowski, M., Johnson, D., and Weiner, H. L. Antineuronal antibodies in sera from patients with amyotrophic lateral sclerosis. Neurology *34* (Suppl. 1): 238, 1984.
39. Gurney, M. E. Suppression of sprouting at the neuromuscular junction by immunoassay sera. Nature *307:* 546–548, 1984.
40. Gurney, M. E., Belton, A. C., Cashman, N.,, and Antel, J. P. Inhibition of terminal axon sprouting by serum from patients with amyotrophic lateral sclerosis. N. Engl. J. Med. *311:* 933–939, 1984.
41. Apatoff, B., Antel, J., and Gurney, M. Autoantibodies in amyotrophic lateral sclerosis. Ann. Neurol. *16:* 109, 1984.
42. Antel, J. P., Arnason, B. G. W., Fuller, T. C., and Lehrich, J. R. Histocompatibility typing in amyotrophic lateral sclerosis. Arch Neurol. *33:* 423–425, 1976.
43. Antel, J. P., Horonha, A. B. C., Oger, J. J. F., and Arnason, B. G. W. Immunology of amyotrophic lateral sclerosis. In: *Human Motor Neuron Diseases*, edited by L. P. Rowland. Raven Press, New York, 1982, pp. 395–401.
44. Bartfeld, H., Pollack, M. S., Cunningham-Rundle, S., and Donnenfeld, H. HLA frequencies in amyotrophic lateral sclerosis. Arch. Neurol. *39:* 270–271, 1982.
45. Krieger, C., and Melmed, C. Amyotrophic lateral sclerosis and paraproteinemia. Neurology *32:* 896–892, 1982.
46. Zil'ber, L. A., Bajdakova, Z. L., Gardasjan, A. N., Konovalov, N. V., Burina, T. L., and Barabadze, E. M. Study of the etiology of amyotrophic lateral sclerosis. Bull. W.H.O. *29:* 449, 1963.
47. Gibbs, C. J., and Gajdusek, D. C. Kuru-A prototype subacute infectious disease of the nervous system as a model for the study of amyotrophic lateral sclerosis. In: *Motor Neuron Diseases*, edited by F. H. Norris and L. T. Kurland. Grune & Stratton, New York, 1969, pp. 269–279.
48. Gibbs, C. J., and Gajdusek, D. C. An update on long term in vivo and in vitro studies designed to identify a virus as the cause of ALS, parkinsonism dementia, and Parkinson's disease. In: *Human Motor Neuron Diseases*, edited by L. P. Rowland. Raven Press, New York, 1982, pp. 342–351.
49. Weiner, L. P., Stohlman, S. A. and Davis, R. L. Attempts to demonstrate virus in amyotrophic lateral sclerosis. Neurology *30:* 1319–1322, 1980.

50. Kayser Gatchalian, L. Late muscular atrophy after poliomyelitis. Eur. Neurol. *10:* 371–380, 1973.
51. Mulder, D. W., Rosenbaum, R. A., and Layton, D. D. Late progression of poliomyelitis or forme fruste amyotrophic lateral sclerosis. Mayo Clin. Proc. *27:* 756–761, 1972.
52. Oshiro, L. S., Cremer, N. E., Norris, F. H., and Lennette, E. H. Viruslike particles in muscle from a patient with amyotrophic lateral sclerosis. Neurology *26:* 57–60, 1976.
53. Kohne, D. E., Gibbs, C. J., White, L., Tracy, S. M., Meinke, W., and Smith, R. A., Virus detection by nucleic acid hybridization: examination of normal and ALS tissues for the presence of polio virus. J. Gen. Viol. *56:* 223–233, 1981.
54. Roos, R. P., Viola, M. V., Wollmann, R., Hatch, M. H., and Antel, J. P. Amyotrophic lateral sclerosis with antecedent poliomyelitis. Arch. Neurol. *37:* 312–313, 1980.
55. Weiner, L. P. Possible role of androgen receptors in amyotrophic lateral sclerosis—hypothesis. Arch. Neurol. *37:* 129–131, 1980.
56. Jones, T. M., Yu, R., and Antel, J. P. Response of patients with amyotrophic lateral sclerosis to testosterone therapy—endocrine evaluation. Arch. Neurol. *39:* 721–722, 1982.
57. Engel, W. K., Siddique, T., Nicolett, J. T., and Wilber, J. F. TRH levels are reduced in CSF of amyotrophic lateral sclerosis patients and rise with intravenous treatment. Neurology *33* (Suppl. 2): 176, 1983.
58. Jackson, M. D., Munsat, T. L., Taft, J., Lechar, R., and Adelman, L. TRH is normal in ALS spinal cord but cyclic His-Pro DKP is elevated. Neurology *35* (Suppl. 1): 106, 1985.
59. Quick, D. T. Pancreatic dysfunction in amyotrophic lateral sclerosis. In: *Motor Neuron Diseases*, edited by F. H. Norris and L. T. Kurland, Grune & Stratton, New York, 1969, pp. 189–198.
60. Engel, W. K., Hogenhuis, L. A. H., Collis, W. J., Schalch, D. S., Barlow, M. H., Gold, G. N., and Dorman, J. Metabolic studies and therapeutic trials in amyotrophic lateral sclerosis. In: *Motor Neuron Diseases*, edited by F. H. Norris and L. T. Kurland. Grune & Stratton, New York, 1969, pp. 199–208.
61. Charcaflie, R. J., Fernandez, L. B., Perec, C. J., Gonzalez, E., and Marzi, A. Functional studies of the parotid and pancreas glands in amyotrophic lateral sclerosis. J. Neurol. Neurosurg. Psychiatry *37:* 683–867, 1974.
62. Appel, S. H., A unifying hypothesis for the cause of amyotrophic lateral sclerosis, Parkinson's, and Alzheimer's disease. Ann. Neurol. *10:* 499–505, 1981.
63. Bradley, W. G., and Krasin, F. A new hypothesis of the etiology of amyotrophic lateral sclerosis. Arch. Neurol. *39:* 677–680, 1980.
64. Davidson, T. J., Hartmann, H. A., and Johnson, P. C. RNA content and volume of motor neurons in amyotrophic lateral sclerosis: I. The cervical swelling. J. Neuropathol. Exp. Neurol. *40:* 32–36, 1981.
65. Davidson, T. J., and Hartmann, H. A. Base composition of RNA obtained from motor neurons in amyotrophic lateral sclerosis. J. Neuropathol. Exp. Neurol. *40:* 193–198, 1981.
66. Dorman, J. D., Engel, W. K., and Fried, D. M. Therapeutic trial in amyotrophic lateral sclerosis. J.A.M.A. *209:* 257–260, 1969.
67. Norris, F. H. Amantadine in Jakob-Creutzfeldt disease. Brit. Med. J. *2:* 349, 1972.
68. Liversedge, L. A., and Campbell, M. J. Motor neurone diseases. In: *Disorders of Voluntary Muscle*, edited by J. N. Walton, Churchill-Livingstone, London, 1974, p. 790.
69. Liversedge, L. A., Swinburn, W. R., and Yuile, G. M. Idoxuridine and motor neuron disease. Brit. Med. J. *1:* 755, 1970.
70. Brody, J. A., Chen, K. M., Yase, Y., Holden, E. M., and Morris, C. E. Inosiplex and amyotrophic lateral sclerosis: therapeutic trial in patients on Guam. Arch. Neurol. *30:* 322–323, 1974.
71. Percy, A. K., Davis, L. E. Johnston, D. M., and Drachman, D. B. Failure of isoprinosine in amyotrophic lateral sclerosis. New Engl. J. Med. *285:* 689, 1971.
72. Norris, F. H., Calanchini, P. R., Fallat, R. J., Panchari, S., and Jewett, B. The administration of guanidine in ALS. Neurology *24:* 721–728, 1974.
73. Mendell, J. R., Chase, T. N., and Engel, W. K. Amyotrophic lateral sclerosis: A study of central monoamine metabolism and a therapeutic trial of levo dopa. Arch. Neruol. *25:* 320, 1971.
74. Olarte, M. R., and Shafer, S. Q. Levamisole is ineffective in the treatment of amyotrophic lateral sclerosis. Neurology *35:* 1063–1066, 1985.
75. Munsat, T. L., Easterday, C. S., Levy, S., Woolff, S. M., and Hiatt, R. Amantidine and guanidine are ineffective in ALS. Neurology *31:* 1054–1055, 1981.
76. Kelemen, J., Hedlund, W., Murray-Douglas, P., and Munsat, T. L. Lecithin is not effective in amyotrophic lateral sclerosis. Neurology *32:* 315–316, 1982.
77. Jackson, I. M. D. Thyrotropin-releasing hormone. N. Engl. J. Med. *306:* 145–154, 1982.
78. Nicoll, R. A. Excitatory action of TRH on spinal motoneurones. Nature *265:* 242–43, 1977.

79. Engel, W. K., Siddique, T., and Nicoloff, J. T. Effect on weakness and spasticity in amyotrophic lateral sclerosis of thyrotropin-releasing hormone. Lancet 2: 73–75, 1983.
80. Engel, W. K., and Spiel, R. H. Prolonged at home treatment of motor neuron disorders with self administered subcutaneous high dose TRH. Neurology 35 (Suppl. 1): 106, 1985.
81. Munsat, T. L., Mora, J. S., Robinton, J. E., Jackson, I., Lechan, R., Hedlund, W., Taft J., Reichlin, S., and Scheife, R. Intrathecal TRH in amyotrophic lateral sclerosis: preliminary observations. Neurology 34 (Suppl. 1): 239, 1984.
82. Brooke, M. H., Florence, J. M., Heller, S. L., Kaiser, K. K., Phillips, D., Gruber, A., Babcock, D., and Miller, J. P. Controlled trial of thyrotropin releasing hormone in amyotrophic lateral sclerosis: Neurology (in press).
83. Imoto, K., Saida, K., Iwamura, K., Saida, T., and Nishitani, H. Amyotrophic lateral sclerosis: a double-blind cross over trial of thyrotropin releasing hormone. J. Neurol. Neurosurg. Psychiatry 47: 1332–1334, 1984.
84. Mitsumoto, H., Salgado, E. D., Negroski, D., Hanson, M. R., Salanga, V. D. and Wilbourn, A. Double-blind cross over trials with acute intravenous thyrotropin releasing hormone infusion in patients with amyotrophic lateral sclerosis: negative studies. Ann. Neurol. 16: 109, 1984.
85. Conrad, J., Clough, J., Sufit, R. L., and Brooks, B. R. Isokinetic assessment of muscle torque in amyotrophic lateral sclerosis patients after administration of saline and thyrotropin releasing hormone (TRH). Neurology 35 (Suppl. 1): 73, 1985.
86. Gracco, V. L., Caligiuri, M., Abbs, J. H., Sufit, R. L., and Brooks, B. R. Placebo controlled computerized dynametric measurements of bulbar and somatic muscle strength increase in patients with amyotrophic lateral sclerosis following intravenous infusion of 10 mg/kg thyrotropin releasing hormone. Ann. Neurol. 16: 110, 1984.
87. Taft, J., Munsat, T., Jackson, I., Robinson, J., Benedict, C., Kaplan, M., and Schiefe, R. A constant infusion pump for intrathecal delivery of TRH in ALS. Neurology 35 (Suppl. 1): 107, 1985.
88. Olarte, M. R., Schoenfeldt, R. S., McKiernan, G., and Rowland, L. P. Plasmapheresis in amyotrophic lateral sclerosis. Ann. Neurol. 8: 644–645, 1980.
89. Rissanen, A., Palo, J., Myllyla, G., and Cantell, K. Interferon therapy for ALS. Ann. Neurol. 7: 392, 1980.
90. Brooks, B. R., Engel, W. K., Sode, J., et al. Cyclic nucleotide phosphodiesterase inhibitor: therapy with phthalazinol in ALS. Neurology 28: 402–404, 1978.
91. Rivera, V. M., Grabois, M., Deaton, W., and Hiner, M. Modified snake venom in ALS. Lack of clinical effectiveness. Arch. Neurol. 37: 201–203, 1980.
92. Tyler, H. R. Double-blind study of neurotoxin in motor neuron disease. Neurology 29: 77–81, 1979.
93. Calcaterra, T. C., Kadell, B. M., and Ward, P. H. Dysphagia secondary to cricopharyngeal muscle dysfunction. Arch. Orolaryngol. 101: 726–729, 1975.
94. Lebo, C. P., U, S. K., and Norris, F. N. Cricopharyngeal myotomy in amyotrophic lateral sclerosis. Laryngoscope 86: 862–868, 1976.
95. Loizou, L. A., Small, M., and Dalton, G. A. Cricopharyngeal myotomy in motor neuron disease. J. Neurol. Neurosurg. Psychiatry 43: 42–45, 1980.
96. Sivak, E. D., Gipson, W. T., and Hanson, M. R. Long term management of respiratory failure in amyotrophic lateral sclerosis. Ann. Neurol. 12: 18–23, 1982.
97. Mulder, D. W., and Howard, F. M., Jr. Patient resistance and prognosis in amyotrophic lateral sclerosis. Mayo Clin. Proc. 51: 537–541, 1976.
98. Singh, N., Sachdev, K. K., and Susheela, A. K. Juvenile muscular atrophy localized to arms. Arch. Neurol. 37: 297–299, 1980.
99. Sobue, I., Saito, N, Lida, M., and Ando, K. Juvenile type of distal and segmental muscular atrophy of upper extremities. Ann. Neurol. 3: 429–432, 1978.
100. Hirayama, K., Tokokura, Y., and Tsubaki, T. Juvenile muscular atrophy of unilateral upper extremity. Neurology 13: 373–380, 1963.
101. Gajdnsek, D. C. Foci of motor neuron disease in high incidence in isolated populations of East Asia and the Western Pacific. In: *Human Motor Neuron Disease*, edited by L. P. Rowland. Raven Press, New York, 1982.
102. Brody, J. A., and Chen, K. M. Changing epidemiological patterns of amyotrophic lateral sclerosis and parkinsonism-dementia on Guam. In: *Motor Neuron Diseases*, edited by F. H. Norris and L. T. Kurland. Grune & Stratton, New York, 1969.
103. Hirano, A., Malamud, N., Kurland, L. T., and Zimmerman, H. M. A review of the pathologic findings in amyotrophic lateral sclerosis. In: *Motor Neuron Diseases*, edited by F. H. Norris and L. T. Kurland. Grune & Stratton, R New York, 1969, pp. 51–60.
104. Garruto, R. M., Gajdusek, D. C. and Chen, K.-M. Amyotrophic lateral sclerosis and Parkinsonism dementia among Philippino migrants to Guam. Ann. Neurol. 10: 341–350, 1981.

105. Garruto, R. M., Gajdusek, C., Chen, K.-M. Amyotrophic lateral sclerosis among Chamorro migrants from Guam. Ann. Neurol. *8:* 612–619, 1980.

106. Gajdusek, D. C. Foci of motor neuron disease in high incidence in isolated populations of East Asia and the Western Pacific. In: *Human Motor Neuron Disease*, edited by L. P. Rowland. Raven Press, New York, 1982, pp. 363–393.

107. Perl, D. P., Gajdusek, D. C., Gariuto, R. M., Yanagihara, R. T., and Gibbs, C. J., Jr. Trace element analysis of neurofibrillary tangle bearing neurons in amyotrophic lateral sclerosis and parkinsonism dementia of Guam. An electron probe x-ray microanalytical study. Science *217:* 1053–1055, 1982.

108. Garruto, R., Yanagihara, R., and Gajdusek, D. C. Disappearance of high incidence amyotrophic lateral sclerosis and parkinsonism-dementia on Guam. Neurology *35:* 193–198, 1985.

109. Kurtzke, J. F. Comments on the epidemiology of amyotrophic lateral sclerosis. In: *Motor Neuron Diseases*, edited by F. H. Norris and L. T. Kurland. Grune & Stratton, New York, 1969, pp. 85–89.

110. Shiraki, H. The neuropathology of amyotrophic lateral sclerosis (ALS) in the Kii peninsula and other areas of Japan. In: *Motor Neuron Diseases*, edited by F. H. Norris and L. T. Kurland. Grune & Stratton, New York, 1969, pp. 80–84.

111. Kimura, K., et al. Epidemiological and geomedical studies on amyotrophic lateral sclerosis. Dis. Nerv. Syst. *24:* 155–159, 1963.

112. Gajdusek, D. C., and Salazar, A. M. Amyotrophic lateral sclerosis and Parkinsonsim syndromes in high incidence among the Auyu and Jakai people of West New Guinea. Neurology *32:* 107–126, 1982.

113. Kondo, K., Tsubaki, T., and Sakamoto, F. The Ryukyuan muscular atrophy: an obscure heritable neuromuscular disease found in the islands of southern Japan. J. Neurol. Sci. *11:* 359–382, 1970.

114. Gomez, M. R., Clermont, V., and Bernstein, J. Progressive bulbar paralysis in childhood. Arch. Neurol. *6:* 317–323, 1962.

115. Alexander, M. P., Emery, E. S., and Koerner, F. C. Progressive bulbar paresis in childhood. Arch. Neurol. *33:* 66–68, 1976.

116. Kaeser, H. E. Scapuloperoneal muscular atrophy. Brain *88:* 407–418, 1965.

117. Furukawa, T., Tsukagoshi, H., Sugita, H., and Toyokura, Y. Neurogenic muscular atrophy simulating facioscapulohumeral muscular dystrophy. J. Neurol Sci. *9:* 389–397, 1969.

118. Emery, E. S., Fenichel, G. M., and Eng, G. A spinal muscular atrophy with scapuloperoneal distribution. Arch. Neurol. *18:* 129–133, 1968.

119. Meadows, J. C., and Marsden, C. D. Scapuloperoneal amyotrophy. Arch. Neurol. *20:* 9–12, 1969.

120. Feigenbaum, J., and Munsat, T. L. A neuromuscular syndrome of scapuloperoneal distribution. Bull. Los Angeles Neurol. Soc. *35:* 47–57, 1970.

121. Fenichel, G. M., Emery, E. S., and Hunt, P. Neurogenic atrophy simulating facioscapulohumeral dystrophy. Arch. Neurol. *17:* 257–260, 1967.

122. Harding, A. E. and Thomas, P. K. Hereditary distal spinal muscular atrophy: a report on 34 cases and a review of the literature. J. Neurol. Sci. *45:* 337–348, 1980.

123. Pearn, J., and Hudgson, P. Distal spinal muscular atrophy: a clinical and genetic study of 8 kindreds. J. Neurol. Sci. *43:* 183–191, 1979.

124. O'Sullivan, D. J., and McLeod, J. G. Distal chronic spinal muscular atrophy involving the hands. J. Neurol. Neurosurg. Psychiatry *41:* 653–658, 1978.

125. Young, I. D., and Harper, P. S. Hereditary distal spinal muscular atrophy with vocal cord paralysis. J. Neurol. Neurosurg. Psychiatry *43:* 413–418, 1980.

126. Ringel, S. P., Lava, N. S., Treihaft, M. M., Lubs, M. L., and Lubs, H. A. Late onset x-linked recessive spinal and bulbar muscular atrophy. Muscle Nerve *1:* 297–307, 1978.

127. Johnson, W. G. Genetic heterogeneity of the hexosaminidase deficiency diseases. Res. Publ. Assoc. Res. Nerv. Ment. Dis. *60:* 215–237, 1983.

128. Yaffe, M. G., Kaback, M., Goldberg, M., Miles, J., Itabashi, H., McIntyre, H., and Mohandas, T. Amyotrophic lateral sclerosis-like syndrome with hexosaminidase A deficiency: a new type of GM2, gangliosidosis. Neurology *29:* 611, 1979.

129. Dale, A. J. D., Engel, A. G., and Rudd, N. L. Familial hexosaminidase A deficiency with Kugelberg-Welander phenotype and mental change. Ann. Neurol. *14:* 109, 1983.

130. Sliman, R. J., Mitsumoto, H., Schafer, I. A., and Horwitz, S. J. A study of hexosaminidase A deficiency in a patient with atypical amyotrophic lateral sclerosis. Ann. Neurol. *14:* 148–149, 1983.

131. Mitsumoto, H., Sliman, R. J., Schafer, I. A., Sternick, C. J., Kaufman, B., Wilbourn, A., and Horwitz, S. J. Motor neuron disease and adult hexosaminidase A deficiency in two families: Evidence for multisystem degeneration. Ann. Neurol. *17:* 378–385, 1985.

132. Poll-The, B., Aicardi, J., Girot, R., and Rosa, R. Neurological findings in triosephophate isomerase deficiency. Ann. Neurol. *17:* 439–443, 1985.

3 diseases of the neuromuscular junction

MYASTHENIA GRAVIS

In 1672 Thomas Willis, writing upon palsies, made the following comments:

> There is another kind of this disease depending on the scarcity and fewness of the Spirits, in which the motion fails wholly in no Part or Member, yet it is performed weakly only, or depravedly by any;—those who be in trouble with a scarcity of Spirits, will force them as much as they may to local Motions, are able at first rising in the Morning to walk, move their Arms this way and that, or to lift up a weight with strength; but before Noon, the stores of the Spirits which influenc'd the Muscles being almost spent, they are scarce able to move Hand or Foot.
>
> I have now a prudent and honest Women in cure, who for many years has been obnoxious to this kind of bastard Palsey not only in the Limbs, but likewise in her Tongue; this person for some time speaks freely and readily enough, but after long, hasty, or laborious speaking, presently she becomes mute as a fish and cannot bring forth a word, nay, and does not recover the use of her Voice till after an hour or two (1).

In the intervening three centuries our knowledge of the disease has increased considerably, although our descriptive eloquence seldom matches that of Willis. The illness that he chronicled is likely to have been that which we now know as myasthenia gravis. It is a reflection upon the puzzling nature of the disease that not only has it baffled physicians throughout the course of history but even today presents many diagnostic problems.

Clinical Aspects

The characteristic signs and symptoms of myasthenia are consequent upon the abnormal susceptibility of the patient's muscles to fatigue. Fatigability is a normal phenomenon, as may be witnessed by anyone who has tried to carry a 100-lb suitcase for more than a few blocks. The hand grip cannot be sustained as the muscles of the forearm become exhausted. The degree of fatigue varies enormously from individual to individual. The trained athlete is capable of sustained exertion far beyond the reach of the rest of us. Patients with myasthenia gravis, however, may find the effort of holding up their eyelids to be overwhelming. In the ranges between these two extremes lie the hysterics whose asthenia overwhelms them when the pressures of their lives become too great and the myasthenic whose disease is slight enough that his symptoms are present only under situations of exertion. It is a small wonder that the one is frequently confused with the other and that the myasthenic can spend many months or years being labeled a hysteric, whereas the hysteric may equally unfairly enjoy the mistaken diagnosis of myathenia gravis. In spite of those in whom the diagnosis is difficult, there are certain characteristics of the disease and of the laboratory abnormalities associated with it that may reliably lead to the diagnosis.

The illness is seen more frequently in women than in men, by a ratio of about 3:2. It usually occurs in sporadic fashion with an incidence of approximately 1 in 20,000 (2). From 5 to 7% of the cases have a family history, although there is no clear-cut pattern of inheritance. This perhaps indicates a genetic predisposition for myasthenia rather than a Mendelian pattern of inheritance. This impression is reinforced by the finding of electromyographic (EMG) anomalies and increased acetylcholine receptor protein antibody levels in 60% of asymptomatic relatives of myasthenic patients (3). The onset may be at any time, but there are two ages of peak incidence: for women the third decade and in men the fifth decade. The onset is sometimes difficult to date, and I have seen patients with an apparently recent history of myasthenia who insist that their strength after treatment with thymectomy and steroids is better than at any time in their lives; they may have had subclinical myasthenia for many years. This is particularly true of the younger myasthenic.

Generally, the symptoms begin in one of three groups of muscles: those of the eyes, of the bulbar musculature, or of the limbs and trunk (Figs. 3.1–3.3). In about half of the patients the eyes are initially involved, in about a quarter the disease presents with difficulty in speaking, swallowing, or chewing, and in about one-fifth of the patients the predominant early symptoms are of generalized weakness of the limbs (4, 5).

When ptosis is an early sign, it may be quite variable. It is frequently very asymmetric and on occasions is unilateral. Like the other symptoms of

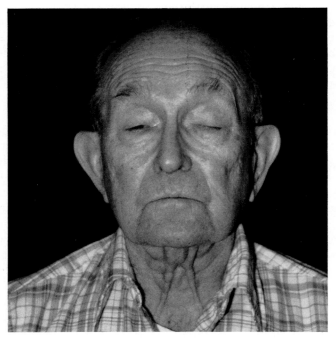

Figure 3.1. Myasthenia gravis. Notice the severe ptosis and the compensatory elevation of the eyebrows as evidenced by wrinkling of the forehead.

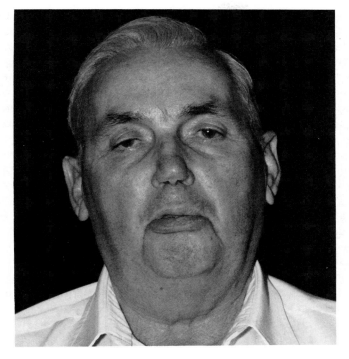

Figure 3.2.   In addition to the ptosis, this myasthenic patient is attempting to whistle but cannot purse the lips.

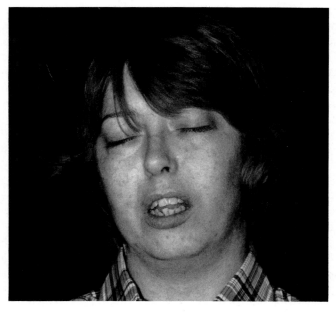

Figure 3.3.   This young woman has severe ptosis and is unable to close her mouth because of the weakness of the face and jaws associated with her myasthenia.

myasthenia gravis, it may be worse towards the end of the day and improve after a night's rest. Another curious feature of the myasthenic ptosis is that it can alternate from one side to the other on successive examinations. It may also be exacerbated by a sudden exposure to bright light. The other muscles of the eyes, with the exception of the pupillary muscles, are frequently involved. The abnormalities may be so slight as to produce ony a blurring of vision, or they may be severe enough that bizarre and dramatic paralyses are seen. It is usually easy to differentiate the myasthenic extraocular palsies from those due to peripheral nerve lesions because the pattern of the weakness does not conform to any anatomical distribution of peripheral nerves.

The bulbar muscles also suffer. The facial muscles are often weak, and a peculiar difficulty with the muscles of the lower part of the face converts the normally pleasant smile into a unsightly snarl. This may be so embarrassing that the patient will hide his mouth behind his hand while laughing. Weakness of the palate and tongue can render speech unintelligible. The patient's enunciation may be distinct as he begins to talk, but after some time the voice becomes hollow, echoing, and totally without consonants. Difficulty with swallowing and choking spells are noted, but a more frequent problem is found in chewing food. When chewing meat, particularly if it is tough, the patient may have to support the chin with the hand in order to complete the task. Weakness of the muscles of the neck is not at all uncommon and is generally of the neck extensors so that the head tends to flop uncontrollably forward. This leads to a characteristic posture adopted by such patients who support the head with the hand tucked under the chin.

The symptoms of the disease when it involves the limbs and the trunk differ only by the nature of the fatigability from symptoms seen in other diseases in which weakness occurs. The weakness may be exacerbated by heat, and many patients complain that taking a hot shower or bath is a debilitating experience. Others notice that their swallowing is worse after taking hot liquids. The respiratory muscles are often involved, particularly when the illness is advanced, and respiratory distress is a very real problem for the myasthenic. Sensory symptoms are unusual, although aching of the muscles can occur, bearing some relationship to the introspection which is natural to such patients.

Frequently the myasthenic tends to be demanding or rather querulous, particularly when the disease has been long-standing. It should be remembered, however, that the terrors of this disease are appreciated only by those who have suffered from it. The patient with myasthenia awakes to an uncertain day, not knowing whether some mild increase in weakness may not be the harbinger of a devastating crisis. It is not surprising in such situations that patients may lose their equanimity.

Myasthenia gravis is an agreeable exception to the general rule in neuromuscular disease. There are medications available and surgery is believed to be effective. Unfortunately such treatment has never been subject to the rigorous testing of a prospective trial. We now find ourselves in the bizarre position of not knowing if treatment changes the natural history while believing that deliberately witholding therapy would be unethical. This makes the study of populations of patients before the advent of steroids and the widespread use of thymectomy of great importance. One such study (5) found a remission rate of about 10% and a death rate of about 35% in 360 patients. It is not clear how this death rate compares with the expected death rate from life insurance tables but it is obviously higher. Over one-half of the deaths occurred within the first 3 years. Between the two extremes were 20% of the patients who improved, 30% who remained the same, and about 5% who were worse. Some confusion may arise because "better," "same," or "worse" was referred to the individual patient's weakest state during the first 3 years of the measurement. The study thus shows that, for most myasthenics, the point of maximum symptoms is to be expected within 3 years.

In the same study, a second group of 676 patients seen between 1960 and 1980 were described. The death rate dropped to below 15%, and 2% of the patients were "worse." Around 40% were better, 40% unchanged, and in 5% the illness disappeared. The authors point out that this change in the natural history occurred before the introduction of steroids and was probably due to better respiratory care.

One subcategory of myasthenia deserves special mention. In about 15% of the patients, the eye muscles alone are affected, although electrical evidence of neuromuscular junction blockade is noted in many. It is a relatively benign disease, slightly commoner in men than women. Of 414 patients whose myasthenia was limited to the eyes during the first month, 40% continued to have the localized variety. Of the others who went on to develop the generalized illness, 90% did so within the first year. Thus, ocular myasthenia of over 1-year's duration seems to have a good prognosis. At the opposite end of the scale, some patients with generalized myasthenia experience such a rapid progression that they decline from perfectly normal health to severe weakness with respiratory insufficiency in a matter of weeks.

Fluctuations in the severity of the disease occur unpredictably, but certain situations are so consistently associated with worsening of myasthenia that it is wise to consider their possibility in any patient who presents with an exacerbation. Perhaps the commonest cause of an apparent worsening of myasthenia gravis is due not to the disease but to the medication used in its treatment. Those who feel that their strength is not as it should be often take increasing doses of anticholinesterase medications. An overdose of these may itself induce weakness which the patient interprets as further indication of the need for more medicine. A vicious cycle is then established in which the patient takes increasing amounts of drug, eventually provoking a cholinergic crisis. Other causes that precipitate a worsening of myasthenia are infections, either viral or bacterial, and either hypo- or hyperthyroidism. Pregnancy is commonly associated with changes in myasthenia gravis. These may be in the direction of either improvement or deterioration. There is no constant relationship but, in general, the disease tends to exacerbate more frequently in the first trimester and may improve in the last two trimesters. Occasionally there is a postpartum myasthenic crisis. Emotional disturbances of all kinds make the patients feel weaker. It is not uncommon to find myasthenics whose immediate reaction to such stress is to take increasing amounts of medication to the point of overdosage. Electrolyte imbalance, particularly hypokalemia or hypocalcemia, may markedly worsen myasthenic symptoms.

Even without the influence of some provocative factor, myasthenics may experience a rapid decline in their strength, increasing difficulty in swallowing and breathing, and find themselves falling through the chute at the end of which lies the myasthenic crisis. In years past, this event was dreaded by both physician and patient, but improvement in respiratory care has changed the outlook. The only way a myasthenic can actually die from the disease is if he stops breathing. Nowadays with positive pressure ventilators and the maintenance of the airway, death is no longer a common result of the myasthenic crisis. The mortality rate from crisis has declined from almost 50% in the early 1960s to 6% between 1975 and 1979 (6). The onset of crisis was within 2 years of the onset of the illness in 51% of the patients with an average of 21 months.

Myasthenia may occur in childhood, when it presents with the same signs and symptoms as in the adult. An unusual form of myasthenia is seen in approximately 15% of babies born to mothers with myasthenia gravis. This neonatal myasthenia is present at birth but lasts no more than 12 weeks. For this reason, the diagnosis and treatment of the illness are extremely important. The baby usually presents as a hypotonic child with difficulty breathing. The baby may have considerable difficulty sucking, and his chin may have to be supported while nursing in the same way as the adult myasthenic has to support his own chin while chewing. The disease may be due to the influence of maternal antibodies and disappears when the infant's own immune system supervenes. Passive transfer of myasthenia from patients to the mouse has been accomplished (7). Neonatal myasthenia may be a natural equivalent to this experiment. Its appearance immediately at birth and its disappearance over the succeeding few weeks might well suggest that the condition results from transfer of the receptor protein antibody from mother to fetus. In outline this is true, but there are interesting anomalies. Neonatal myasthenia cannot be related to the duration or the severity of the maternal disease (8). In infants born to myasthenic mothers, many have high levels of the antibody in the blood, but few develop neonatal myasthenia. At the other extreme, one child developed neonatal myasthenia when the mother was in complete remission, although her blood antibody levels were also high (9). The development of the illness may be related to the rate of destruction of the antibody in the infant. This disappears rapidly from the blood of healthy children, whereas levels persist for far longer in the myasthenic infant (10). Analysis of the type of antibody suggests that the affected infants may be manufacturing their own antibody which differs slightly from their mothers'. Perhaps some other cell or factor is passed from mother to child causing a temporary abnormal immune response in the body.

The diagnosis of myasthenia gravis may be suspected from the clinical examination by the demonstration of pathological fatigability. A fatigable ptosis is demonstrated by asking the patient to sustain upward gaze. The eyelids begin a slow drift downwards with the passage of time. This test is often used in conjunction with an edrophonium (Tensilon) test by timing the point at which the lids cross the border of the pupil. Fatigability of the limbs can be demonstrated by having the patient sit with outstretched arms or by having him grasp a dynamometer repetitively and measuring his grip strength.

A phenomenon, sometimes known as the Walker phenomenon, has been described in patients with myasthenia. When a cuff is inflated around the upper arm and the arm exercised ischemically, the muscles fatigue. This fatigability is limited to the arm. When the cuff is released, a subsequent dramatic deterioration in the myasthenic signs in the rest of the body has been reported (11). Thus a patient may develop a marked ptosis following such arm exercise. This does not seem to be a constant finding, and many physicians have never seen it. Some investigators have suggested that the worsening may be due to production of lactate and the subsequent reduction of available calcium (12).

If pathological fatigue is demonstrated, the effect of edrophonium should be investigated. This anticholinesterase drug when injected intravenously acts within 30 seconds to 1 minute. Its effect is over within 5–10 minutes. After establishing the level of fatigue in the untreated patient, a test injection of 1 mg of edrophonium is given intravenously. If there is no untoward effect from this test injection, up to 10 mg may be given, although a clear-cut result is usually seen with 6 mg if any effect is to be found. Obviously, in children the dose should be appropriately smaller. The patient's fatigability is then tested again to determine any change. It is particularly important to quantitate such testing since relying on the patient's, or even the examiner's, impression can be misleading. A control injection of normal saline is useful on occasions, although once the patient has experienced the effect of edrophonium and its side effects, he is in no doubt as to which is the active drug and which is the control. If there is no response to edrophonium it is important to evaluate the effect of neostigmine, since some patients, especially those with ocular myasthenia, may not improve with edrophonium.

Patients with myasthenia may have marked atrophy of muscles, but this is unusual and is seen only in those whose myasthenia is long-standing.

Laboratory Studies

Electrical testing of myasthenia gravis patients is designed to demonstrate the defect in neuromuscular conduction. When surface recording electrodes are placed over a muscle belly, the electrical potential which is evoked following stimulation of the motor nerve gives some measure of the number of muscle fibers which are being activated. If there is a progressive failure in neuromuscular transmission, the amplitude of the evoked potential will become progressively smaller. In normal subjects, repetitive stimulation at frequencies below 10 cycles per second produces little change in the amplitude of the evoked potential (less than 10%). In myasthenia gravis there is a decrement of more than 10% in the amplitude of evoked potentials at such frequencies. This reduction in potential reaches its maximum on the fourth evoked potential, and further decrement is not seen after the sixth evoked potential (13). Indeed, with sustained repetitive stimulation there may be some increase in the amplitude, or fluctuations may occur which are difficult to interpret. The abnormality may be seen in only one of several muscles. The proximal muscles are more likely to be affected than the distal ones. This presents a practical problem, since the proximal muscles are not as easy to stimulate. However, with some practice, stimulation over the brachial plexus at Erb's point can be used to produce evoked potentials in the deltoid muscles. It is important to keep the limb warm when testing for the myasthenic response since the transmission defect increases with an increase in body temperature. Although intracellular recordings have given much information as to the nature of myasthenia gravis, the standard needle EMG is really of little help in the diagnosis of this disease.

With the development of single fiber EMG, a phenomenon known as "jitter" has been analyzed (14). Muscle fibers innervated by the terminal branches of the same motor unit will be depolarized more or less synchronously. It is the investigation of this "more or less" aspect which has given rise to the concept of jitter. Because of slight differences in the lengths of the terminal nerve branches and because of some differences in conduction properties, the individual muscle fibers of a motor unit are not actually depolarized simultaneously. If one takes the action potential from a single muscle fiber as a reference, a similar potential from a muscle fiber in the same motor unit will occur a fraction of a second after the first. In normal muscle, this second motor unit potential will always occur when the first is seen. The time interval between the two motor unit potentials can be relatively constant, but there is a variability in this interval. This is known as "jitter." In patients with myasthenia gravis not only is the jitter increased, but there may be occasions on which the second motor unit may disappear entirely, presumably because of a failure of neuromuscular transmission (15).

Patients are particularly susceptible to the paralyzing action of curare, from which phenomenon the curare test was developed (16, 17). The regional curare test is the only one which is now employed, but for the sake of completeness, the full curare test will also be described here. The latter was never done unless intubation and respiratory support could be carried out immediately. Thus, the test was usually performed with an anesthesiologist in attendance. EMG was carried out concurrently and the evoked potential from a suitable muscle obtained. In addition, various tests of the patient's strength were obtained. Approximately 0.15 mg curare per kilogram body weight was diluted in 50 ml saline; 1 ml of this was given intravenously, and the patient's strength and evoked potential were studied after 1 minute. After 2 minutes a second injection of 2 ml is given then repeated. Similarly, 3 ml are injected after a further 2 minutes, and finally 4 ml. The test is discontinued at any stage if the patient's strength deteriorates or the evoked potential starts to fall.

Because of hazards of a severe paralysis associated with the standard curare test, the regional curare test is usually used (16, 17), if the diagnosis requires this type of confirmation.

In this test 0.125 mg of curare is diluted in 20 ml of saline. A cuff is placed around the upper part of the forearm and inflated above systolic pressure, the arm being held vertically in such a way as to promote venous drainage. The curare is then injected intravenously at the wrist, and this injection is followed by 5 ml of saline. The total time of the injection is 1 minute; the cuff is deflated after a further 4.5 minutes. The repetitive evoked potentials are then recorded from the abductor pollicis brevis at 5, 15, and 20 minutes after the injection. Normally there is little or no diminution of the evoked potentials compared to those obtained before the injection. In patients with myasthenia there is considerable reduction in the amplitude of the evoked potential (usually more than 20%), and this reduction persists longer than in the normal subject. The amount of curare reaching the rest of the circulation will not be sufficient to cause a generalized paralysis. Many patients experience a slight tingling in the hand during the injection. This can be used as an indication that the drug is being injected intravenously, if there is any doubt.

In the past the decamethonium test has been recommended as useful for the diagnosis of myasthenia gravis. Patients with myasthenia seem to be resistant to the effects of this drug. However, an article which commented on the necessity of general anesthesia during this test did little to reassure physicians about its utility (18).

Routine muscle biopsy has been of less use in the diagnosis of myasthenia gravis, although electron microscopy has revealed much about pathological mechanisms underlying the disease. The routine muscle pathology usually shows signs of Type 2 fiber atrophy, which is sometimes focal, or of mild denervation. Lymphorrhages were orginally thought to be commonly associated with myasthenia gravis, but in my experience they have been quite rare and are seen in no more than 10% of the patients.

Because of the coincidence of myasthenia gravis and thymomas, a chest x-ray and, perferably, chest CAT scans are an important part of the evaluation. Approximately 10–15% of myasthenic patients have a thymoma, and the prognosis in these patients is significantly worse than in those without tumor. Determination of the level of antibodies may be of great diagnostic help in difficult cases. These are of two classes, the antiacetylcholine receptor antibodies and that directed against the contractile component of muscle or the striational antibody. Eighty-five to 90% of patients with generalized myasthenia gravis have elevated titers of the receptor protein antibody. Striated muscle antibody is present in up to 40% of patients with generalized myasthenia, mainly those over 40 years. In myasthenic patients with thymoma, 90% have elevated levels of the striational antibody (19–21). A much smaller percentage of patients with purely ocular myasthenia have detectable antibodies in the blood.

The receptor protein antibodies are a heterogenous group and there does not seem to be any particular correlation of one type of antibody with one type of myasthenia (21).

Pathology and Etiology

The abnormality which causes the symptoms in myasthenia gravis lies at the neuromuscular junction, the fundamental process causing these changes is slowly being unraveled. In order to provide a background against which the abnormalities may be understood, it is necessary to review the normal neuromuscular junction (Fig. 3.4). Where the motor nerves contact the muscle, they lose their myelin and the terminal expansions of the axons come into direct contact with the muscle. At an ultrastructural level, many small vesicles are found in the terminal expansions. These vesicles contain acetylcholine, and it is their discharge through the presynaptic membrane that releases the small quanta of acetylcholine. The gap between the nerve terminal and the underlying endplate region is known as the primary synaptic cleft. Acetylcholine must travel across this gap to reach the receptor sites in the postjunctional part of the apparatus. Postjunctionally, the membrane is dimpled and folded producing secondary synaptic clefts. In addition to the acetylcholine receptor sites, the endplate zone also contains acetylcholinesterase. When an electrical impulse travels down the motor nerve, the terminal

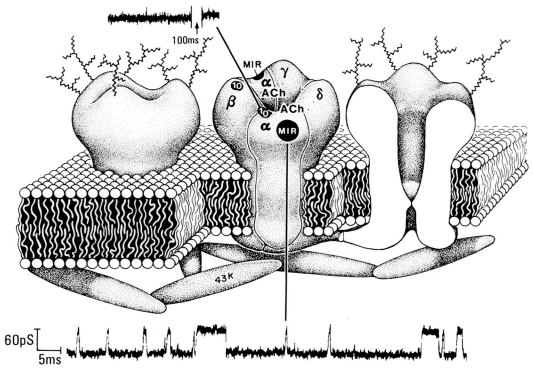

Figure 3.4. The acetylcholine receptors are illustrated embedded in the membrane and arrayed around the central ion channel. The main immunogenic region (*MIR*) is indicated on the α subunit. The branched structures protruding from the surface are glycosyl residues. The objects labeled "*43K*" are structural components of the cell cytoskeleton. The order of the subunits may be slightly incorrect, and the δ unit should probably change places with the contiguous α unit. Electrical recordings of reconstituted ion channels are also indicated above and below the drawing. The lower tracing demonstrates that monoclonal antibodies binding to the main immunogenic region are without effect. The upper trace shows that a different monoclonal antibody (*10*) blocks the channel opening completely. (Reproduced with permission from J. Lindstrom, S. Tzartos, W. Gullick, et al.: Cold Spring Harbor Symposium on Quantitative Biology, *48:* 89–99, 1983.)

expansions are depolarized, causing a massive release of acetylcholine from the presynaptic vesicles. This transmitter substance travels across to the postsynaptic receptors and causes a depolarization at the endplate region, which results in a propagated electrical potential and eventual contraction of the muscle fiber. The acetylcholine is broken down by acetylcholinesterase and the depolarization reserved. Even during the resting state there is a continuous discharge of the presynaptic vesicles, although not in sufficient quantities to cause a propagated depolarization of the entire muscle fiber. It can, however, be recorded by intracellular electrodes as miniature endplate potentials (MEPPS).

The acetylcholine receptor protein is a molecule of about 250,000 daltons which is an integral part of the muscle membrane and associated with heparan sulfate proteoglycan on the basal lamina. The receptor protein is made up of several subunits (α, β, γ, and δ), a portion of the α subunit is inherently immunogenic and is known as the main immunogenic region. The receptor protein structure resembles a donut of about 100 A diameter with a hydrophilic core (22). The cation channel passes through the middle of the donut and is triggered by the action of acetylcholine. The acetylcholine binding site is only one small part of the acetylcholine receptor molecule. The density of acetylcholine receptor molecules in the end plate region has been estimated at between 10,000 and 30,000/μm^2 (23–26).

α-Bungarotoxin is a component of snake venom with a particular affinity for the acetylcholine receptor protein. When bungarotoxin is conjugated with peroxidase, it may be visualized using a simple histochemical technique and can be used to demonstrate the distribution of acetylcholine receptors in tissue sections. The majority of the receptor protein is on the terminal expansions—the "peaks"—of the postjunctional folds (27).

Receptor proteins are not set into the membrane in perpetuity but undergo a steady turnover. Some are synthesized by the cell and inserted into the muscle membrane while others are degraded and digested within the cell. Their half-line is measured in days.

Normal neuromuscular function depends upon many things. It is necessary that acetylcholine be synthesized and stored. Substances such as calcium and cyclic AMP are implicated in both the release of acetylcholine and the synthesis of the receptor protein (28). Cyclic AMP may be linked with calcium in its action in neuromuscular transmission since the compound is important in the mobilization of calcium in living cells (29). Cyclic AMP as well as stimulators of adenyl cyclase such as noradrenaline and ephedrine (which increase the cellular level of cyclic AMP by increasing its formation) may facilitate neuromuscular transmission (30).

Abnormalities of the motor endplates were noted by Coers and Woolf (31) in their study of motor point biopsies from the patients with myasthenia gravis. Both the endplates and the subneural apparatus were found to be elongated. Engel and Santa (32), in a careful study of the ultrastructure of the endplate region, found that the nerve terminals were rather small, that the primary cleft between the nerve and the subneural apparatus was widened, and, most strikingly, that the secondary synaptic clefts were shallow and sparse. They showed that the area which was reactive for acetylcholinesterase was reduced in size, with multiple small reactive areas appearing along an extended length of the fiber. There was no abnormality in the number or size of synaptic vesicles. This last finding was important because other studies had shown a decrease in the amplitude of the miniature endplate potentials and the suggestion had been made that the packets of acetylcholine released from the synaptic vesicles were abnormally small (33).

Myasthenic endplates demonstrate reduced binding of α-bungarotoxin (34), indicating that the amount of receptor proteins on the postjunctional surface is reduced. Early studies showed that serum globulin present in myasthenic patients inhibited the binding of α-bungarotoxin to the endplate receptor site (35, 36), suggesting that there was a circulating compound inhibiting the normal functioning of the postsynaptic part of the neuromuscular junction. This same immunoglobulin was believed to be involved in the passive "transfer" of myasthenia from man to mouse which was accomplished by injecting the animal with an ammonium sulfate-precipitated immunoglobulin fraction (7).

In any patient taking medication, the possibility exists that this may produce some of the changes seen in the muscle. Engel et al. (37) studied the effect of long-term anticholinesterase therapy in rats. Changes in the endplates, which were similar to those in human myasthenia, were noted but were limited to the soleus and the diaphragmatic muscles. The postsynaptic pinocytotic vesicles became quite abundant and the primary synaptic cleft became wider. The Schwann cell processes proliferated terminally, partially covering up the presynaptic membrane. The same type of changes were thus produced as seen in myasthenia gravis but with important differences. In myasthenia gravis all muscle fiber types are involved. Additionally the nerve terminal area in myasthenia gravis is reduced as well as the postjunctional part of the endplate. However, the experiment did suggest that prolonged administration of anticholinesterase may have an adverse effect on the neuromuscular junction. Others have commented on a similar adverse effect with both physiological and anatomical changes (38). The administration of acetylcholine agonists in experimental animals reduced the number of receptors at the endplate and thereby impaired neuromuscular transmission (39). The administration of neostigmine also produced ultrastructural alterations in the neuromuscular junction (40). The reduction of neuromuscular transmission produced by cholinergic drugs is independent of the effect produced by antibody and indeed summates with it (28).

The search for the actual cause of myasthenia has been a fascinating study over the years. The studies occupied two separate eras, the one before, and the other after, the discovery of experimental allergic myasthenia gravis. The possible relationship of myasthenia gravis to "autoimmune" diseases was pointed out by Simpson (41). Although rheumatoid arthritis is the commonest of these and occurs in 4% of patients, many others including systemic lupus erythematosus, Sjogren's syndrome, and pernicious anemia have been described. It is not entirely clear, because of the small numbers involved, whether such associations are more than coincidental. A fifth of myasthenics have a positive test for antinuclear antibodies and, in the presence of one other autoimmune disease, this antibody is found in all patients (42). Strauss and others (43) showed that in almost one-half of the patients with myasthenia gravis there was a circulating antibody (a 7S gammaglobulin) which bound to the A bands of skeletal muscle. It is difficult to understand why this striational antibody should be significant, since the pathology of myasthenia gravis lies not in the A bands but in the neuromuscular junction. Careful attempts to demonstrate binding of this antibody to the neuromuscular junction were unsuccessful (44). This same antibody, however, showed reactivity to cells in the thymus, and this may have been a more important finding. As noted previously, the great majority of myasthenic patients with thymomas demonstrate such antibodies, whereas it is found in only a third of other myasthenics.

The whole concept of the role of immunity in myasthenia gravis widened following the purification of the nicotinic acetylcholine receptor protein from the electric eel, a technical tour de force in itself. When the receptor protein was injected into rabbits in conjunction with Freund's adjuvant, the animals became sensitized. A second injection of receptor protein, after 15 days, caused the majority of the animals to develop severe weakness, very similar to that of myasthenia gravis, which was responsive to anticholinesterase medications (45). An antibody to the receptor protein was demonstrated in the serum of these animals. Experimental myasthenia gravis has also been produced in monkeys (46) and in rats and guinea pigs (47). Experimental allergic myasthenia gravis of guinea pigs may be transferred to other animals by the injection of washed lymph node cells from the affected animal indicating that cellular immune factors are important (48).

As mentioned previously, the receptor protein is a complex structure and, because of its complexity, it may elicit several different antibodies. With the development of hybridoma techniques for the production of monoclonal antibiodies, it is now possible to characterize some of these. Some will increase the rate of destruction of the receptor protein (antigenic modulation). Others block the flux of carbamylcholine in an artifical preparation of reconstituted endplate vesicles, suggesting that they may have a blocking effect on the in vivo binding of the analogous acetylcholine (22). Antigenic modulation requires cross linking of parts of the receptor by the antibody. Drachman et al. (49) used fragments of antibody to demonstrate that only the divalent fragments, capable of cross linking, accelerated the degradation of the endplate. The monovalent fragments were without effect (49).

It would seem to be common sense that antibodies capable of increasing the degradation of the receptor protein in a mammalian endplate might well result in myasthenia gravis secondary to this increased destruction. Unfortunately, as is so often the case, an explanation whose simplicity can instantly appeal to the clinician has little place in nature's scheme. Acetylcholine receptor turnover was studied by injecting peroxidase labeled α-bungarotoxin in animals with experimental allergic myasthenia gravis as well as in normal controls (27). The animals were sacrificed some time later and there was indeed increased internalization of the acetylcholine receptor in the myasthenic animal. On the other hand, it appeared that a compensatory increased synthesis of acetylcholine receptors by the cell was quite capable of replenishing the population on the membrane. The severity of the experimental myasthenia correlated not with the internalization of membrane receptors, but with the actual destruction of membrane. Membrane lysis results from activation of the complement system adding another dimension to the pathogenesis of myasthenia in both animals and humans. Experimental allergic myasthenia gravis (EAMG) is easily produced in rats. Animals, in which the complement C3 levels were depleted, developed only minor electrophysiological abnormalities, whereas control rats were moribund. Similarly, guinea pigs deficient in C4 were protected against the development of EAMG (23).

Activation of the complement cascade appears essential and the attachment of the antibody to the receptor protein does not alone cause myasthenia. There has been controversy over this point with Drachman maintaining that, although the depletion of C3 reduces the effect of the myasthenic antibody in mice, it does not eliminate it (49). There is general agreement that antigenic modulation of receptor proteins increases the degradation, the disagreement centers around whether the rate of synthesis keeps pace with this degradation.

Thus far, the situation in animals has been described, but there are many parallels in the human disease. Endplates from patients with myasthenia have long been known to bind only small amounts of α-bungarotoxin, suggesting that there is a reduced amount of receptor protein on the postjunctional surface membrane. The demonstration of binding of immunoglobulin G (IgG) to the endplates in myasthenia was effected by labeling staphylococcal protein A, a substance which binds to the Fc portion of IgG. This IgG binding was proportional to the amount of acetylcholine receptors remaining. The severity of the disease was related not to the amount of IgG bound, as might be the case if the binding of IgG altered the function of the endplates, but to the *loss* of acetylcholine receptors (27). No difference in acetylcholine receptor protein antibodies exists in the different clinical varieties of generalized myasthenia. The destruction of membrane in the human disease is also dependent upon the presence of the complement C5b-9 membrane attack complex. C9 has been nicely demonstrated in immunocytochemical preparations. The localization of both IgG and the complement cascade system is concentrated, as would be predicted, around the crests of the postjunctional folds. Eventually, in myasthenia, the endplate region is markedly altered as described in previous paragraphs.

An experimental model to investigate miniature endplate potential and the effect of myasthenic serum upon these potentials was devised using the mouse diaphragm. The miniature endplate potential amplitude was reduced by exposing the diaphragm to whole myasthenic serum, indicating a blocking factor in the serum. This reduction in amplitude was reversed by washing which would suggest that it was not due to actual lysis of the membrane. If the serum was heated to 56°C before application to the diaphragm, no blocking effect was seen. Such treatment of myasthenic serum would inactivate the complement, but would not destroy the antireceptor protein antibody. More curious was the fact that the addition of normal human serum to the heated myasthenic serum did not restore the blocking effect suggesting that there is a heat labile factor in myasthenic serum which is not present in the normal serum. It is not easy to invent an explanation for these findings, but it once again emphasizes the complexity of the whole situation (50).

Taking into account the intricacies of the mechanisms so far known, it is not surprising that there is no simple correlation between the acetylcholine receptor protein antibodies found in the blood of 80–90% of patients with myasthenia and the severity of their myasthenia. It was, perhaps, naive to expect that the status of endplate function and neuromuscular transmission could be deduced from levels of antibodies in the blood which may be governed by totally different factors. Nevertheless, there is a general correlation between the two. Seybold et al. (51) studied myasthenics who were unchanged after 1 year and found that four-fifths of them showed less than a 50% change in the antibody titers, whereas 3 of 6 patients who were improved after 1 year showed a greater than 50% change. Seybold and other workers have concluded that there is an overall relationship between the clinical course and antibody levels, during prednisone or immunosuppressive treatment but it is everybody's experience that, in the individual case, correlation is woefully lacking (52–55).

In a study of patients treated with immunosuppression (azathioprine) it was noted that 50% of the patients who were in remission on this drug relapsed following its withdrawal. The receptor protein antibodies in the blood increased in 7 out of 8 relapses (56).

Some have suggested that modifying the technique of assay, using rat acetylcholine receptor instead of human to seek out the antibody or the evaluation of monoclonal antibodies rather than of antibodies to the entire complex, might sharpen the clinical correlation. This remains to be seen. Early results are not encouraging (57).

Enlargement of the thymus has long been recognized as a feature of myasthenia gravis. Its role in the pathogenesis of the disease is still unclear. There is normally a progressive involution of the thymus after the first decade, but in about 70% of patients with myasthenia gravis, thymic hyperplasia is found (58) and in about 10% of patients, a thymoma is present. The hyperplastic changes of the lymphoid tissue are associated with the presence of germinal centers.

An increased number of IgM carrying B cells has been noted in the peripheral blood in myasthenic patients. A tentative suggestion was made that the increased number of B cells and the new antigenic determinants on their surface might represent persistent stimulation by a virus (59), and clinical myasthenia is not infrequently noted for the first time following a viral infection. Careful attempts to detect a persistent viral infection of the thymus using a number of different techniques showed no evidence of such an infection (60).

The thymus contains other tissue including epithelial elements which are thought to be the source of the thymic hormones, thymosin-1 and thymopoietin. These hormones play a part in the maturation of the immature prothymocytes to the immunocompetent thymocytes. Thymic epithelium may also instruct the prothymocytes by direct cell to cell contact, perhaps allowing them to acquire surface antigens, especially those which are important to self-recognition such as the histocompatibility antigens HLA—A, B, and the Ia types (61). It has been proposed that the excessive hormonal activity in the enlarged thymus might lead to an overproduction of helper T cells, especially those sensitized to acetylcholine receptor protein (62).

The other unusual cell in the thymus is the myoid cell. Only a few of these are present, but they are intriguing because their resemblance to muscle cells includes not only the cross striations but also the property of binding peroxidase labeled bungarotoxin, presumably indicating receptor protein.

The thymocytes from patients with myasthenia gravis behave differently from normal in a number of ways. An earlier observation showed that stimulation with phytohemagglutinin causes some thymic lymphocytes to be cytotoxic to cultured muscle (63). Phytohemagglutinin and pokeweed are both nonspecific agents but cause a greater stimulation of thymocytes from myasthenic patients than from others (64). Thymocytes themselves may produce antiacetylcholine receptor antibody but probably in insignificant amounts in terms of any possible role in the human disease. When irradiated thymocytes (radiation prevents any antibody formation from the thymocytes themselves) are cocultured with peripheral blood lymphocytes, a specific stimulation of the lymphocytes occurs and acetylcholine receptor antibody is produced without any associated production of other antibodies (65). The stimulation of lymphocytes by exposure to purified acetylcholine receptor protein has also been reported (66, 67). All of these studies indicate that, in the myasthenic, the autoimmune mechanisms are turned on to react to acetylcholine receptor proteins with a high degree of sensitivity and that the thymus plays an important part perhaps in initiating this stimulation. Newsom-Davis et al. (65) suggested that acetylcholine receptor specific helper T cells may be responsible for mediating these effects.

The use of monoclonal antibodies against lymphocytes allows the definition of subpopulations of these cells. Thus, helper T cells, suppressor and cytotoxic T cells, B cells, monocytes, and Ia (immunoglobulin A) positive cells were all identified. When cell suspensions obtained from the thymus of patients with myasthenia gravis were compared with the same cells obtained during cardiac surgery on control patients, the only significant difference was an increase in the percentage of Ia positive cells in the thymic cell suspensions from myasthenia gravis patients (but not in the peripheral blood cells). The nature of the Ia bearing cells in unclear. B cells are Ia positive, but there were more Ia positive cells than B cells identified using surface Ig as an indicator. Thymic epithelial cells are also Ia positive although morphologically the cells did not appear to be epithelial (68). Although the thymus has been implicated as the major culprit in the immunologic pathology, other sites may also be responsible for acetyl choline receptor antibody production. Cultured bone marrow lymphocytes from a 65-year-old man with myasthenia spontaneously produced the antibodies (69).

Because myasthenia gravis is obviously a disturbance in the body's immunity, a search has been made for abnormalities of the histocompatibility antigens. There are certain patterns associated with myasthenia, an increase of HLA-A1, B8, and DR3 in younger Caucasian women; A1, B8, and DR5 in American blacks, and A3, B7, and DRw2 in older men. In Chinese and Japanese patients, none of these is increased. It is not clear what interpretation to give these findings (70, 71).

Whatever the initial event which triggers the mechanisms directed against the neuromuscular junction, it is likely to be a complicated story and certainly far removed from the initial explanation of myasthenia gravis being due to a circulating curare-like compound.

Treatment

Anticholinesterase Medications. The early observations that myasthenia gravis resembled curare poisoning led Walker to try the use of anticholinesterase medications. The two most common ones are neostigmine bromide (Prostigmin) and pyridostigmine (Mestinon). Pyridostigmine is probably the choice of most physicians and patients because it has less of the cholinergic side effects and a slightly longer action. It is more likely to give patients relief from bedtime until morning than is neostigmine. The drug begins to act within half an hour of oral administration, and the length of its action is about 4 hours. It is commonly administered at 4–6-hour intervals. There is really no "corrrect" dose. Enough of the drug is given to counteract the effects of myasthenia as nearly as possible. In some patients this may be as little as 30 mg (½ tablet) every 6 hours. Others take 20, 30, or more pills per day. Methods are available to monitor blood levels of pyridostigmine but there is little correlation between the values obtained and the clinical response (72). Pyridostigmine is also available in a slow release form (Timespan). This contains 180 mg of the medication and is well tolerated by some patients. Many, however, find the effect of this preparation to be somewhat unpredictable.

Another anticholinesterase drug which is less frequently used is ambenonium (Mytelase). This drug is said to be more effective in peripheral weakness. It should be started in low doses (5 mg), and it may have to be discontinued because of the development of headaches. If a patient is being given ambenonium, he should be cautioned against the use of phospholine iodine, a long-term esterase inhibitor which is used in glaucoma and which markedly potentiates the effect of ambenonium (2). Other useful preparations are liquid preparations of pyridostigmine, which are easily administered by nasogastric tube in patients who cannot swallow, and parenteral preparations of neostigmine. The following are roughly equivalent doses: 15 mg neostigmine, 60 mg pyridostigmine, and 25 mg ambenonium by mouth, and 1 mg neostigmine by intramuscular injection. The patient who is being given anticholinesterase medication should be warned about the cholinergic side effects and the possibility of overdosage. It should be stressed that weakness is one of the chief side effects. It is often impossible to distinguish the weakness due to myasthenia from that due to overmedication. Although the latter is frequently associated with abnormal cramping pains and diarrhea as well as with widespread fasciculations, the absence of these side effects does not necessarily mean that the patient is having an exacerbation of myasthenia.

Anticholinesterase medications may not be an unmixed blessing, since there is evidence that they may cause structural abnormalities at the neuromuscular junction (37, 38). With the increasing use of thymectomy and of immunosuppression, the use of anticholinesterase medication is less popular.

Adjuvant medications which are used from time to time are all agents which directly or indirectly affect neuromuscular transmission. Ephedrine is used in doses of 25 mg thrice daily. Aldactone, spironolactone, guanidine, and the veratrum derivatives, germine mono- and diacetate (73) have all been used in the treatment of myasthenia gravis, although the results have been equivocal.

Steroids. The use of steroids in myasthenia gravis is logical in view of the etiology of the disease. ACTH was formerly recommended in short intensive courses which were sometimes repeated at intervals (74). The usual course consisted of daily injections of 100 units of ACTH for 10 days. Frequently an initial worsening of the disease was seen, followed by a gradual recovery which was usually not sustained. Early reports on the use of oral corticosteroids emphasized the worsening of the disease which may occur with such medication. With recent years, however, the emphasis has changed. Although it is well recognized that the use of prednisone or similar steroids may cause an initial increase of the weakness, this is often outweighed by the dramatic improvement which may be seen with the long-term use of suppressive doses of these medications. Prednisone may be given on alternate days as a single morning dose of 50–100 mg. This is combined with the administration of a low-sodium high-protein diet and 20–30 meq of potassium daily as replacement therapy (75–78). In most series marked benefit or remission was achieved in 80% of the patients with remission rates varying between 25% and 35%. The tendency of patients to relapse as the steroids are withdrawn is a recurrent problem. In our experience, the commonest serious side effect has been the development of cataracts. Other side effects include weight gain, skin changes, hypertension, diabetes and osteoporosis, but they are usually accepted by the patient in view of the improvement in the illness.

Before starting treatment, skin tests and chest x-ray should be obtained to rule out the possibility of tuberculous infection, and respiratory function should be evaluated. If the patient is undergoing anticholinesterase therapy, the dose of this medication should be halved or, if possible, discontinued. Close watch is kept on the respiratory function and assisted respiration is started if the patient appears to be deteriorating in the early stages of steroid therapy. The most usual time for exacerbations to occur has been during the first 3 weeks. Engel and coworkers (58) believe that part of this exacerbation may be due to increased sensitivity of the patient to his anticholinesterase medication. Others have implicated an enhancement of lymphocyte reactivity.

Perhaps because we have been treating patients in the early stages of myasthenia, we have not had to assist respirations during the initial period of treatment and have noticed very little worsening. We usually monitor the vital capacity every 4 hours and have not had to institute any other measures. Attempts should be made to discontinue the anticholinesterase medication as soon as this is feasible. Very frequently the patient notices a difference in muscle strength between the day off prednisone and the day on prednisone. The patient is usually weaker on the "off" day but occasionally may be stronger. This difference disappears after 3–4 weeks on prednisone; if it persists beyond the fourth week of treatment, it may be helpful to add a small amount of prednisone on the "off" day. In patients with severe myasthenia, in whom the potential dangers of the phase of worsening may be life threatening, Seybold and Drachman (79) have recommended slowly increasing the dose of prednisone from 25 mg every other day to 100 mg by 12.5 mg steps at each third dose. There are patients whose response to steroids is better when the drug is given at a daily dose of 60 mg prednisone rather than on an alternate day schedule. Suppressive steroid therapy is also quite effective in the form of myasthenia which is limited to the eyes (80).

When steroids alone are used in the management of myasthenia, they should be continued for 2 years or more; otherwise, relapses are common. Withdrawal of the medication should be very gradual. I have maintained patients on very low doses of prednisone (5–10 mg) for indefinite periods to try to prevent relapses. Whether this almost homeopathic dose is sensible or not, I would not care to say, but relapses seem to have been less frequent in this group.

Immunosuppression. Azathioprine in doses of 150–250 mg daily is also an effective medication in many myasthenics (81). Since, in some patients, the side effects of prednisone may be disfiguring, it is often more popular with patients. Side effects of azathioprine include leukopenia, pancytopenia, cholestasis, unusual infections, and an idiosyncratic response with fever and vomiting. Blood counts should be carefully monitored and during the initial phase of treatment, a complete blood count is obtained every few days. Later it is sufficient to obtain these on a weekly or every other week basis. In a recent series of 78 patients treated with azathioprine, 40% of the patients went into remission and 53% showed improvement.

There is disagreement among myologists about the relative benefits and perils associated with prednisone and azathioprine and which to use. My own view is that it is not so much the drug as the state of the disease that governs the response. Both are effective early, and often neither drug will affect the late stages of the illness. Those who commence treatment with one of the drugs will be impressed by its efficacy. When the other drug is used to treat cases resistant to the first, it will often also fail. Thus, the "prednisone first" clinicians will be sanguine about azathioprine and the azathioprine enthusiasts will likewise see more failure with prednisone (81).

Thymectomy. Removal of the thymus gland has been used as a form of therapy for myasthenia gravis since the changes of hyperplasia and thymoma were noted in the thymus. Several series attest to the benefit obtained from such a procedure (52, 82–87). Both patients with and without thymoma are helped. Although the presence of a tumor is associated with a less favorable outcome, there is an additional indication for surgery in patients with a thymoma, namely the necessity of removing the tumor. Patients with congenital myasthenia do not seem to benefit from thymectomy and these patients probably have a different form of illness. At least three-quarters of patients with myasthenia improve after thymectomy and, in over one-third, the improvement continues all the way to a total remission of the disease.

The technique for surgery has also been debated. A transcervical approach has been suggested to have less postoperative complications and to be cosmetically more appealing. The majority, though, have favored a transternal approach, maintaining that this allows for complete exposure of the thymus gland and an exploration of remote sites for possible anomalous thymus tissue. Proponents of the transcervical approach have countered that full exploration is possible through the transcervical route, and that those who criticize the procedure have never actually done it. It seems a reasonable premise that all of the thymus must be removed if the surgery is to be successful. As a nonsurgeon, it seems to me the widest possible exposure would allow the detection of bits of thymus stuck in unexpected places. The only patients I have followed have all had the transternal procedure.

Although postoperative complications were at one time a major deterrent to thymectomy, as to all intrathoracic surgery, modern techniques have eliminated these and serious postoperative complications are seen in less than 1% of the patients.

In one series of 40 patients with generalized myasthenia (excluding those with thymoma and congenital myasthenia gravis), the remission rate was 38%. Ten percent were asymptomatic and a further 45% were improved. There was a fall in acetylcholine receptor antibodies in 21 of 35 patients. Nine of these 21 were in complete remission, suggesting the general relationship between antibody levels and the clinical improvement, but individuals proved to be exceptions to this rule (61).

An unusual aspect of the improvement after thymectomy is that it may continue up to 7–10 years. Perhaps the prolonged recovery time is due to the survival of long lived abnormal lymphocytes in the circulation. There has been a suggestion that the presence of germinal centers in the thymus may be association with a good prognosis, although again the literature is inconsistent with regard to this (61, 82–85, 88). The use of radiation in addition to surgical removal of the thymus has been suggested (89), but this practice has now been largely abandoned.

The benefit from thymectomy seems to be greatest in those patients who have had the disease for a shorter period of time.

Plasmapheresis. In 1976 a report appeared which documented the improvement of myasthenia gravis following plasma exchange (90). The wisdom of removing the patient's plasma contaminated as it is by abnormal antibodies directed against the endplates would seem incontrovertible. Subsequent reports of the use of this technique have ranged from the cautious to the hortatory (91, 92). The exchange consists of the removal of between 2 and 4 liters of the patient's plasma. This is often done on a daily or alternate daily basis usually for a total of between 6 and 10 treatments and reduces the level of the antiacetylcholine receptor antibody by about 60%. Unfortunately the levels return to pretreatment values in most patients within 28 days (91). A dramatic improvement may be seen within a few days of plasmapheresis and provided the basis for the early enthusiasm. There are both practical and theroetical problems associated with the technique. First of all, the patient must either have adequate veins for repeated plasmapheresis or must have such access provided surgically by means of a shunt or similar device. Second, plasmapheresis is not entirely without risk. Thrombophlebitis, embolus, endocarditis, and hemolysis leading to renal failure have all been recorded. Such complications are rare enough that they seldom will be a deterrent when the indications for plasmapheresis are otherwise clear. A theoretical disadvantage of plasmapheresis is that it actually accelerates the production of the antibody against the receptor. This is due to removal of an apparent inhibitory feedback as the levels of antiacetylcholine antibody in the blood fall (51, 93). Treatment of this rebound has shown no synergism between plasma exchange and immunosuppressive therapy carried out at the same time (91). Once again the picture is confused because the clinical response demonstrated by the patient does not necessarily mirror the fall in the antibody levels. Patients with no significant decline in the antibody level may demonstrate clinical improvement, others are clinically unchanged despite a fall in the antibody levels.

In the early days of plasmapheresis, there was some difference of opinion about its clinical effect. Part of the confusion may have been due to the background against which it was used. It seemed to be most effective in clinics where patients were treated primarily by means of anticholinesterase medication and where steroids were used only when the patient became worse or resistant to these medications. Plasmapheresis seemed to have least effect in those clinics where thymectomy and immunosuppressive treatment was popular in the early stages of the disease. It may simply reflect once again the propensity of myasthenics to respond to different forms of treatment more readily when they are in the early stages.

Interpretation of the effects of plasmapheresis is further distorted by the fact that many patients are also taking immunosuppressive drugs, leading to arguments as to which part of the clinical picture is attributable to which treatment. All are agreed, however, that the improvement is temporary and if one attempts to treat a patient by pheresis alone, it is likely that the patient will spend much of his time and a lot of his money in the hospital.

What then are the indications for plasmapheresis in the light of our present knowledge? There seems to be general agreement that plasmapheresis is worthwhile as a temporary boost in patients whose illness has taken a turn for the worse. It can be used in preparing the patient for thymectomy or in the treatment of the relatively rare patient with myasthenic crisis. It may also be used following thymectomy in patients who develop increasing weakness if the physician does not wish to restart anticholinesterase medication. It is also used in patients whose reponse to thymectomy and immunosuppression has been disappointing. In this last situation, we have seen only one or two patients who have benefited from plasmapheresis.

It should again be emphasized that control trials of plasmapheresis are lacking and clinical anecdotes should not be considered an adequate replacement for such trials.

Combined Therapy. There is as much discussion over the selection of patients for thymectomy as there is for those to be treated with steroids. In former days one did not use either of these two forms of treatment until the patient had moderately severe difficulty from the myasthenia gravis. There was hidden in this pearl more than a grain of illogic. In thymectomy and immunosuppressive treatment we have two forms of therapy which are ultimately of benefit but which may initially make the patient worse. Instead of using these early in the disease, when the patient's general condition enables him better to withstand the threat of major surgery and the side effects of potentially dangerous medications, we waited until the patient was already severely debilitated and frequently in respiratory crisis. It was not surprising that the complications involved in such treatment were pronounced. It seems much more logical to use both thymectomy and steroids early in the disease. If myasthenia gravis or treatment with anticholinesterase drugs produces permanent changes in the muscle, it would be unwise to allow the disease to continue if its eradication is a practical possibility. The question whether the treatment with thymectomy and steroids dose, in fact, eradicate the disease during its early stages is not yet answered. In our clinic we have used the combined approach of thymectomy and steroids as soon as the diagnosis of myasthenia is made, unless the myasthenia is limited totally to the eyes. After a complete evaluation of the patient's disease, thymectomy is performed. The anticholinesterase medications are reduced or discontinued before surgery. As soon as is practical after the surgery (usually on the fourth or fifth day) the patient is started on high dose, daily prednisone therapy, and this is continued for approximately 6 months to a year.

Patients who were placed on steroids without thymectomy often had a relapse of their illness if steroids were withdrawn within the year. The worsening usually occurred within 6–12 months after cessation of the medication. Patients who have had a thymectomy can often have their steroid dosage reduced at an earlier date without such relapse and, therefore, the side effects of steroids are reduced. In comparison to the large series of patients reported elsewhere, our own experience is small, but the therapy seems particularly effective in the young myasthenic with a short history of the illness. Of 21 such patients under 30 all except 5 are in remission and the remaining patients are only mildly handicapped. The longest period during which we have followed such patients is 12 years but most have been followed for less than 8.

Management of Crisis. Patients with myasthenia gravis occasionally arrive in the emergency room with an acute exacerbation of weakness. It may be difficult to know whether they are in myasthenic crisis or cholinergic crisis. The edrophonium test has been recommended as a means of distinguishing between the two. The advantage of edrophonium is that if the patient is, in fact, in cholinergic crisis, its action is short-lived and any worsening of the patient's condition is rapidly reversed. If there is a clear-cut improvement with edrophonium, the patient's medication can be adjusted accordingly and sometimes the patient will be well enough to return home. This, however, is the exception and it is often difficult to decide whether there has been any improvement with edrophonium; if improvement is noted, this may be slight. In such a situation, the best course is to discontinue all medication. The only way of dying from myasthenia gravis itself is from respiratory failure, and assisted respirations are a routine procedure in the intensive care unit. The patient should be admitted to such a unit and intubated, or a tracheostomy should be carried out if necessary. All medications are withdrawn and a suction machine provided to remove the saliva that pools in the nasopharynx. The patient is maintained in this fashion for between 4 and 10 days and then anticholinesterase medications are reinstated in small doses. Very often, there is a dramatic increase in the sensitivity of the patient to cholinergic medications after this "drying out" period, and management may once again be instituted on an outpatient basis. The use of plasmapheresis should also be considered in the treatment of crisis.

Usually the patient undergoes cycles of these crises so that he seems to need more and more anticholinesterase medicines to control his disease and eventually he will once again be resistant to the effects of the medicine.

Obviously, any patient who is seen in myasthenic crisis may be suffering from some other condition (such as intercurrent infection) which may be exacerbating the condition as discussed earlier.

Penicillamine-induced Myasthenia. Myasthenia gravis seems to occur as a complication of the treatment of rheumatoid arthritis with D-penicillamine. Approximately 1% of those taking the drug develop clinical myasthenia. It is more common in women than in men by a ratio of 6 to 1 and, in all the reported cases, starts in the ocular muscles, although it later becomes generalized (71, 94). The age range, as might be expected in a population of patients with rheumatoid arthritis, is higher than the usual age distribution of myasthenia. This complication to D-penicillamine treatment has also been seen in Wilson's disease and is not limited to rheumatoid arthritis. The reaction cannot be thought of as simply a side effect of the drug since it disappears only slowly when the drug is withdrawn. It seems that the same immunologic factors are involved in the process as in true myasthenia gravis. Antiacetylcholine receptor antibodies are found in these patients and the HLA distribution in 3 of 7 patients in whom it was measured indicated the presence of HLA A1 and B8 as in the spontaneously occurring myasthenia. The administration of the drug in patients with rheumatoid arthritis is associated with the development of the antistriational antibody in about 20%. Ordinarily, the antibody is associated with thymoma, but this does not seem to be true in patients reported thus far. If there is severe myasthenia, plasmapheresis has also been used and gave temporary improvement (95).

Drugs to Be Used with Caution. Many commonly used drugs have an adverse effect on neuromuscular transmission and should be used with caution in patients with myasthenia (96). Among the antibiotics, the aminoglycosides such as neomycin, streptomycin, kanamycin, gentamycin and tobramycin have been shown to decrease neuromuscular transmission and may have both pre- and postsynaptic actions at the neuromuscular junction. Other peptide antibiotics such as polymyxin B and colistin may have similar effects. All of this has led to the common advice given to house officers that one does not prescribe a drug ending in "mycin" for a patient with myasthenia gravis.

Drugs which are active on the cardiovascular system may also act on striated muscles. Quinine, quinidine and procainamide (97), propranolol and other β-adrenergic blockers (98), may interfere with neuromuscular transmission. Diphenylhydantoin may also cause an increase in the myasthenic's symptoms (99). The psychotrophic drug lithium carbonate may act on transmission at the presynaptic site by substituting lithium ions for sodium. It also seems to have a post synaptic action and prolongs the neuromuscular blockade produced by succinylcholine or curare (100).

In view of the necessity for performing CAT scans of the chest in patients with myasthenia gravis, it is of interest that 2 patients were reported as experiencing an acute exacerbation of their myasthenia after the intravenous injection of the contrast material meglumine diarizoate during this procedure (101).

REFERENCES

1. Guthrie, L. B. Myasthenia gravis in the 17th century. Lancet *1:* 330, 1903.
2. Osserman, K. E., and Genkins, G. Studies in myasthenia gravis: a review of a 20-year experience in over 1,200 patients. Mt.Sinai J. Med. N.Y. *38:* 497–537, 1971.
3. Priskanen, R., Bergstrom, K., Hammarstrom, L., et al. Neuromuscular safety margin: genetical, immunological, and electrophysiological determinants in relatives of myasthenic patients: a preliminary report. Ann. N.Y. Acad. Sci. *377:* 606–613, 1981.
4. Perlo, V. P., Poskanzer, D. C., Schwab, R. S., Viets, H. R., Osserman, K. E., and Genkins, G. Myasthenia gravis: evaluation of treatment in 1,355 patients. Neurology *16:* 431–439, 1966.
5. Grob, D., Brunner, N. G., and Namba, T. The natural course of myasthenia gravis and effect of therapeutic measures. Ann. N.Y. Acad. Sci. *377:* 614–639, 1981.
6. Cohen, M. S., and Younger, D. Aspects of the natural history of myasthenia gravis: crisis and death. Ann. N.Y. Acad. Sci. *377:* 670–677, 1981.
7. Toyka, K. V., Drachman, D. B., Pestronk, A., and Kao, I. Myasthenia gravis: passive transfer from man to mouse. Science *190:* 397–399, 1975.
8. Lefvert, A. K., and Osterman, P. O. Newborn infants to myasthenic mothers: a clinical study and an investigation of acetylcholine receptor antibodies in 17 children. Neurology *33:* 133–138, 1983.
9. Elias, S. B., Butler, I., and Appel, S. H. Neonatal myasthenia gravis in the infant of a myasthenic mother in remission. Ann. Neurol. *6:* 72–75, 1979.

10. Keesey, J., Lindstrom, J., Cokely, H., and Herrmann, C. Antiacetylcholine receptor antibody in neonatal myasthenia. N. Engl. J. Med. *296:* 55, 1977.
11. Walker, M. B. Myasthenia gravis: case in which fatigue of forearm muscles could induce paralysis of extraocular muscle. Proc. Roy. Soc. Med. *31:* 722, 1938.
12. Patten, B. M., Oliver, K. L., and Engel, W. K. Effect of lactate infusions on patients with myasthenia gravis. Neurology *24:* 986–990, 1974.
13. Ozdemir, C., and Young, R. R. Electrical testing in myasthenia gravis. Ann. N.Y. Acad. Sci. *183:* 287–302, 1971.
14. Ekstedt, J., Nilsson, G., and Stahlberg, E. Calculation of the electromyographic jitter. J. Neurol. Neurosurg. Psychiatry *37:* 526–539, 1974.
15. Stahlberg, E., Ekstedt, J., and Broman, A. Neuromuscular transmission in myasthenia gravis studied with single fiber electromyography. J. Neurol. Neurosurg. Psychiatry *37:* 540–547, 1974.
16. Brown, J. C., Charlton, J. E., and White D. J. K. A regional technique for the study of sensitivity to curare in human muscle. J. Neurol. Neurosurg. Psychiatry *38:* 18–26, 1975.
17. Brown, J. C., and Charlton, J. E. A study of sensitivity to curare in myasthenia disorders using a regional technique. J. Neurol. Neurosurg. Psychiatry *38:* 27–33, 1975.
18. Meadows, J. C., Ross-Russel, R. W., and Wise, R. P. A re-evaluation of the decamethonium test for myasthenia gravis. Acta Neurol. Scand. *50:* 248–256, 1974.
19. Lindstrom, J. M., Seybold, M. E., Lennon, V. A., Whittingham, S., and Duane, D. D. Antibody to acetylcholine receptor in myasthenia gravis. Clinical correlates and diagnostic values. Neurology *26:* 1054–1057, 1976.
20. Lennon, V. Myasthenia. Diagnosis by assay of serum antibodies. Mayo Clin. Proc. *57:* 723–724, 1982.
21. Vincent, A., and Newsom-Davis, J. Acetylcholine receptor antibody characteristics in myasthenia gravis: 1. Patients with generalized myasthenia or disease restricted to ocular muscles. Clin. Exp. Immunol. *49:* 257–265, 1982.
22. Lindstrom, J., Tzartos, S., and Gullick, W. Structure and function of the ACh receptor molecule studied using monoclonal antibodies. Ann. N.Y. Acad. Sci. *377:* 1–19, 1981.
23. Lennon, V. A., and Lambert, E. H. Monoclonal auto antibodies to acetylcholine receptors: evidence for a dominant idiotype and requirement of complement for pathogenicity. Ann. N.Y. Acad. Sci. *377:* 77–95, 1981.
24. Grohovaz, F., Limbrick, A. R., and Miledi, R. Acetylcholine receptors at the rat neuromuscular junction revealed by deep etching. Proc. R. Soc. Lond [Biol.] *215:* 147–154, 1982.
25. Heuser, J. E., and Salpeter, S. R. Organization of acetylcholine receptors in quick-frozen, deep-etched, and rotary replicated torpedo postsynaptic membrane. J.Cell. Biol. *82:* 150–173, 1979.
26. Hirokawa, N., and Heuser, J. E. Internal and external differentiation of the postsynaptic membrane at the neuromuscular junction. J. Neurocytol. *11:* 487–510, 1982.
27. Engel, A. G., Sahashi, K., and Fumagalli, G. The immunopathology of acquired myasthenia gravis. Ann. N.Y. Acad. Sci. *377:* 158–174, 1981.
28. Appel S. H., Blosser, J. C., McManaman, J. L., and Ashizawa, T. Acetyl choline receptor turnover in myasthenia gravis. Am. J. Physiol. *243:;* E31–36, 1982.
29. Takamori, M., Ishii, N., and Mori, M. The role of cyclic 3'5'-adenosine monophosphate in neuromuscular disease. Arch. Neurol. *29:* 240–242, 1973.
30. Hokkanen, E., Vapaatalo, H., and Anttila, P. On the possible role of cyclic AMP in the neuromuscular transmission and in the treatment of myasthenia gravis. Acta Neurol. Scand. (Suppl.) *51:* 375, 1972.
31. Coers, C., and Woolf, A. L. *The Innervation of Muscle.* Blackwell, Oxford, 1959.
32. Engel, A. G., and Santa, T. Histometric analysis of the ultrastructure of the neuromuscular junction in myasthenia gravis and in the myasthenic syndrome. Ann. N.Y. Acad. Sci. *183:* 46–63, 1971.
33. Elmqvist, D., Hoffmann, W. W., Kugelberg, J., and Quastel, D. M. J. An electrophysiological investigation of neuromuscular transmission in myasthenia gravis. J. Physiol. *174:* 417–434, 1964.
34. Fambrough, B. M., Drachman, D. B., and Satyamurti, S. Neuromuscular junction in myasthenia gravis: decreased acetylcholine receptors. Science *182:* 293–295, 1973.
35. Almon, R. R., Andrew, C. G., and Appel, S. H. Serum globulin in myasthenia gravis: inhibition of alphabungarotoxin binding to acetylcholine receptors. Science *186:* 55–57, 1974.
36. Bender, A. N., Ringel, S. P., Engel, W. K., Daniels, M. P., and Vogel, Z. Myasthenia gravis: a serum factor blocking acetylcholine receptors of the human neuromuscular junction. Lancet *1:* 607–608, 1975.
37. Engel, A. G., Lambert, E. H., and Santa, T. Study of long term anticholinesterase therapy:

effects on neuromuscular transmission and motor end plate fine structure. Neurology *23:* 1273–1281, 1973.

38. Ward, M. D., Forbes, M. S., and Johns, T. R. Neostigmine methylsulfate: does it have a chronic effect as well as a transient one? Arch. Neurol. *32:* 808–814, 1975.
39. Noble, M. D., Brown, T. H., and Peacock, J. H. Regulation of acetyl choline receptor levels by cholinergic agonists in mouse muscle cell cultures. Proc. Natl. Acad. Sci. *75:* 3488–3492, 1978.
40. Hudson, C. S., Rash, J. E., Tiend, T. N., and Albuquerque, E. X. Neostigmine-induced alteration at the mammalian neuromuscular junction: II. Ultra structure. J. Pharmacol. Exp. Ther. *205:* 340–356, 1978.
41. Simpson, J. A. Myasthenic gravis and myasthenic syndromes. In: *Disorders of Voluntary Muscle*, Ed. 3, edited by J. N. Walton. Churchill Livingstone, London, 1974, pp. 653–692.
42. Rule, A. H., and Kornfeld, P. Studies in myasthenia gravis: biological aspects. Mt. Sinai J. Med. N.Y. *38:* 538–572, 1971.
43. Strauss, A. J. L., Siegal, B. C., Hsu, K. C., Burkholder, P. M., Nastuk, W. L., and Osserman, K. E. Immunoflourescence demonstration of a muscle binding, complement fixing, serum globulin fraction in myasthenia gravis. Proc. Soc. Exp. Biol. *105:* 184, 1960.
44. McFarlin, D. E., Engel, W. K., and Strauss, A. J. L. Does myasthenic serum bind to the neuromuscular junction? Ann. N.Y. Acad. Sci. *135:* 656–663, 1971.
45. Patrick, J., and Lindstrom, J. Autoimmune response to acetylcholine receptor. Science *180:* 871–872, 1973.
46. Tarrab-Hazdai, R., Aharonov, A., Silman, I., Fuchs, S., and Abramsky, O. Experimental autoimmune myasthenia induced in monkeys by purified acetylcholine receptor. Nature *256:* 128–130, 1975.
47. Lennon, V. A., Lindstrom, J. M., and Seybold, M. E. Experimental autoimmune myasthenia: a model of myasthenia gravis in rats and guinea pigs. J. Exp. Med. *141:* 1365–1375, 1975.
48. Tarrab-Hazdai, R., Aharanov, A., Abramsky, O., Yaar, I., and Fuchs, S. Passive transfer of experimental autoimmune myasthenia by lymph node cells in inbred guinea pigs. J. Exp. Med. *142:* 785–789, 1975.
49. Drachman, D. B., Adams, R. N., Josifek, L. E., Pestronk, A., and Stanely, E. F. Antibody mediated mechanisms of ACh receptor less in myasthenia gravis: clinical relevance. Ann. N.Y. Acad. Sci. *377:* 175–187, 1981.
50. Lerrick, A. J., Vincent, A., and Newsom-Davis, J. Electrophysiological effects of myasthenic serum factors studied in mouse muscle. Ann. Neurol. *13:* 186–191, 1983.
51. Seybold, M. E., and Lindstrom, J. M. Patterns of acetylcholine receptor antibody fluctuation in myasthenia gravis. Ann. N.Y. Acad. Sci. *377:* 292–306, 1981.
52. Oosterhuis, H. J. G. H. Observations of the natural history of myasthenia gravis and the effect of thymectomy. Ann. N.Y. Acad. Sci. *377:* 678–690, 1981.
53. Olanow, C. W., Lane, R. J., and Roses, A. D. Relationship between the acetylcholine receptor antibody titer and the clinical status in myasthenia gravis. Ann. N.Y. Acad. Sci. *377:* 856–857, 1981.
54. Oosterhuis, H. J. G. H., Limburg, P. C., Hummel-Tappel, E., et al. Anti-acetylcholine receptors in myasthenia gravis: II. Clinical and serological follow-up individual patients. J. Neurol. Sci. *58:* 371–385, 1983.
55. Vincent, A., Newsom-Davis, J., Newton, P., et al. Acetylcholine receptor antibody and clinical response to thymectomy in myasthenia gravis. Neurology *33:* 1276–1282, 1983.
56. Hohlfeld, R., Toyka, K. V., Besinger, V. A., Gerhold, B., and Heininger, K. Myasthenic gravis: reactivation of clinical disease and of autoimmune factors after discontinuation of long term azathioprine. Ann. Neurol. *17:* 238–242, 1985.
57. Harrison, R., Lunt, G. G., Morris, H., and Marengo, T. S. Patient specific antiacetylcholine antibody patterns in myasthenia gravis. Ann. N.Y. Acad. Sci. *377:* 332–341, 1981.
58. Engel, W. K., Festoff, B. W., Patten, B. M., Swerdlow, M. L., Newball, H. H., and Thompson, M.D. Myasthenia gravis. Ann. Intern. Med. *81:* 225–246, 1974.
59. Editorial. N. Engl. J. Med. *291:* 1304, 1971.
60. Tomonobu, A., Drachman, D. B., Asher, D. M., Gibbs, C. J., Bahmanyar, S., and Wolinsky, J. S. Attempts to implicate viruses in myasthenia gravis. Neurology *35:* 185–192, 1985.
61. Penn, A. S., Jaretzki, A., Wolff, M., Chang, H. W., and Tennyson, V. Thymic abnormalities: antigen or antibody? Response to thymectomy in myasthenia gravis. Ann. N.Y. Acad. Sci. *377:* 786–803, 1981.
62. Dalakos, M. C., Engel, W. K., McClure, J. E., and Goldstein, A. L. Thymosin in myasthenia gravis. N. Engl. J. Med. *302:* 1092–1094, 1980.
63. Armstrong, R. M., Nowak, R. M., and Falk, R. E. Thymic lymphocyte function in myasthenia gravis. Neurology *23:* 1078–1083, 1973.

64. Abdou, N. I., Liasak, R. P., Zweiman, B., Abrahamsohn, I., and Penn, A. S. The thymus in myasthenia gravis: evidence for altered cell population. N. Engl. J. Med. *291:* 1271–1275, 1974.
65. Newson-Davis, J., Willcox, N., Scadding, G., Calder, L., and Vincent, A. Antiacetylcholine receptor antibody synthesis by cultured lymphocytes in myasthenia gravis: thymic and peripheral blood cell interactions. Ann. N.Y. Acad. Sci. *377:* 393–402, 1981.
66. Abramsky, O., Aharonov, A., and Webb, C. Cellular immune response to acetylcholine receptor rich fraction in patients with myasthenia gravis. Clin. Exp. Immunol. *19:* 11–16, 1975.
67. Richman, D. P., Patrick, J., and Arnason, B. G. W. Cellular immunity in myasthenia gravis. N. Engl. J. Med. *294:* 694–698, 1976.
68. Lisak, R. P., Sweiman, B., Skolnik, P., Levinson, A. I., Moskovitz, A. R., and Guerrero, F. Thymic lymphocytes subpopulations in myasthenia gravis. Neurology *33:* 868, 1983.
69. Fujii, Y., Monden, Y., Hashimoto, J., Nakahara, and K., Kawashima, Y. Acetylcholine receptor antibody production by bone marrow cells in a patient with myasthenia gravis. Neurology *35:* 577–579, 1985.
70. Compston, D. A. S., Vincent, A., Newson-Davis, J., et al. Clinical, pathological, HLA antigen and immunological evidence for disease heterogeneity in myasthenia gravis. Brain *103:* 579–601, 1980.
71. Dawkins, R. L., Christiansen, F. T., and Garlepp, M. J. Autoantibodies and HLA antigens in ocular, generalized and penicillamine induced myasthenia gravis. Ann. N.Y. Acad. Sci. *377:* 372–383, 1981.
72. Davison, J. C., Hyman, N. M., Dehghan, A., and Chan, K. The relationship of plasma levels of pyridostigmine to clinical effect in patients with myasthenia gravis. J. Neurol. Neurosurg. Psychiatry *44:* 1141–1145, 1981.
73. Flacke, W. E., Blum, R. P., Scott, W. R., Foldes, F. F., and Osserman, K. E. Germine monodiacetate in myasthenia gravis. Ann. N.Y. Acad. Sci. *183:* 316–333, 1971.
74. Liversedge, L., A., Yuill, G. M., Wilkinson, I. M. S., and Hughes, J. A. Benefit from adrenalcorticotrophin in myasthenia gravis. J. Neurol. Neurosurg. Psychiatry *37:* 412–415, 1974.
75. Kjaer, M. Myasthenia gravis and myasthenic syndromes treated with prednisone. Acta Neurol. Scand. *47:* 464–474, 1971.
76. Johns, T. R., Crowley, W. J., and Miller, J. Q. The syndrome of myasthenia and polymyositis with comments on therapy. Ann. N.Y. Acad. Sci. *183:* 64–71, 1971.
77. John, T. R. Treatment of myasthenia gravis: long term administration of corticosteroids with remarks on thymectomy. Adv. Neurol. *17:* 99–122, 1977.
78. Warmolts, J. R., and Engel, W. K. Myasthenia gravis: benefit from alternate day prednisone. N. Engl. J. Med. *286:* 17–20, 1972.
79. Seybold, M. E., and Drachman, D. B. Gradually increasing doses of prednisone in myasthenia gravis. N. Engl. J. Med. *290:* 81–84, 1974.
80. Fischer, R. C., and Schwartzmann, R. J. Oral corticosteroid in the treatment of ocular myasthenia gravis. Ann. N.Y. Acad. Sci. *274:* 652–654, 1976.
81. Mertens, H. G., Reuther, P., and Ricker, K. Effect of immunosuppressive drugs (azathioprine). Ann. N.Y. Acad. Sci. *377:* 691–698, 1982.
82. Perlo, V. P., Arnason, B., Poskanzer, D., Castleman, B., Schwab, R. S., Osserman, K. E., Papatestas, A., Alpert, A. L., and Kark, A. The role of thymectomy in the treatment of myasthenia gravis. Ann. N.Y. Acad. Sci. *183:* 308–315, 1971.
83. Cohn, H., E., Solit, R. W., Schatz, N. J., and Schlezinger, N. Surgical treatment of myasthenia gravis. J. Thorac. Cardiovasc. Surg. *68:* 876–885, 1974.
84. Mulder, D. G., Herrmann, C., and Buckberg, G. D. Effect of thymectomy in patients with myasthenia gravis: A 16 year experience. Am. J. Surg. *128:* 202–206, 1974.
85. Genkins, G., Papatestas, A. E., Horowitz, S. H., and Kornfeld, P. Studies in myasthenia gravis: early thymectomy. Am. J. Med *58:* 517–524, 1975.
86. Olanow, C. W., Lane, R. J., and Roses, A. D. Thymectomy in late onset myasthenia. Arch. Neurol. *39:* 82–83, 1982.
87. Olanow, C. W., Wechsler, A. S., and Roses, A. D. A prospective study of thymectomy and serum acetyl choline receptor antibodies in myasthenia gravis. Ann. Surg. *196:* 113–121, 1982.
88. Sambrook, M. A., Reid, H., Mohr, P. D., and Boddie, H. G. Myasthenia gravis: clinical and histological features in relation to thymectomy. J. Neurol. Neurosurg. Psychiatry *39:* 38–43, 1976.
89. Schultz, M. D., and Schwab, R. S. Results of thymic (mediastinal) irradiation in patients with myasthenia gravis. Ann. N.Y. Acad. Sci. *183:* 303, 1971.
90. Pinching, A. J., Peters, D. K., and Newsom-Davis, J. Remission of myasthenia gravis following plasma exchange. Lancet *2:* 1373–1376, 1976.

91. Hawkey, C. J., Newsom-Davis, J., and Vincent, A. Plasma exchange and immunosuppressive drug treatment in myasthenia gravis. J. Neurol. Neurosurg. Psychiatry *44:* 469–475, 1981.
92. Dau, P. C., (Editor). *Plasmapheresis and the Immunobiology of Myasthenia gravis.* Houghton Mifflin, Boston, 1979.
93. Seybold, M. E., Tsoukas, C., Lindstrom, J., Foug, S., and Vaughan, J. Leukoplasmapheresis for myasthenia gravis. Acetylcholine receptor antibody production. Arch. Neurol. *39:* 433–435, 1982.
94. Dawkins, R. L., Garlepp, M. J., McDonald, B. L., Williamson, J., Zilko, P. J., and Carrano, J. Myasthenia gravis and D-penicillamine J. Rheumatol. (Suppl.) *7:* 169–174, 1981.
95. Lang, A. E., Humphrey, J. G., and Gordon, D. A. Plasma exchange therapy for severe penicillamine induced myasthenia gravis. J. Rheumatol. *8:* 303–307, 1981.
96. Argov, Z., and Mastaglia, F. L. Disorders of neuromuscular transmission caused by drugs. N. Engl. J. Med. *301:* 409–413, 1979.
97. Kornfeld, P., Horowitz, S. H., Genkins, G., and Papatestas, A. E. Myasthenia gravis unmasked by antiarrhythmic agents. Mt. Sinai J. Med. *43:* 10–14, 1976.
98. Herishann, Y., and Rosenberg, P. β Blockers and myasthenia gravis. Ann. Intern. Med. *83:* 834–835, 1975.
99. Brumlik, J., and Jacobs, R. S. Myasthenia gravis associated with dyphenylhydantoin therapy for epilepsy. Can. J. Neurol. Sci. *1:* 127–129, 1974.
100. Hill, G. E., Wong, K. C., and Hodges, M. R. Potentiation of succinylcholine neuromuscular blockade by lithium carbonate. Anesthesiology *44:* 439–442, 1976.
101. Chagnac, Y., Hadani, M., and Goldhammer, Y. Myasthenic crisis after intravenous administration of iodinated contrast agent. Neurology *35:* 1219–1220, 1985.

CONGENITAL MYASTHENIC DISORDERS

The original concept of congenital myasthenia gravis was of a disorder occurring at birth, often familial, and more frequently affecting boys than girls. The cardinal symptoms were ptosis and extraocular weakness which remained relatively fixed and which was often associated with facial, bulbar, and, on occasions, mild limb weakness. This illness was obviously different from neonatal myasthenia since the mother showed no evidence of the disease. The weakness responded to Tensilon, although often without the dramatic improvements seen in myasthenia gravis. Fatigability and the other hallmarks of myasthenia accompanied the illness. The illness was assumed to be identical to myasthenia in the adult, although it seldom got worse as the patient grew older. As the puzzle of acquired myasthenia gravis was unravelled, another striking difference was noted. In the congenital myasthenic, acetylcholine receptor antibodies are not noted in the plasma. This perhaps explains why such patients do not respond to thymectomy and prednisone administration as does the more usual variety of myasthenia.

The term, familial infantile myasthenia, was given to a similar disease in which the generalized weakness was much more severe and was associated with respiratory difficulties, particularly spells of apnea in childhood.

A. G. Engel's group has carefully analyzed the immunological, physiological and biochemical abnormalities in this type of patient and has outlined three further categories.

Acetylcholinesterase Deficiency

This is associated with a deficiency of acetylcholinesterase at the neuromuscular junction (1).The patient was a 16-year-old boy who was noted to have ptosis within 5 days birth. As he grew older, he exhibited extraocular weakness, as well as weakness of the facial, bulbar, neck, trunk, and limb muscles, which was made worse by exercising and relieved by rest He also had a scoliosis. Electrical testing showed a decremental response and also a repetitive muscle action potential response to a single nerve stimulus. Treatment with anticholinesterase inhibitors was unrewarding. Receptor antibody titers were normal. The miniature endplate potentials were abnormally prolonged, presumably due to the fact that acetylcholine was not removed by the esterase, resulting in prolonged depolarization and a repetitive muscle action potential. Acetylcholine receptor antibody was normal at the endplate, but there were degenerative changes and the nerve terminals were small. It is possible that the small nerve terminals and the decreased release of acetylcholine, which were also found, were secondary to the total absence of acetylcholine esterase since this seemed to be the most striking defect.

Defect of Acetylcholine

Another variety of congenital myasthenia syndrome was characterized by a decrease in the size of miniature endplate potentials following repetitive stimulation for some minutes. Everything else about the endplate was normal and there was no evidence of antibody formation in the blood. In this condition, a defect in the resynthesis of acetylcholine was postulated (2). The clinical picture was of congenital myasthenia associated with apnea. The illness responded to prostigmine, but not to prednisone, and three other siblings, two of whom had myasthenic symptoms, had died suddenly in infancy. Because the miniature endplate potentials were initially normal and the cytochemical demonstration of acetylcholine receptor was not deranged, the defect must lie in the ability of the presynaptic region to restore its supplies of acetylcholine vesicles, leading to the suggestion of a deficiency in synthesis and packaging.

Slow Ion Channel Defect

The third type was postulated as a defect in the acetylcholine activated ion channel (3). The clinical picture was again similar, but this time there was a selective weakness of the muscles of the face and of the shoulder and forearm, particularly of the wrist and finger extensors. A repetitive muscle action potential was again seen in response to a single stimulus of the nerve and the miniature endplate potentials were again prolonged. Since acetylcholinesterase was normally present, it was suggested that the underlying cause of these physiological abnormalities was that the ion channel activated by acetylcholine remained open for an abnormally long time. There were also degenerative changes at the endplate, but these were felt to be secondary. Of interest in this patient was the presence of tubular aggregates in the muscle biopsy. Similar, although perhaps not identical, cases in which tubular aggregates have been associated with myasthenic features have been described (4). Morgan Hughes et al. (5) also described a patient with myasthenic features and tubular aggregates in whom the affinity of the endplate region for D-tubocurarine was increased approximately 10-fold.

It is difficult to know how best to summarize these various reports. Perhaps the only safe thing to say is that the complexity of neuromuscular transmission is great and that it may go wrong at any step in the sequence. When it does so, unusual syndromes may be produced at birth, emphasizing that, in any patient with an undiagnosed disease, neuromuscular function deserves to be investigated. Repetitive stimulation and a Tensilon test are the beginning, but not the end, of such investigations.

REFERENCES

1. Engel, A. G., Lambert, E. H., and Gomez, M R. A new myasthenic syndrome with endplate acetylcholinesterase deficiency, small nerve terminals, and reduced acetylcholine release. Ann. Neurol. *1:* 315–330, 1977.
2. Hart, Z. H. Sahashi, K., Lambert, E. H., Engel, A. G., and Lindstrom, J. A Congenital familial myasthenic syndrome caused by a presynaptic defect of transmitter resynthesis or mobilization. Neurology *29:* 556–557, 1979.
3. Engel, A. G., Lambert, E. H., Mulder, O. M., Torres, C. F., Sahashi, K., Bertorini, E., and Whitaker, J. N. A newly recognized congenital myasthenic syndrome attributed to a prolonged open time of the acetylcholine induced ion channel. Ann. Neurol. *11:* 553–569, 1982.
4. Dobkin, B. H., and Verity, M. A. Familial neuromuscular disease with type 1 fiber hypoplasia, tubular aggregates, cardiomyopathy, and myasthenic features. Neurology *28:* 1135–1140, 1978.
5. Morgan Hughes, J. A., Lecky, B. R. F., Landon, D. N., and Murray, N. M. . Alterations in the number and affinity of junctional acetylcholine receptors in a myopathy with tubular aggregates: a newly recognised receptor defect. Brain *104:* 274–295, 1981.

MYASTHENIC SYNDROME (LAMBERT-EATON SYNDROME)

The defect of neuromuscular transmission seen in the myasthenic syndrome is quite different from that of myasthenia gravis (1–5). The symptoms of the illness are equally distinct and perhaps the name "myasthenic" syndrome implies more common ground between this disease and myasthenia gravis than actually exists. To set the background for this illness, the next paragraph reviews the role played by presynaptic structures in the transmission of the impulse across the neuromuscular junction.

Acetylcholine is stored in the presynaptic nerve terminal in packets or "quanta" and only a small percentage of these are available for immediate release when the nerve is depolarized. The number of quanta released will determine the size of the endplate potential produced. If the acetylcholine in this releasable fraction is not replenished, neurotransmission will soon fail. Acetylcholine can be mobilized from the other stores in the nerve terminal and transferred to the releasable pool, either in response to high frequency stimulation of the nerve or following a period of voluntary exercise. It is obvious that even this pool of acetylcholine will be depleted unless there is some provision for resynthesis. This is accomplished by an uptake of choline (the product of hydrolysis by the acetylcholinesterase) and the formation of acetylcholine by the enzyme choline acetylase. If any part of this complicated system is abnormal, neuromuscular transmission ultimately fails, leading to the electrophysiological changes of increased "jitter" and the actual blocking of transmission. The evoked potential measured in muscle in this situation will decline as muscle fibers become inactive. The process of mobilization of acetylcholine does not cease as the nerve stimulus ceases. The continuing replenishment of the releasable pool may result in an overabundance of acetylcholine so that a succeeding nerve impulse may release more than the usual amount. This increases the size of the endplate potential thereby increasing the number of actively contracting muscle fibers in the motor unit by boosting more endplates past the critical threshold of depolarization. This effect lasts for several seconds and is in part responsible for the phenomenon of postexercise facilitation in which the motor unit, following a short period of exercise, is slightly larger than that seen at rest. Facilitation may also be due to accumulation or mobilization of calcium at the release sites (6).

Postexercise facilitation of muscle strength may be quite marked in the myasthenic syndrome, in which there is a decrease in the amount of acetylcholine released at the endplate.

The myasthenic syndrome occurs more frequently in men than women by a factor of 5 and is usually found over the age of 40. Its association with small cell carcinoma of the bronchus is well recognized; over half of the patients have such neoplasms. Up to 70% of the patients have a malignancy of one kind or another, although the symptoms of the myasthenic syndrome may occur many months before it becomes apparent.

The initial symptom is usually a feeling of weakness and tiredness around the hips which gives the patient predictable difficulty in arising from a chair or climbing stairs. Mild and nonspecific aching of the back and thighs may be found at this stage. The weakness differs from that of myasthenia gravis in being worst soon after arising in the morning, having a tendency to improve as the day goes on. Exercise may help rather than hinder the patient's strength for a brief time, although fatigue again supervenes after prolonged effort. The weakness may spread to involve muscles of the legs, shoulders, and arms, but rarely does it involve the muscles of the head and neck. While some mild difficulty with swallowing is noted in about third of the patients, and a few have noticed transient blurring of vision or ptosis, the severe involvement of extraocular and bulbar muscles which is so characteristic of myasthenia gravis is lacking in the myasthenic syndrome.

Another unusual symptom is that of a peculiar taste or dryness of the mouth. Perhaps the fact that the majority of patients have small cell carcinoma of the bronchus and that this is associated with cigarette smoking may partly explain this symptom, but other evidence of autonomic dysfunction such as impotence implies that cholinergic transmission in other systems is not normal. One patient with clear dysautonomia was described who had unresponsive pupils and abnormalities of salivation, lacrimation and sweating (7).

The clinical examination may show mild weakness or no weakness at all. Sometimes the increase in strength following exercise is noted on examination. A patient attempting to raise the legs straight off the examining couch may initially be unable to withstand any resistance to the movement on the part of the examiner. After a few attempts, however, the strength gradually returns to the legs and may be almost normal. The increasing strength may impart to the examiner a sensation similar to drawing up water from a well with a hand pump; with each movement the resistance needed to overcome the patient's strength increases. Prolonged sustained activity of the muscles, however, causes the weakness to appear again. The deep tendon reflexes are usually depressed, particularly at the knees. Since the illness is one of the remote effects of cancer, and since the various syndromes associated with cancer seldom occur in isolation, the myasthenic syndrome may coexist with symptoms of cerebellar ataxia, or the fleeting, changing paresthesias and hypesthesias of carcinomatous neuromyopathy.

The diagnosis is confirmed by electrophysiological studies. The miniature endplate potentials, which may reflect the amount of acetylcholine in each quantum, are normal, but too few quanta are released, and the threshold necessary for complete depolarization of the endplate and a propagated muscle action potential may not be reached (8). Increasing the available quanta, either by postexercise facilitation or high frequency electrical stimulation, will improve transmission, restore the motor unit, decrease the amount of jitter, and reverse the neuromuscular blocking. Hence, the most useful test in the diagnosis of the myasthenic syndrome is the EMG, and in particular the response of the evoked muscle action potentials to repetitive stimulation. The amplitude of the initial evoked response is very small when a single stimulus is given. With repetitive stimulation at rates of 3 cycles per second or less there is a further decrease in the amplitude of the evoked potential. However, with repetitive stimulation of from 20 to 50 cycles per second, facilitation of the response occurs and the amplitude may increase to 20 times the resting amplitude. Within 2 seconds after a 10-second period of maximum voluntary contraction, the evoked potential is also markedly increased, up to 12 times the resting level. This increase decays over the next 20–30 seconds and within 2–4 minutes after the contraction the evoked potential is less than the resting value. Single fiber EMG demonstrates a block in neuromuscular transmission that worsens following rest (9).

The abnormality in neuromuscular transmission in the myasthenic syndrome is similar in this regard to that produced by magnesium ions, botulinum toxin, and neomycin. Since the release of acetylcholine is calcium dependent, the possibility of some unknown substance interfering with the utilization of calcium has been entertained. Takamori et al. (10) have suggested that the defective calcium dependent acetylcholine release in the Lambert-Eaton syndrome can be partially corrected by calcium, epinephrine, aminophylline, or caffeine.

The muscle biopsy in myasthenic syndrome shows nonspecific findings with histochemical or light microscopic techniques. Some Type 2 fiber atrophy is seen and an occasional inflammatory response. With electron microscopic examination of the neuromuscular junction, Engel and Santa (11) have shown overdevelopment of the postsynaptic region; this is in contrast to the changes seen in myasthenia gravis. Defective function of calcium is also suggested by electron microscopic studies of freeze fracture preparations of presynaptic membranes. There is a decreased number of "active zones" and active zone particles. The active zones may be the areas through which calcium gains access to the interior of the cell (12).

The illness may have an autoimmune basis. Overall, 45% of patients with Lambert-Eaton Syndrome were found to have organ specific autoantibodies directed against either the thyroid or stomach. If patients who had coexistent tumor were omitted, the incidence was even higher (52%) (13). There are a group of autoimmune diseases including pernicious anemia and thyroiditis which tend to possess such antibodies. The argument for guilt by association is strengthened by the finding of an abnormal IgG in the serum of patients with Lambert-Eaton syndrome that causes the same abnormal electrophysiological and ultrastructural features of the disease in mice treated with this globulin (14). The injection of plasma from a patient with myasthenic syndrome into mice caused a decrease in the release of acetylcholine at the endplate secondary to nerve stimulation. The defect appeared to be a specific interference with transmitter release and was due to a factor in the IgG. This defect developed even in the absence of any clinical weakness occurring in the mice (15). A similar series of experiments continued that IgG was responsible and that the reduction in the quantal content of acetylcholine was also found when C5 deficient mice were used proving that the complement components were not involved (16).

Treatment of the illness begins with a search for malignancy. When one is found, the myasthenic syndrome sometimes improves after treatment of the underlying cancer. Since the myasthenic syndrome may precede the appearance of the tumor, the search for malignancy should be repeated every 3–6 months. The successful use of corticosteroids and immunosuppressive drugs has been reported (17, 18). The fatigue of the myasthenic syndrome is usually only poorly responsive to therapy with the cholinesterase inhibitors. Guanidine may be very effective but its use is limited by potential side effects. Daily doses of from 20 to 30 mg per kilogram of body weight are employed. Usually a third of this dose is administered every 8 hours. It is wise to start the drug out in small doses and gradually to increase them. Possible side effects include nausea, vomiting, dizziness, and tingling of the fingers. Liver and blood toxicity may also be noted. 4-Aminopyridine also increases the release of acetylcholine at the endplate. Although beneficial, the coincidence of side effects (including paresthesias, convulsions and confusion) at the dosage needed for the therapeutic effect limits the usefulness of the drug (19).

REFERENCES

1. Eaton, L. M., and Lambert, E. H. Electromyography and electric stimulation of nerves in diseases of motor units: observations on myasthenic syndrome associated with malignant tumors. J.A.M.A. *163:* 1117–1124, 1957.
2. Elmqvist, D., and Lambert, E. H. Detailed analysis of neuromuscular transmission in a patient with the myasthenic syndrome sometimes associated with bronchogenic carcinoma. Mayo Clin. Proc. *43:* 689–713, 1968.
3. Lambert, E. H., and Rooke, E. D. Myasthenic state and lung cancer. In: *The Remote Effects of Cancer on the Nervous System,* edited by W. Brain and F. H. Norris. Grune & Stratton, New York, 1965.
4. Herrmann, C. Myasthenia gravis and the myasthenic syndrome. Calif. Med. *113:* 27–36, 1970.
5. Lambert, E. H. Defects of neuromuscular transmission in syndromes other than myasthenia gravis. Ann. N.Y. Acad. Sci. *135:* 367–384, 1966.
6. Swift, T. R. Disorders of neuromuscular transmission other than myasthenia gravis. Muscle Nerve *4:* 334–353, 1981.
7. Rubenstein, A. E., Horowitz, S. H., and Bender, A. N. Cholinergic dysautonomia and Eaton-Lambert syndrome. Neurology *29:* 720–723, 1979.
8. Lambert, E. H., and Elmqvist, D. Quantal components of end plate potentials in myasthenic syndrome. Ann. N. Y. Acad. Sci. *183:* 183–199, 1971.
9. Schwartz, M. S., and Stalberg, E. Myasthenic syndrome studied with single fiber electromyography. Arch. Neurol. *32:* 815–817, 1975.
10. Takamori, M., Ishii, N., and Mori, M. The role of cyclic 3′,5′-adenosine monophosphate in neuromuscular disease. Arch. Neurol. *29:* 420–424, 1973.
11. Engel, A. G., and Santa, T. Histometric analysis of the ultrastructure of the neuromuscular junction in myasthenia gravis and in the myasthenic syndrome. Ann. N.Y. Acad. Sci. *183:* 46–63, 1971.
12. Fukunaga, H., Engel, A. G., Osame, M., et al. Paucity and disorganization of presynaptic membrane active zones in the Lambert-Eaton myasthenic syndrome. Muscle Nerve *5:* 686–697,1982.
13. Lennon, V. A., Lambert, E. H., Whittingham, S., and Fairbanks, V. Autoimmunity in the Lambert-Eaton syndrome. Muscle Nerve *5:* S21–S25, 1982.
14. Lang, B., Newsom-Davis, J., Prior, C., et al. Antibodies to motor nerve terminals:

an electrophysiological study of a human myasthenic syndrome transferred to mouse. J. Physiol. (Lond.) *344:* 335–345, 1983.

15. Kim, Y. I. Passive transfer of the Lambert-Eaton myasthenic syndrome neuromuscular transmission in mice injection with plasma. Muscle Nerve *8:* 162–172, 1985.
16. Prior, C., Lang, B., Wray, D., and Newsom Davis, J. Action of Lambert Eaton myasthenic syndrome IgG at mouse motor nerve terminals. Ann Neurol *17:* 587–592, 1985.
17. Streib, E. W.,and Rothner, A. D. Eaton-Lambert myasthenic syndrome: long-term treatment of three patients with prednisone. Ann. Neuro. *10:* 448–453, 1981.
18. Lang, B., Newsom-Davis, J., Wray, D., et al. Auroimmune etiology for myasthenic (Eaton-Lambert) syndrome. Lancet *2:* 224–226, 1981.
19. Murray, N. M. F., and Newsom-Davis, J. Treatment with oral 4-aminopyridine in disorders of neuromuscular transmission. Neurology *31:* 265–271,1981.

BOTULISM

It is a testimony to the potency of the botulinum toxin that its fame is celebrated in the lay literature as much as in medical texts. Botulism is caused by the exotoxin of *Clostridium botulinum,* an anaerobic organism which may contaminate improperly canned food. Home canned vegetables have been the most common culprits; of these, peppers seem particularly noteworthy. Outbreaks have been caused by commercially canned foods, and fish products have also been known to harbor toxin. Since the bacillus and the exotoxin it produces are destroyed by heat, proper boiling of food before canning and during the preparation of the food for the table should eliminate attacks. At high altitudes water boils at a lower temperature, and this may account for a greater frequency of botulism (1, 2). The use of a pressure cooker at such altitudes may solve the problem. Contaminated food may be suspected if the can is buckled or "blown," or if home prepared food has a strong and unpleasant smell. A second source of the botulinum toxin is the infection of a wound by the organism. Most cases of wound botulism occur between spring and fall and are generally subsequent to wounds sustained in open fields or on farms.

There are eight distinct types of *C. botulinum* (A, B, C_1, C_2, D, E, F, and G), but the three major ones associated with botulism are A, B, and E. Types A and B are more frequently found in cases from the Eastern United States and are more often the causal agent in botulism due to canned vegetables, whereas outbreaks due to Type E have been due to contaminated fish products. The mortality following Type B botulism may be less than in Types A and E (3). The majority of cases of wound botulism have been due to Type A.

The toxin is extremely potent; a neuromuscular junction can be blocked by a few molecules. It impairs acetylcholine release from the nerve terminal perhaps by blocking exocytosis (4).

Clinically the symptoms begin within 2 hours to 7 days of ingestion of contaminated food. With wound botulism the incubation time is somewhat longer, up to 14 days (5). This is probably due to the time lag necessary for the development of the bacillus in the wound.

The symptoms usually begin in the bulbar muscles. Blurring of vision, diplopia, and difficulty with chewing and swallowing are noted. When the disease is due to ingested toxin, nausea, gastric discomfort, or vomiting may occur. The weakness becomes rather rapidly widespread, and paralysis of the arms, legs, and the respiratory muscles ensues. Death occurs from respiratory failure, and the mortality rate is as high as 25%. If the patient does not die, full recovery may be expected, although this may take many months. Examination reveals a flaccid and areflexic patient; the extraocular muscles are involved, and there may be paralysis of the pupil. Such pupillary paralysis was long considered to be the hallmark of the disease, but it may be by no means as common as was previously thought (2). Sensory abnormalities are not seen. The normal spinal fluid protein serves to differentiate botulism from the Guillain-Barré syndrome, which it may closely resemble.

Mild cases of botulism have additional interesting features. Although fatigability of the type seen in myasthenia gravis is not usually art of the clinical picture, it sometimes exists and may even respond to anticholinesterase drugs. Electrophysiologically, the defect in botulism approximates that of the Lambert-Eaton syndrome. Nerve conduction velocities, both motor and sensory, are normal. A small evoked muscle action potential is found in response to a single stimulus in a muscle which is clinically weak. Post-tetanic facilitation is noted, although not as dramatic as the facilitation seen in the Lambert-Eaton syndrome. In 38% of the patients, there was no facilitation. It is said to persist longer, up to 5 min, and it is more common with the Type B botulism than in the other varieties (6). The decremental response may be absent at a slow rate of stimulation. That Type A botulinum toxin does not cross the placental barrier may be deduced from the reported cases of an unaffected child delivered by a mother who suffered from botulism at the time.

The diagnosis and the type of botulinum toxin involved is established by its lethal effect on mice and by neutralization of the toxin with the specific antitoxin. From 10 to 20 ml of the patient's serum should be sent to the nearest competent laboratory. Further information can be obtained from the Center for Disease Control in Atlanta, Georgia. Samples of the gastric content should also be examined for the toxin, and 50 g of feces should also be collected and similarly analyzed.

The main principles of treatment are the same as for any patient with a severe respiratory paralysis. Proper care and respiratory support, including tracheostomy, will give the patient the best chance of recovery. After the collection of specimens, botulinum antitoxin may be administered to the patient. Divalent antitoxin is active against A and B, trivalent against A, B, and E. The efficacy has not really been proven and the incidence of side effects associated with the administration of a foreign protein is frequent enough to cause some hesitation in its use. It has also been suggested that gastric lavage and the administration of enemas will help eliminate the bacillus and the toxin from the gastrointestinal tract. The use of guanidine and germine has been suggested and may have been of benefit in some patients, but their usefulness requires confirmation.

Infant Botulism

Infantile botulism is different both in its origin and symptoms from the adult form. First reported in 1976, it causes an illness in which the babies become listless and weak, often with severe constipation (7, 8). Bulbar muscles are involved and there is difficulty feeding and the children have uncontrolled drooling. In the severe form of the disease, there may be complete paralysis with ptosis, and large dilated pupils which react poorly to light. The disease is not due to the ingestion of the botulinum toxin, but to ingestion of the clostridium itself, which grows in the gut elaborating the toxin. The source of these organisms may be from food or the environment. In particular, honey has been implicated (7, 8). Most cases have been due to the Type A or B toxin, but Type F toxin has also been implicated. The width of the clinical spectrum is not quite certain. On the one hand, infant botulism has been implicated as a cause of the crib syndrome (8). On the other hand, patients whose only symptoms were constipation or feeding difficulties have been shown to be harboring *C. botulinum* organisms in the gut (9). Electrophysiological changes include the typical incremental response following stimulation at 20 and 50 Hz (10).

REFERENCES

1. Cherington, M. Botulism: clinical and therapeutic observations. Rocky Mt. Med. J. *69:* 55–58, 1972.
2. Cherington, M. Botulism: ten year experience. Arch. Neurol. *30:* 432–437, 1974.
3. Merson, M. H., Hughes, J. M., Dowell, V. R., Taylor, A., Barker, W. H., and Gangarosa, E.J. Current trends in botulism in the United States. J.A.M.A. *229;* 1305–1308, 1974.
4. Kao,I. Drachman, D. B., and Price, D. L. Botulinum toxin:mechanism of presynaptic blockade. Science *193:* 1256–1258, 1976.
5. de Jesus, P. V., Slater, R., Spitz, L. K., and Penn, A. S Neuromuscular physiology of wound botulism. Arch. Neurol. *29:* 425–431, 1973.
6. Cherington, M. Electrophysiologic methods as an aid in diagnosis of botulism. A review. Muscle Nerve *5:* S28–S29, 1982.
7. Pickett, J., Berg, B., Chaplin, E., and Brunstetter-Shaefer, M. A. Syndrome of botulism in infancy. Clinical and electrophysiological study. N. Engl. J. Med. *295:* 770–772, 1976.
8. Arnon, S. S. Infant botulism. Annu. Rev. Med. *31:* 541–560, 1980.
9. Thompson, J. A., Glasgow, L. A., Warpinski, J. R. and Olson, C. Infant botulism. Clinical spectrum and epidemiology. Pediatrics *66:* 936–942, 1980.
10. Cornblath, D. R., Sladky, J. T., and Sumner, A. J. Clinical electrophysiology of infantile botulism. Muscle Nerve *6:* 448–452, 1983.

TICK PARALYSIS

The association of a progressive symmetrical paralysis with a tick bite is a rare occurrence, but if the possibility is not considered the patient's life may be unnecessarily placed in hazard. There are over 40 species of ticks lurking in the brush capable of inflicting such damage but only 3 are common in human tick paralysis. They are *Dermacentor andersoni* and *D. variabilis*, both in North America, and *Ixodes holocyclus* in Australia (1–3). Ticks in the higher elevations and in dry parts of the country thrive in the spring and early summer when they may occasionally be ubiquitous. As the summer's heat advances and the vegetation dries, the creatures disappear until the next year. In more humid areas they persist throughout the summer. It is probably not illuminating to say that ticks may be recognized by the fact that they look like ticks, but verbal descriptions are not very helpful. They have eight legs as opposed to flies, beetles, and other insects, and a flattened hard abdomen almost impossible to crush in the nonengorged state. Most cases of tick paralysis are in children and the majority of these are girls. It is necessary for the tick to be embedded for 5–6 days before the paralysis begins. Although social habits are continually changing, many young girls have long hair and the tick, which is usually embedded near the hairline, is unnoticed.

The paralysis often begins in the legs and it rapidly becomes generalized. Bulbar symptoms include difficulty with speech and swallowing, weakness of the face, and, occasionally nystagmus and blurring of vision. The paralysis of arms and legs is associated with areflexia and with numbness and tingling of the extremities and of the face. The paralysis is probably due to a neurotoxin which the tick injects while embedded in the skin. The mode of action is not precisely known and neurophysiological studies, although frequently reported, are often not well controlled (3). In the case of paralysis caused by *D. andersoni*, the muscle action potential evoked by nerve stimulation was markedly reduced returning to normal after removal of the tick. Motor nerve conduction velocity was also slightly decreased and returned to normal. Sensory fibers were also affected. There was no indication of an abnormality in acetylcholine release. The site of action was postulated as being the terminal branches of the nerves (4). Not all tick paralysis is due to the same mechanism and the only justification for including this in a section on neuromuscular junction disorders is that the Australian tick, *I. holocyclus*, may exert its effect by interfering with acetylcholine release.

When an engorging tick is found it should be removed. The emergency room physician who finds himself faced with an embedded tick and is new to the situation should resist the temptation to grasp the abdomen of the insect and yank it out. This will probably leave the head firmly embedded in the patient, and the danger of secondary infection is apparent. There are many ways of removing ticks but the initial step is to cause the tick to withdraw from the skin. This may be done by applying a lighted match or cigarette to the tick. I disapprove of this method since it seems a little incendiary and the risk to the patient's hair is a real one. Another favorite method is to cover the creature with Vaseline. Presumably the anoxia produced by this causes the tick to withdraw. The abdomen may then be grasped with forceps and the tick may be withdrawn by turning it gently. A hot debate rages in Colorado as to whether the tick should be turned clockwise or anticlockwise to permit the easiest withdrawal. As far as I know, no controlled study has been done.

REFERENCES

1. Editorial: Tick paralysis. Br. Med. J. *3:* 314–315, 1969.
2. Cherington, M., and Snyder, R. D. Tick paralysis: neurophysiologic studies. N. Engl. J. Med. *278:* 95–97, 1968.
3. Gothe, R., Kunze, K., and Hoogstraal, H. The mechanisms of pathogenicity in the tick paralyses. J. Med. Entomol. *16:* 357–369, 1979.
4. Swift, T. R., and Ignacio, O. J. Tick paralysis: electrophysiologic studies. Neurology *25:* 1130–1133, 1975.

4

muscular dystrophies

DUCHENNE MUSCULAR DYSTROPHY
(PSEUDOHYPERTROPHIC MUSCULAR DYSTROPHY)

"I thought humanity to be inflicted with enough evils already. I do not congratulate you, sir, upon the new gift that you have made to it." In these words, one of Duchenne's acquaintances commented upon the description in 1868 of the "Pseudohypertrophic Muscular Paralysis" (1). In the intervening century his friend would have been dismayed by the number and variety of other neuromuscular ailments that have been uncovered. Yet Duchenne dystrophy remains the best known of all of them to the extent that its name has become almost synonymous with muscular dystrophy.

Clinical Aspects

The disease is usually inherited as an X-linked recessive gene; the disease is passed to boys by their relatively unaffected mothers. Between 20 and 30 out of every 100,000 boys born will suffer from the disease and the prevalence rate in the total population is about 3 per 100,000 (2, 3). Perhaps up to one-third of the cases are due to a spontaneous mutation either in the patient or his mother, a point which has been disputed by those who believe that almost all of the mothers can be shown to be carriers if the search for abnormalities is diligent enough (4). Although there is histological and laboratory evidence that the disease exists in children from birth, the clinical manifestations are usually seen in the second year of life. The child's early development and such milestones as his ability to raise his head while lying prone and to sit upright are normally attained. It is when he begins to stand and to walk that his difficulty becomes apparent. At first, this is so slight that he is thought to be clumsy. His frequent falls, the slightly waddling walk, or the accentuation of the normal thud of the heel upon the ground are not considered abnormal in a child who has just recently started walking. There may some early difficulty in arising from the floor, but the transient hand support upon his knee is shrugged off as an idiosyncrasy by parents and physician alike. The boy is often well muscled with the oddly compact and rubbery muscles characteristic of the illness. It is, therefore, hard to believe that any trouble with his strength could arise from abnormalities of the muscle. Shortly after the first difficulties are noted, the child begins to walk with his heels slightly off the ground, often with the feet externally rotated and wide based (Figs. 4.1–4.3). Sometimes an orthopaedic problem is suspected and corrective shoes are provided. However, the inevitable discovery of the child's weakness comes by the time he is 3–4 years of age and is betrayed by his inability to keep up with his peers, by the difficulty he has climbing stairs (which are taken one at a time, usually with the same foot leading for each step) and by an increasing rolling movement to the hips while walking. Running is never

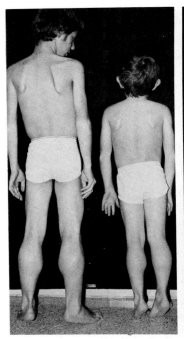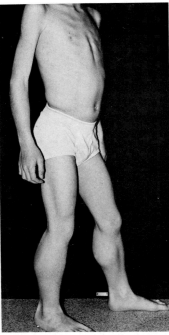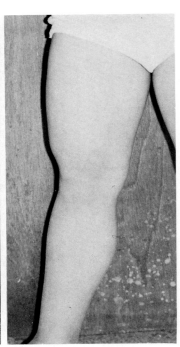

Figures 4.1 (*left*) and 4.2 (*center*).   Two brothers who had pseudohypertrophy of the calf muscles and stood and walked on their toes. The mother felt this was a "habit" since both boys could stand with their heels on the ground when so instructed, as in Figure 4.2.
Figure 4.3 (*right*).   Pseudohypertrophy is not limited to calf muscles. In this boy, the quadriceps were enlarged.

well accomplished and, at best, the patient achieves a clumsy lope. Jumping is also impossible. He tries, but the feet remain glued to the ground.

Often in the early stage of the illness, the patient will complain of leg pains. The history of these pains is seldom volunteered but can be elicited on questioning. They are usually in the calf muscles, come on fairly abruptly, and last for 2–3 days, after which time, they gradually subside. They do not resemble the night cramps of patients with motor neuron disease and their cause remains obscure.

Between 3 and 6 years of age, the family may be encouraged by an apparent improvement in the child's ability. He may walk faster, climb stairs more readily, and arise from the floor more easily. False hopes are raised that the diagnosis is in error, or that he is responding to some particular therapy. Such an improvement is short lived and the disease resumes its downward march. Progressive difficulty occurs in arising from the floor and the boy uses increasing amounts of hand support to push himself to an upright position. The accentuation of the lumbar lordosis associated with the forward thrust of the abdomen, the tendency to lock the knee backwards to prevent the collapse of that joint, and the shortening of the posterior muscles of the calf combine to give the child appearance of being perched precariously on his toes, even during quiet standing (Figs. 4.4 and 4.5). Frequent falls are no

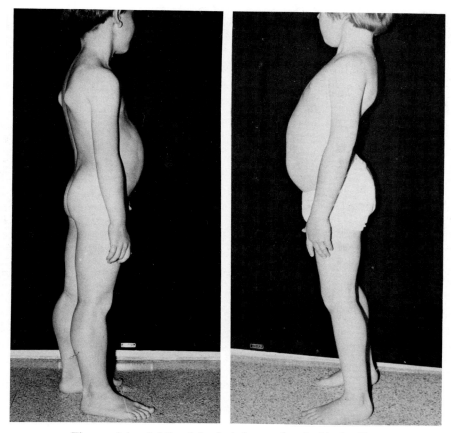

Figures 4.4 and 4.5.   A lordosis is associated with the illness.

longer dismissed as the ordinary tumbles of a clumsy child and now become a serious problem. If the boy gets off balance, the leg muscles lack the strength to make correcting movements and the knees collapse abruptly, pitching the patient to the ground. The boy ceases to be able to climb stairs, and shortly thereafter, he is no longer able to walk independently and needs a wheelchair. Once in the wheelchair, contractures develop and joints may freeze in the position in which the boy sits. The hips, knees, and elbows are flexed. The feet turn downwards and inwards with a marked curve to the instep which prevents the child from wearing normal shoes (Fig. 4.6). A progressive kyphoscoliosis develops, further hampering an already weakened respiratory system. In the terminal stages, the boy sits in his wheel chair twisted like a pretzel, barely able to move any of his muscles (Fig. 4.7). Even the face muscles are involved and lack of neck support causes the head to loll against the back of the chair. The tongue is often enlarged and may protrude from a slack mouth. Because of poor pulmonary excursions, simple colds have a tendency to be complicated by secondary infection and pneumonia is the terminal event. Rarely, cardiac failure may be seen; when it does occur, it is in the terminal stages of the illness and may not respond to digitalization.

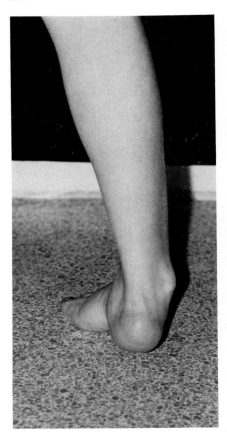

Figure 4.6. The foot assumes a position of inversion and plantar flexion. This is associated with tightening of the heel cords although it is not necessarily caused by that.

The ankle edema seen in the late stage of Duchenne dystrophy is probably due more to venous stasis in inactive legs than to congestive failure.

It may have occurred to some that I have not documented the ages at which these various stages occur. This evasion is deliberate because of several factors. The first is the relative scarcity of studies on the natural history of illness, a situation which, to some extent, has been remedied by current reports (5, 6). There remains a further problem which concerns the influence of therapy on the natural history of the disease. All of the centers which have published information on the natural history are known for being fairly aggressive in their treatment of the disease and the published series reflect this. If, indeed, treatment has an effect on the outcome of the disease, then the natural history studies are by no means as "natural" as one would suppose. It is necessary, though, to provide some framework on which to arrange these concepts and what follows presents our experience, blemishes and all. Some of the findings are presented in graphic form (Figs. 4.8–4.16) and it would be repetitious to detail them here.

Most families are interested in knowing how long their child may be expected to walk. In a combined study of over a 100 patients, we found that there were no children who lost their ability to walk unaided or to climb

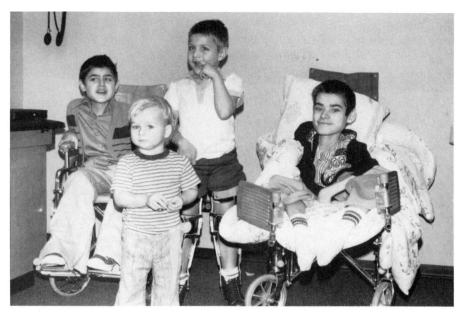

Figure 4.7. A family of 4 brothers all with Duchenne dystrophy at various stages of the illness. The boy on the extreme right represents a stage of the disease which we try to avoid by means of proper bracing and positioning in a wheelchair.

stairs under the age of 8 years. The average age at which children have increasing difficulty with stair climbing, so that they take more than 12 seconds to climb 4 standard stairs, is 9 years of age. At about 10 years of age, they cease to climb stairs or to stand up from the floor independently. By 11.5 years, on the average, the boy can no longer walk a distance of 30 feet, and shortly after the age of 12, the patient will be confined to a wheelchair (see Table 4.1). The disease appears to be quite heterogeneous in its clinical course, with boys of the same age having widely differing abilities (see Fig. 4.15). Whether this represents a genetic heterogeneity or is simply a representation of two ends of the same spectrum is not clear, but it does make any prognostication difficult. In an attempt to identify the "outliers," those children who may be expected to do better than their peers, we analyzed a large number of variables in the collaborative study. Approximately 15% of the patients were either climbing stairs without perceptible difficulty at the age of 8 or were climbing stairs easily, but with support from the railing, over the age of 11. These were identified as "outliers," and in addition to their average muscle strength, there were three other parameters which set them apart from the rest of the population. Pulmonary function tests were above the 90th percentile for the group (i.e., closest to the normal values). The creatine to creatinine ratio in a 24-hour urine specimen was closest to normal and the neck flexor strength was close to sufficient to sustain the head against resistance, as well as gravity. This last finding requires a little explanation. In the Duchenne patient, the neck flexors, when evaluated with the patient in a supine position, are not strong enough to lift the head from a fully extended

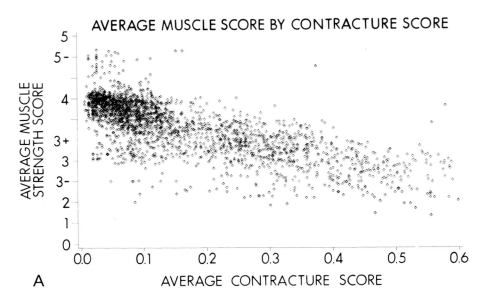

AVERAGE MUSCLE SCORE BY CONTRACTURE SCORE

A

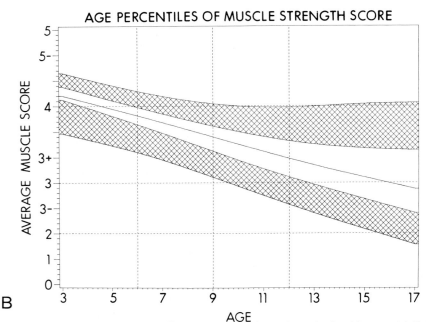

AGE PERCENTILES OF MUSCLE STRENGTH SCORE

B

AGE

Figures 4.8 through 4.17. These figures are taken from data obtained in a multiclinic study of 150 patients with Duchenne muscular dystrophy (5). The figures have been updated from those published and include data generated in the population of 140 boys with Duchenne dystrophy followed over a period of between 3 and 4 years. The scattergrams are representations of the data points obtained on all boys on every visit at which they were evaluated. Since each boy was evaluated approximately 15 times, a large number of points appear on each graph.

Figure 4.8A. Change in muscle strength with the age of the child. The "average muscle score" is derived by examining 34 muscles and giving each muscle a score which may vary between 0 (no movement) and 5 (normal strength). This is based on the medical research council grading scale (5) (see Chapter 1), 3 represents the strength of a muscle which can move the joint against gravity but not against resistance. A muscle which is weak but can exert a moderate degree of resistance is equivalent to 4 on the scale. The score is then the average of all of the muscles examined.

Figure 4.8B. Data of Figure 4.8A presented in a percentile fashion. The center line of the graph represents the 50th percentile. The lower shaded area spans from the 5th to 25th percentile, the upper area from the 75th to 95th percentile. The values for the muscle strength are the same as in the previous graph.

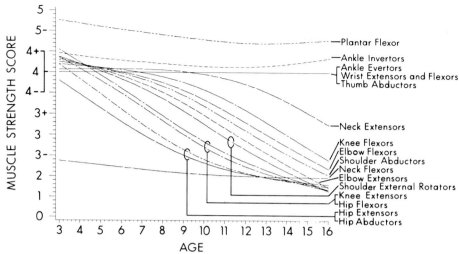

Figure 4.9. In this graph, the 50th percentile lines for the muscle strength for each individual muscle are plotted against the age of the children.

position. This occurs even in the younger children and does not change very much with the course of the illness. Thus, the finding of relative preservation of the neck flexor strength in the outlier population is significant.

Mentally, Duchenne children are often somewhat dull, although occasionally a boy may be above average intelligence. The verbal IQ seems to be particularly affected and many were found to be handicapped in reading. In general, the overall IQ is below the level of matched controls and is usually found to be around 85 (7, 8). We found it curious that, in our own collaborative study, the average IQ, as tested by the Peabody Picture Vocabulary Test, was normal, but this may well be an accident due to the unconscious selection of the more cooperative patients or the nature of the test. More detailed testing of our population has shown a particular difficulty with arithmetic and with the Raven matrices. The latter tests many factors including abstraction and design perception. Although some of the retardation could be due to physical handicap preventing the child from being in a proper learning situation, children with spinal muscular atrophy who are equally disabled do not suffer the same mental retardation and, if anything, seem usually bright.

The child with Duchenne dystrophy often goes through two phases during which he may be anxious and depressed. Perhaps the surprising thing about the depression is not that it occurs, but that it does not occur more often. Around the age of 5, the child realizes for the first time that there is something wrong with him and he may become withdrawn and shy. This is not helped by the fact that his playmates at school often delight in pushing him over in the playground merely for the interest of seeing him get up again. The second phase during which children may become very depressed is shortly after they start using a wheelchair. To some extent, this depends on the manner in which the wheelchair is offered to the boy. If the entire aim of treatment is presented to the child as keeping him out of the wheelchair, then the necessity

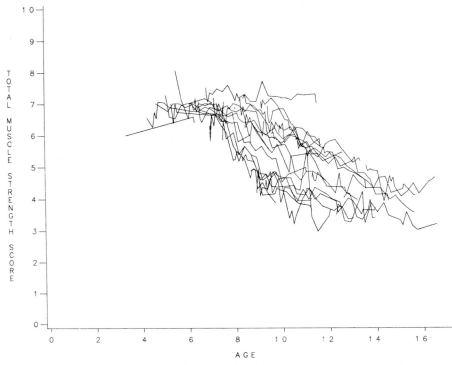

Figure 4.10. These plots are of the strength of 40 of the patients during the course of the protocol. The average muscle score of each patient is plotted against the age of the patient. The points for an individual patient are then joined. This graph illustrates that there is some variability in the progression of each patient and that the "slope" of the line may vary between patients.

for this device represents failure. If, on the other hand, the wheelchair is approached simply as another form of treatment, the problems associated may be less. I often tell boys that there is nothing wrong with using a bicycle if it helps you get from one place to another quickly and a wheelchair is simply a bicycle with the wheels side by side. However, there is frequently some depression at this stage and many of the children respond with a period of bowel and bladder incontinence. This is only partially due to the fact that the help they need in going to the bathroom is sometimes unavailable. Usually, parents can be reassured that this incontinence will disappear in a few months.

The findings on examination will vary, of course, depending upon the stage of the disease. In young boys, mild proximal weakness, more of the hips than of the shoulders, is associated with rubbery hard muscles. Contractures may be noted as early as 3–4 years of age. They are first detected in the hip flexors, iliotibial bands, and the heel cords. Deep tendon reflexes tend to disappear early. Later in the illness, more florid changes are seen and the weakness may involve all the muscles of body except the extraocular muscles. When the patient is confined to a wheelchair, contractures of the elbows and wrist flexors become prominent and the hips and knees are often fixed at 90° unless

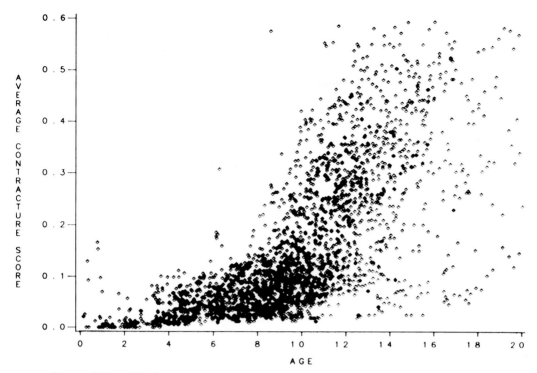

Figure 4.11. This is a scatter plot of patients' joint contractures against their age. The average contracture score is a derived number that becomes higher as contractures become worse. Note that as the children become older there is a wide range in the degree of contractures which they may have. Presumably some of this is due to physical therapy and the effects of surgery.

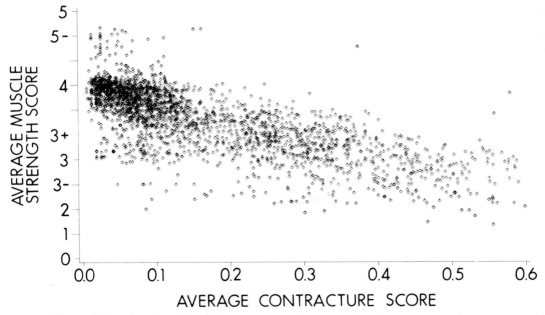

Figure 4.12. A scatter plot of the average muscle score against the average contracture score. This indicates that the weaker the patient, the worse are the contractures. The correlation coefficiency for this plot is 0.70, $p < 0.0001$.

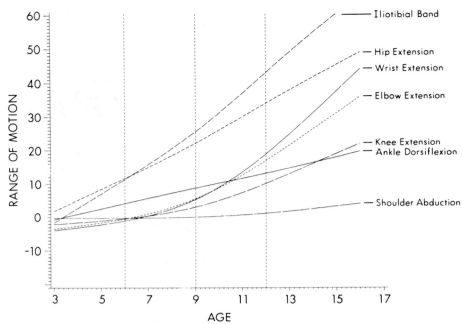

Figure 4.13. Individual joint contractures expressed as the value of the 50th percentile of the population plotted against the age of the patient. Note the early development of contractures in the hip extension, iliotibial bands, and ankles and the subsequent development of contractures of the knees, elbows and wrists. Note that, with the exception of the iliotibial bands, the labels indicate the movement which is restricted not the muscle. Thus, the hip extensions restriction is due to contractures occurring in the hip *flexors*. The *y* axis is the degrees of *limitation* from full range.

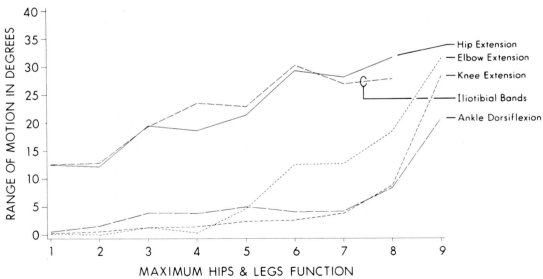

Figure 4.14. Mean values of the contractures at individual joints plotted against the grade of the patients' hip and leg function (see Chapter 1) at the time the contractures were measured (the measurement increases as the contractures get worse). The functional grade varies from 1, which is normal function, to 9, which is a patient who is confined to a wheelchair. Functional grade 6 is the patient who can walk only with assistance or by using long leg braces. At some time between functional grade 6 and 8 the patient spends the major part of the day in the wheelchair. Elbow and knee contractures develop as the patients become increasingly wheelchair dependent.

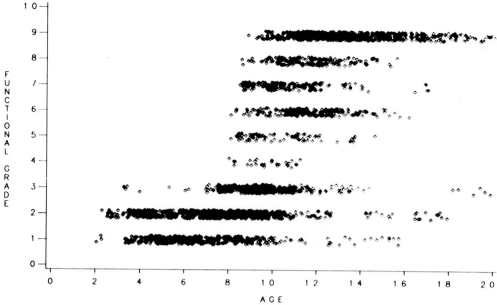

Figure 4.15. The functional grade of the patients plotted against their age. Although, in general, the functional grade increases as the boy gets older, (i.e., the child goes from normal walking and stair climbing to being confined to a wheelchair) some anomalies should be noted. There are a number of older children who maintain functional grade 1 (climb stairs rapidly). These are not necessarily Becker dystrophy patients, but may be the "outliers," children who do much better than the average child with Duchenne dystrophy. Similarly, there is a wide range of ability between the ages of 9 and 11 with some children being confined to a wheelchair (functional grade 9), whereas others can still climb stairs (functional grades 1, 2 and 3; see Chapter 1). This graph simply points out that the disease is not as sterotyped as commonly thought.

some effort is taken to prevent this. Children in the advanced stages of Duchenne dystrophy tend to be either very thin or very fat. The latter stage is easy to understand in view of the muscular inactivity and the undiminished appetite, but the cause of loss of weight in Duchenne dystrophy is less simple. It is not due to loss of muscle bulk alone and the mechanical difficulties with swallowing are rarely severe enough to provide an adequate explanation. Attacks of acute gastric dilatation, manifest by copious effortless vomiting, may result in dehydration. The treatment is to withhold oral feeding and to provide intravenous fluid replacement.

Laboratory Studies

Laboratory tests, which are of value in Duchenne dystrophy, include the serum creatine kinase (CK), the EKG, EMG, and muscle biopsy.

Elevated levels of CK and myoglobin are always seen in the early stages of the illness. When the patient is manifesting a slight waddle and is having mild difficulty in arising from the floor, one may expect to see CK levels of many thousands. The values may be even higher in the first year of life when the disease is not yet clinically manifested. There is no well documented case of

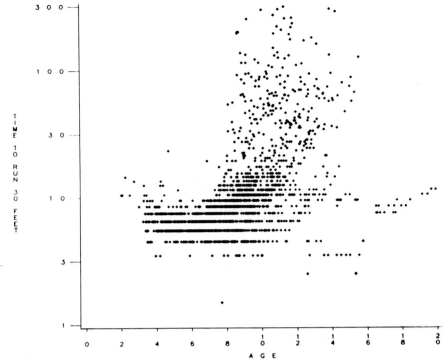

Figure 4.16. A scatter plot of the time in seconds taken to traverse 30 feet against the age of the child. The instructions given to the boy were simply to cross the 30 feet as fast as possible. Note the initial phase of "improvement" indicated by J shape to the scatter plot.

Table 4.1. Follow-up of Boys with Duchenne Dystrophy[a]

Milestone	Average Age in Years (± S.D.)
Climbs stairs >12 seconds	9.4 ± 1.8 ($N = 54$)
Ceases to stand from chair	9.4 ± 1.3 ($N = 53$)
Ceases to arise from floor	10.2 ± 1.3 ($N = 42$)
Ceases to climb stairs	10.4 ± 1.5 ($N = 53$)
Walks only with assistance or with brace	10.8 ± 1.5 ($N = 45$)
Ceases to walk 30 feet	11.4 ± 1.8 ($N = 44$)
Wheelchair confined	12.3 ± 1.7 ($N = 46$)

[a] Boys with Duchenne dystrophy have been followed for several years in a multiclinic study (5). During the course of the study, many of them passed certain "milestones." The average ages at which each of these is attained are listed here.

a patient with a normal CK during the first year of life who later develops Duchenne muscular dystrophy; thus, a normal CK is strong presumptive evidence against the possibility of the disease. As the disease progresses, the levels of CK and myoglobin fall (see Fig. 4.17), although they never attain a normal value. The CK remains in the hundreds even in the patient who is severely disabled and in a wheelchair.

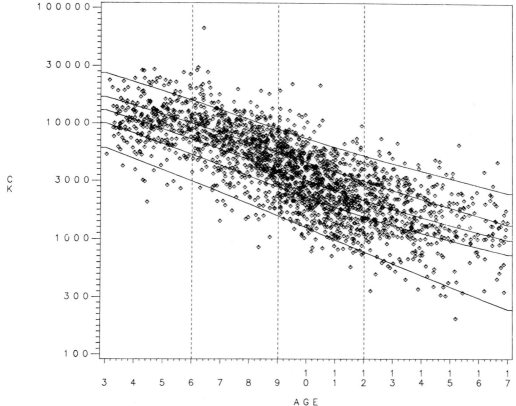

Figure 4.17. Scatter plot of CK values against the patients' age expressed on a logarithmic scale. The lines represent the 5th, 25th, 50th, 75th, and 95th percentiles.

In the normal untrained adult, quite striking elevation of CK and myoglobin may occur following exercise. There is a delay in the response particularly in the case of CK, with peak values of the enzyme occurring several hours after the period of exercise. Similar findings are noted in Duchenne dystrophy. The daily fluctuations in the level of CK in the child are not random. Both the CK and the myoglobin vary in close correlation to minor changes in the children's activity level (9). This response differs from the normal adult response in its time course which is much shorter and in the very minor amount of activity which induces this change. Bed rest results in a progressive decrease of CK levels, although there has been no study to show whether the CK would ever return to normal, since the prolonged bed rest which would be necessary is not justified in a child with muscular dystrophy.

Abnormalities in the EKG are common in Duchenne muscular dystrophy in the neighborhood of 70–90% (10, 11). There are tall right precordial R waves and deep limb lead and precordial Q waves (12). This results in an abnormally high value for the algebraic sum of R and S waves (R − S) in V_1 (13). Arrhythmias and persistent tachycardias have been noted in patients with Duchenne dystrophy. Many different explanations have been postulated for all of these changes, but none has been entirely satisfactory. The suggestion of right ventricular hypertrophy or abnormal right ventricular conduction were not confirmed by vectorcardiographic analyses (14). Correlation of EKG, echocardiogram, and autopsy studies on the heart demonstrated replacement fibrosis of the free wall of the left ventricle associated with diminished excursion of the left ventricular posterior wall and altered left ventricular dimension shortening (10).

Electromyography shows the small polyphasic potentials and increased recruitment of motor units with effort associated with all of the myopathies. In the advanced disease, there may be additional changes of fibrillations.

The muscle biopsy is characteristic, even early in the disease (Figs. 4.18–4.24). There is increased fibrosis. Most of the fibers are circular rather than the usual polygonal shape. There is evidence of necrosis and phagocytosis, and in particular, small groups of basophilic fibers are noted. Often large circular fibers demonstrating very dark staining, the so-called "opaque" fibers, are noted. These are, in fact, hypercontracted fibers and when followed in serial sections, it is found that other portions of the same fibers are ruptured. Many Type 2C or undifferentiated fibers are noted, often leading to poor separation into Type 1 and Type 2 fibers with the routine ATPase stains.

Etiology

The interests of brevity and accuracy are both properly served by the simple statement that the etiology of Duchenne muscular dystrophy is unknown. It is inherited as an X-linked recessive disorder and the gene is located on the short arm of the X chromosome at position Xp21 (the first part of the second major band on the short arm) (15, 16). Most of the neuromuscular community is wedded to the idea that muscle itself is the primary site of the defect, although a brief flirtation with other theories provided an interesting diversion some years back at a time when nothing much seemed to be happening on the muscle front.

An early suggestion that circulatory difficulties might be responsible for some of the findings in muscular dystrophy (17) was reinforced by the description of an experimental myopathy appearing in rabbit muscle subsequent to the injection of the femoral arteries with small dextran particles. The pathological changes which were produced by this were strikingly similar to those seen in Duchenne dystrophy (18). A combination of aortic ligation and the intraperitoneal injection of 5-hydroxytryptamine in rats produced a similar change (19). Parker and Mendell (20) used 5-hydroxytryptamine in combination with imipramine, a compound capable of blocking the uptake of biogenic amines. They felt that the similarity between the experimental myopathy so produced and Duchenne dystrophy was substantiated not only by the pathological change in the muscle, but also by increase of CK in the serum. The effect of imipramine and serotonin may be a direct one on the muscle membrane, however, rather than due to any interruption on blood supply (21). The search for abnormalities in catecholamine metabolism was accelerated by the finding of a reduced initial rate of accumulation of serotonin in platelets from patients with Duchenne muscular dystrophy (22).

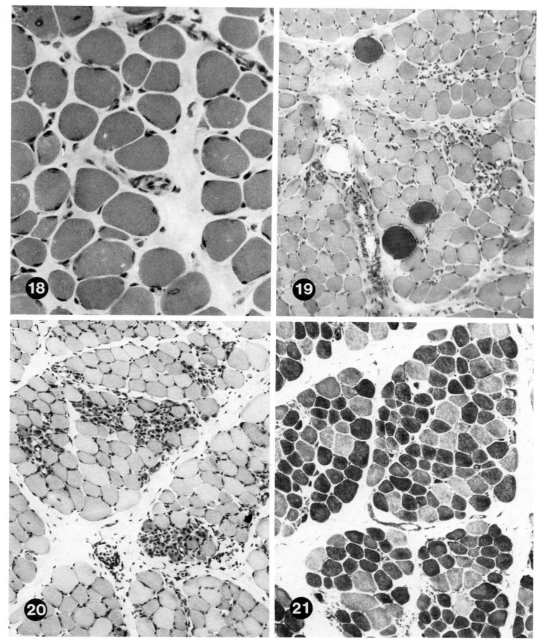

Figure 4.18. Duchenne muscular dystrophy. The appearance of the routine stains is characteristic. The fibers vary widely in size and tend to be circular or polygonal rather than angulated. Individual fibers are separated by an abnormal amount of fibrous tissue.

Figure 4.19. "Opaque" fibers are scattered throughout the biopsy. These fibers stain intensely with a number of different reactions including the hematoxylin and eosin stain. They are, in fact, hypercontracted fibers which have pulled apart so that if they are viewed in longitudinal section they have the appearance of an hourglass where the bell of the hourglass is the hypercontracted region and the neck of the hour glass is an area of rupture. Internal nuceli are not profuse in this disorder.

Figure 4.20. Another characteristic change of Duchenne dystrophy is the presence of small groups of basophilic fibers which stain a darker blue with the hematoxylin and eosin stain.

Figure 4.21. Oxidative enzyme reactions reveal no particular change in the intermyofibrillar network pattern and merely demonstrate changes that are easily seen in the hematoxylin and eosin stain (NADH-tetrazolium reductase).

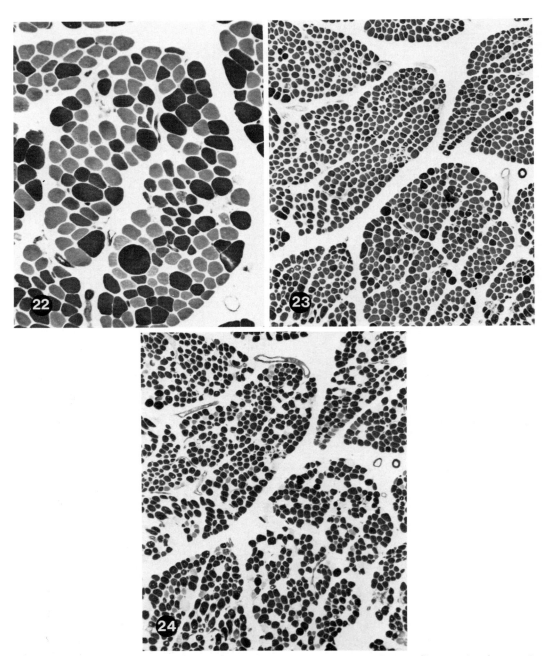

Figures 4.22 through 4.24. The ATPase stains show a tendency to Type 1 fiber predominance. In addition it is often difficult to determine the type of many of the fibers. This poor differentiation is due to the presence of many undifferentiated or Type 2 fibers. These fibers are characteristic of degeneration and regeneration. They are also seen in reinnervating diseases and so are not specific for Duchenne muscular dystrophy. The Type 2 fibers can be recognized because they retain an intermediate intensity of staining when the biopsy is preincubated at pH 4.3 before the ATPase reaction is carried out. This is illustrated in Figures 4.23 and 4.24. These are serial sections from the same muscle. Figure 4.23 is of a routine ATPase reaction pH 9.4 in which the Type 1 fibers stain lightly and the Type 2 fibers darkly. The section on the right has been preincubated at pH 4.3. Following this preincubation the stain is reversed. Type 1 fibers now stain darkly and the stain is absent in Type 2 fibers. Notice, however, that there are many fibers with an intermediate staining pattern (look at the fascicle on the lower left of the photograph). These are the so called Type 2C fibers and very often correspond to the basophilic fibers seen with the hematoxylin and eosin stain.

Morphological identity does not, however, prove etiologic identity and studies of the actual blood flow in muscles of patients with Duchenne dystrophy failed to demonstrate any abnormality (23). Electron microscopic and morphometric studies of the capillaries in the muscles in Duchenne patients have been similarly unrevealing (24). In a variation on the vascular theory for Duchenne, it has been suggested that, although the resting blood flow may be relatively normal, there is an abnormal response to adrenaline (25).

McComas and associates (26) suggested that the muscle fibers in Duchenne dystrophy were not being lost in a random fashion, but were disappearing in groups associated with the loss of motor units. They proposed that the disease might have it origin in the malign influence of a sick motor neuron upon the muscle fibers. Unfortunately, other laboratories have been unable to duplicate McComas' findings in Duchenne dystrophy (27, 28) and the "sick motor neuron" theory of dystrophy has few adherents at the present time.

The belief that muscle itself is the site of the primary defect has gathered momentum as a result of more recent studies. One of the earliest known abnormalities in Duchenne dystrophy is the extraordinary increase in the level of CK in the serum. The enzyme seems to be released from the muscle and, because it shows a progressive decrease with age and the severity of the disease, it is reasonable to suppose that the amount of enzyme in the blood is proportional to the muscle mass. The release of CK is accompanied by a release of myoglobin. This is not, in itself, an abnormal situation since normal muscle may be provoked into releasing large amounts of CK and myoglobin under the influence of various types of exercise. The same influences are at work in patients with Duchenne dystrophy in whom major flucuations of CK levels occur in association with very mild exercise. Although some have suggested that there is no correlation between the myoglobin and CK in Duchenne muscular dystrophy (29), more recent studies have shown a very close correlation between CK and myoglobin levels and the level of muscle activity (9). The leak of CK from the interior of the muscle cell has not been explained either in the normal subject or in the dystrophic muscle. Since the cell surface membrane is the structure which keeps the inside from becoming the outside, it is natural to look there for evidence of any abnormality. The electron microscope shows small lesions in the sarcolemma with adjacent wedge-shaped areas of cell destruction. These are the so-called "delta" lesions (30). Their importance is amplified by their presence in children as young as 2 weeks of age (A. G. Engel, personal communication) at a time when the muscle is only mildly abnormal. Such a breach in the cell's surface must be disastrous for its function. Large molecules, such as peroxidase and procion yellow (30, 31), can pass into the cell which almost certainly means that calcium will have uncontrolled access to the interior of the muscle fiber. High concentrations of intracellular calcium could initiate a whole series of catabolic reactions leading to the destruction of the muscle fiber. Increased calcium has been found in muscle fibers in Duchenne dystrophy by both histochemical and other techniques (32). Calcium is increased when measured by atomic absorption spectrophotometry and magnesium content is reduced (33). The calcium blocker diltiazem decreased the deposition of calcium in the heart of dystrophic hamsters as well as reducing the level of CK in the animals (34). Unfortunately, the hamster model may not be a good representation of Duchenne muscular dystrophy and it remains to be seen whether the drug will have any effect in the human illness. Preliminary studies have not been very encouraging.

It does not seem reasonable that a catastrophic breach in the sarcolemmal membrane would suddenly appear without some prior change. There must be other abnormalities in the membrane which render it susceptible to such damage. The search is thus continued at an ultrastructural level for other evidence of membrane anomalies. The best known of these is apparent in freeze fracture electron microscopic preparations of dystrophic muscle. Freeze fracture is a technique which splits the surface membrane, peeling the outer surface away from the inner surface along a line which passes through the interior of the membrane. Both of the faces can be looked at under the electron microscope and are found to be covered with particles of various types, some of which are arranged with a rectangular distribution, so-called square or orthogonal arrays. In Duchenne muscular dystrophy, there is a significant diminution in the number of orthogonal arrays (35, 36). There may also be a decrease in the intramembranous particles on both surfaces, although one study failed to detect this (37).

The cell surface membrane is not homogeneous. Embedded in it are proteins and other compounds subserving different aspects of membrane activity. The glycoproteins and glycolipids of cell membranes perform important functions including a role in the receptor sites. Probes are available to identify these constituents by virtue of the selective binding of the probe to a specific compound. One such probe is concanavalin A, a member of a group of plant proteins called lectins which have a specific affinity for sugar residues. Concanavalin A binds specifically with mannose, glucose, and fructose residues. In Duchenne dystrophy the pattern of concanavalin A binding is patchy and irregular, contrasting with the regular and continuous pattern seen in the normal muscle and suggesting an abnormality in the cell membrane (38).

There are, of course, other ways of studying muscle membrane. Both Na-K-ATPase and adenyl cyclase are enzymes associated with the cell surface membrane. Both have been reported as abnormal in Duchenne dystrophy, although the evidence is still controversial (39). The reasons behind the controversy are mostly methodologic. The direct study of the properties of isolated membranes is always difficult since any attempt to isolate the membrane results in a disturbance of the complex relationships between it and the cell which it surrounds. A careful analysis of the variables which affect the adenylate cyclase assay seems to confirm the original observations of Mawatari et al. (40) and indicates that both the basal activity of this enzyme and its response to isoproterenol stimulation is subnormal in the Duchenne patient (41).

In addition to the problems involved in preparing the membrane in a form intact enough to permit sensible inferences to be made, there is a more serious problem. It is akin to arriving home and finding that your house has been destroyed by a tornado and then trying to prove that the neighbor's cat was actually responsible for destroying your favorite Ming vase. Even if you could find the cat, incriminating it of a minor breakage amidst the general awfulness is not going to be easy. So it is with the Duchenne muscle. There is so much necrosis, degeneration, fibrosis, and other secondary changes attendant upon the disease, that it may be excessively optimistic to hope to find the primary change among the general havoc. This has lead to other attempts to unravel the puzzle. If Duchenne dystrophy is a primary abnormality in the muscle, then one would suppose that the change might be reproduced by culturing muscle cells from patients with the illness. Some abnormalities have been described, ranging from abnormalities in the growth pattern, to changes in the isoenzyme patterns of CK in the myotubes (42, 43), but for the most part, cultured muscle is suspiciously normal. Freeze fracture techniques do not reveal any abnormalities in the intramembranous particles. The cultured cells seem to behave normally electrophysiologically (44, 45) and although an abnormality in adenyl cyclase was described (46), it was not the same as that found in the dystrophic muscle itself.

The possibility that the hypothetical membrane abnormality might affect other tissues than muscle alone has been raised. Duchenne dystrophy is, after all, a genetic disease and different cell surface membranes share many similar properties. A relatively inexhaustible supply of membrane is found in the red blood cell and this has led to a legion of studies. A quintessential review by Rowland (47) (which is also quintessential Rowland) is an excellent place to start a review of the literature.

In summary, red cell membranes have been both inculpated and exculpated of all of the following: changes in size, shape, deformability and other physical properties, abnormalities in various ATPases, changes in calcium transport, abnormalities of electrolyte content and permeability, abnormal phosphorylation of protein, abnormalities of adenyl cyclase, and a general reluctance to behave consistently in the hands of various investigators (48–52). About the only thing that has not been shown is any abnormality in the function of the red blood cell in vivo.

Not everyone has joined in the stampede to the leaky membrane theory. Abnormalities in neurofilaments have been postulated as part of the abnormality in Duchenne muscular dystrophy (53) and have been refuted by others (54, 55). Ionasescu et al. (56) have long studied a possible abnormality in collagen synthesis in the Duchenne patient and more recently described an abnormal response in Duchenne dystrophy to a protein called the muscle ribosome detachment factor. This protein released more ribosomes from Duchenne patients' membranes than from normal subjects, although the study awaits confirmation. A possible plasma factor is implicated in some of the early changes described in red blood cells (57). This factor has recently been resurrected in another form in a study of the temperature sensitivity of sodium potassium ATPase in the red blood cell membrane. In the normal red blood cell, the temperature sensitivity of sodium potassium ATPase has a biphasic pattern, but is linear in Duchenne dystrophy. The plasma from Duchenne patients converts the normal plot to the Duchenne type (58). An abnormality in low density lipoproteins in the plasma was found in Duchenne boys leading to a suggestion that their transport capacity was impaired (59).

Fibroblasts cultured from the skin of patients with the illness have also been harvested in an attempt to detect abnormalities. Even here the situation remains murky. A decreased adhesiveness between fibroblasts has been described using a technique in which the cells are encouraged to collide with each other and the "stickiness" is measured following such collisions. The adhesiveness is reduced in the fibroblasts from Duchenne patients, but there is an overlap between normal subjects and the Duchenne patients. Cultured skin fibroblasts also contain CK which might make this a useful tool for studying the enzyme in disease states, but no difference was found either in the total amount of enzyme or in the proportion of the isozyme content (60).

Using a double labeling technique and two-dimensional electrophoresis, Wrogemann described a missing protein in fibroblasts cultured from patients with Duchenne dystrophy. This was seized upon as a possible key to the unlocking of the mystery more by others than by the original authors who maintained a cautious approach (61). The caution was justified since later it became apparent that the protein abnormality was due to the site from which the skin biopsy was taken rather than to the disease itself (62).

Considering all the necrosis, phagocytosis, and release of CPK and myoglobin that is is occurring, one would suppose that a great deal of muscle degeneration is taking place. The excretion of 3-methylhistidine, an unusual amino acid that is present in actin and myosin, has been used as an indicator of muscle breakdown. Not unexpectedly, its excretion is increased in Duchenne muscular dystrophy (63). This logic may be flawed because, although muscle contains the largest amount of 3-methylhistidine in the body, other actin containing tissues, such as skin and gut, may turn over 3-methylhistidine much faster. Sources other than muscle may account for as much as 50% of the total 3-methylhistidine excretion (64).

The Duchenne patients' muscles do not visibly waste away from week to week; which simple observation means that protein synthesis must be keeping pace with protein degradation, even though over the long haul, degradation wins out. Measuring degradation is less practical than measuring muscle protein synthesis by the incorporation of leucine into the muscle pool. Surprisingly, this technique showed that protein synthesis in the muscle of patients with Duchenne dystrophy was reduced, not increased. This would imply that protein degradation in the child was also decreased, a seemingly paradoxical situation (65). Several abnormalities in the metabolism of muscle have been described. An increased turnover of adenine nucleotides was found suggesting that somehow muscle levels of ATP might be compromised (66).

An abnormality in the oxidation of palmitic acid, one of the major energy sources for muscle was found, which may indicate a defect in intramitochondrial fatty acid oxidation. Although the oxidation of palmitic acid labeled in the 1-C position was normal, $[U\text{-}^{14}C]$palmitic acid oxidation was deficient (67). This suggests that the defect was not an overall reduction in the activity of all enzymes but was specifically of that part of the beta oxidation process that splits off two carbon fragments further down the skeleton than the terminal carbon. If there is indeed a defect in handling the fuel supply in the muscle this might explain why the Duchenne boy experiences such a rise in myoglobin and CK with mild exercise.

Genetics and Carrier Detection

The production of specific "bits" of chromosomes by restriction endonucleases and the incorporation of these pieces into hybrid cell lines using recombinant DNA techniques has resulted in an explosion in our knowledge of the human genome (68). Duchenne muscular dystrophy is inherited as an X-linked disorder. The theory proposed by Haldane (69) would suggest that, in a disease whose incidence in the general population does not seem to be changing, the proportion of new mutant cases necessary to sustain the pool can be calculated from the formula $(1 - F) \mu/(2\mu + \nu)$. F is the reproductive fitness of the affected boy, which in the case of Duchenne approaches 0 since none of the children sire offspring of their own. "μ" and "ν" represent the mutation rate in the female and male cells, respectively. If we assume that μ and ν are equal, then it follows that one-third of the cases of Duchenne dystrophy arise from new mutations. This point has been disputed by those who believe that only a minority of the boys are the result of new mutations and that if the entire pedigree is screened for females at risk, some of the women will have an abnormally high CK (70). This begs the question of what is a normal CK, as discussed below. The same group found that when they evaluated boys who were isolated cases, in those families who had a subsequent son, the younger son had the illness in a higher proportion of cases than would be predicted by the Haldane theory (70, 71).

Location of the Duchenne gene on the short arm of the X-chromosome was suggested by the occurrence of several cases of muscular dystrophy appearing in girls. These patients were found to have a translocation of the short arm of the X chromosome with one of the other chromosomes. The break almost always occurred at locus Xp21. The only problem is the assumption that the girls did indeed have Duchenne dystrophy since the evidence was not always convincing. However, they certainly all shared a common locus for the translocation.

Turner's syndrome with an XO-chromosome pattern is another rare situation which may coexist with Duchenne dystrophy in an apparent girl since the abnormal X is not suppressed by its normal twin chromosome. The only girl I have seen whose clinical appearance, laboratory studies, and muscle histochemistry looked identical to Duchenne dystrophy had neither a translocation nor Turner's syndrome nor any other genetic abnormality that we could discover.

Genetic probes are now available for unlocking some of the mysteries of the chromosomes. These probes can recognize short lengths of the chromosome (restriction fragment length polymorphisms or RFLPs) having a specific nucleic acid sequence. Such short pieces of the chromosome may exhibit polymorphism in the general population. The probe may then lable one segment but may fail to lable the polymorphic corresponding segment. If the possibility of recombination is ignored for a moment, then a probe which recognized a segment of the X chromosome in a boy with Duchenne dystrophy could be used for identifying any other boy in the family with the illness and more importantly for detecting any possible carrier females who share the affected "dystrophic" X chromosome. Obviously this is an ideal situation which ignores the possibility of recombination. During cell division, breaks may occur randomly anywhere along the entire length of the chromosome thus an RFLP which is a considerable distance away might easily get separated during cell division. One which is immediately adjacent would most probably travel with the affected gene and not be subject to recombination. So, the closer the probe is to the actual disease gene locus, the less will be the chance that recombination will occur. Although there are no ideal probes at the present time some are available that are very close. Probe 754, B24 and the probe for ornithine transcarbamylase may be as close as 3 centimorgans from the Duchenne gene (72). "Close" is perhaps a misnomer when a centimorgan may represent as much as 10^6 base pairs.

The next step occurred when a boy with a combination of Duchenne dystrophy, chronic granulomatous disease, retinitis pigmentosa and McLeod's syndrome was revealed to have a small deletion in the X chromosome at Xp21 (73). Because part of the chromosome was missing, when its DNA was hybridized with normal human DNA the DNA from the latter which failed to match up and was "left over" would have to correspond to the DNA from Xp21. This "enriched" DNA was used to make probes consisting of short fragments of DNA, (16) shorter than the total length of the deleted region, which are thus precisely targeted at lengths of DNA within Xp21. Using one of these pERT 87, a deletion was found in 5 of 57 unrelated boys with Duchenne dystrophy. This included the segment indicated by pERT 87 and a minimum of 38 kb of surrounding DNA.

All of this makes it likely that by the time this book is in print we will be using several such genetic probes in carrier detection, and the use of CK tests will be relegated to a minor role.

The Lyon hypothesis suggests that random inactivation of either of the two X chromosomes occurs in all cell lineages (74). In females carrying an X-linked recessive trait, the abnormal X may remain active in a proportion of the cells, particularly early in life. This is the basis of prior efforts at carrier detection in Duchenne muscular dystrophy. The assumption is that the carrier female may show, in small part, some of the characteristics of the illness. This is, again, an area of great debate. Some believe that all carriers have overt weakness (75). Other reports find the incidence to be less than 5% (76). Asymmetric gastrocnemius hypertrophy has been described, but a careful study showed no difference between 19 carriers and 32 normal female controls (77). Occasionally, all the carriers in a given family will demonstrate mild weakness, giving rise to the suspicion that there may be some additional genetic factor which allows the disease to surface in the females.

If the Lyon hypothesis holds true, one would expect some evidence of a population of abnormal cells particularly in the early years. This is the basis of the CK test for carrier detection. Standard practice is to obtain samples on 3 or 4 separate occasions at least a week apart. If any one of these values is abnormally high, the mother is advised that she is most probably a carrier. If all the values are normal, there is still a 10–20% possibility of the patient being a carrier. It is important to obtain blood samples from possible carriers before the age of 10 years whenever feasible, because the levels of CK are likely to be more abnormal in the first decade (78). During pregnancy the CK levels may fall, limiting the usefulness of the test at this stage (79, 80). All of this sounds reasonable until one comes to deciding what is a "normal" CK. Certainly values which are derived by the clinical laboratory from a large number of hospital inpatients, many of whom will be elderly and the majority of whom will be at bed rest, cannot be used to compare with a population of young active women. Furthermore, normal levels of CK fluctuate with age (81). When women who are proven carriers of Duchenne dystrophy (i.e., a mother of a child with the illness related by maternal linkage to another affected member of family) were evaluated, between 70 and 80% were said to have an elevated CK, as compared to unrelated normal women in the general population. Other serum constituents, such as pyruvate kinase (PK), hemopexin, and lactic dehydrogenase (LDH) have also been found helpful in carrier detection (82, 83). Many factors including age, exercise, and genetic predisposition seem to influence the levels of CK. For this reason, a multiclinic study compared the levels of CK and PK in definite carriers of the illness with the levels found in female relatives on the *paternal* side. When this was done, the most accurate correlation between the carrier state and the enzymes was found by using the mean of three determinations of both CK and PK. In this large study, the percentage of definite carriers detected was only 45%. The higher detection rate in other studies was due to a different population of control patients (84).

The use of muscle biopsy has been suggested in carrier detection and foci of necrotic fibers, moth-eaten and whorled changes in the intermyofibrillar network pattern, and an abnormal number of internal nuclei have been described (85, 86). The problem is that these changes may be noted in normal patients who are not carriers, particularly if the gastrocnemius muscle is biopsied. Whereas these changes may identify a *group* of carriers, in the individual patient, it is hard to know what significance to attach to them.

The electrocardiogram may also be abnormal. The algebraic sum of the R and S waves in V_1 has been found to be greater in carriers than in normal women (87). Once again, at least one study has failed to confirm this finding (11). Thus, at present, the EKG is not used in carrier detection.

Abnormalities of the EMG in the carrier state have been described with the focal appearance of short and low amplitude polyphasic potentials. The use of routine EMG in this fashion, however, has not increased the possibility of carrier detection (88, 89). A refinement of the technique with frequency analysis of the potentials may sharpen the accuracy of this method (90), but again has not found wide acceptance.

The search for biochemical abnormalities has ranged far and wide, not only in the disease itself, but also in the carrier state. Substances as esoteric as rubidium have been implicated only to have later studies refute the findings (91). Abnormalities in the intramembranous particles have been sought, but not found (92). An abnormality in ribosomal protein synthesis was described in Duchenne dystrophy (56). Isolated ribosomes were found to synthesize increased amounts of collagen. A similar finding was noted in carriers in whom an abnormally large amount of noncollagenous protein, as well as collagen, was synthesized (87). Adequate confirmation of this observation is needed and its use in carrier detection has remained regional.

The increased ability of the erythrocyte membrane to phosphorylate protein, which has been described as a feature of Duchenne dystrophy, is also found in carriers of the illness (4). The mean values for the groups of definite, probable, and possible carriers were similar and were different from the mean value from matched controls. This suggested that the spontaneous mutation rate must be very low, since if there were noncarrier mothers in the "possible" and "probable" groups, their normal values of protein kinase should have reduced the mean value of these two groups compared to definite carriers. An alternate interpretation is that the finding was unrelated to the carrier state. Once again the individual variability made the test unsuitable for use in carrier detection at a practical level.

There is one basic problem in the detection of the carrier state that should always be borne in mind. There are three levels of certainty of the carrier state: definite, probable, and possible. For a woman to be a proven carrier, she must have an affected son as well as the appropriate family history. Probable carriers have two or more affected sons, but there are no other affected members in the maternal family. Possible carriers are mothers of isolated cases or female relatives (e.g., sisters) of affected males. The definite carriers, and to a lesser extent, the probable carriers are the group of women used to obtain data about the chemical abnormalities of the carrier state. Bearing an affected son is an essential part of the definition of definite and probable carriers. Many of these children are quite severely disabled and require considerable physical exertion in their care. Morphologically, this is expressed by an increase in the size of Type 2 fibers from the biopsies of carriers (94) and perhaps it may also account for some of the differences between carriers and the population of mothers with normal children.

So what does the clinician do with regard to genetic counseling at the present time? There are probably two choices. One is to obtain CK and PK values on as many maternal relatives as possible, as well as on the suspected carrier herself. Considering the total picture within the entire pedigree will modify the chances depending upon the number of female relatives who have had normal CK values, the number of male relatives who were at risk and yet did not develop the disease, and the proximity of the known cases of muscular dystrophy to the girl whose carrier state is being evaluated. Using the Bayesian theorem, one may then predict with some degree of accuracy the percentage changes of the mother-to-be having a child with the illness. In difficult cases, these percentages often lie between 3 and 15%.

Changing the odds of having a child with Duchenne dystrophy from 15% to 5% really makes little difference to the possible carrier's decision about family planning. Those who have a close acquaintance with dystrophic children usually retain their reluctance to embark upon a possible tragic pregnancy, whereas those whose acquaintance with muscular dystrophy is more remote proceed undeterred. The second alternative is to wait! With the explosive progress in genetics it is likely that we will have a more reliable test by the time this book is in print.

Another problem arises when a possible or proven carrier becomes pregnant. The question then revolves around prenatal diagnosis. Again, to summarize, there is no known way of making the intrauterine diagnosis of Duchenne muscular dystrophy. For a while it appeared that fetoscopy (95) and the sampling of fetal blood would allow us to detect the affected male fetus. Unfortunately, these expectations were dashed when a child was born with the illness whose fetal CK was normal (96, 97). Intrauterine diagnosis will be a reality as soon as genetic probes can identify the abnormal gene.

Treatment

At the present time Duchenne muscular dystrophy is an incurable disease. In spite of many therapeutic trials of substances, as diverse as estrogens, steroids, vitamin E, allopurinol (98, 99), superoxide dismutase (100), vera-pamil (101), leucine (102), and nifedipine (103), no effective drug is available. The use of protease inhibitors such as leupeptin and pepstatin has been proposed based on a possible effect in tissue culture and in animal dystrophy (104, 105). There has been little enthusiasm, so far, for their use in humans. In the first place, proteases play a part in removing unwanted degradation products and it might not be wise to interfere with their function. Studies on cathepsin-D, a protease which can be identified by immunocytochemical techniques, showed an increased staining of the small regenerating muscle fibers in tissue from patients with Duchenne muscular dystrophy. If these fibers are, in fact, regenerating and cathepsin-D is playing a part, then the use of protease inhibitors might not be entirely beneficial. It is, of course, difficult to tell under the microscope when a fiber is regenerating or degenerating, and the argument is still not settled. Also, if the problem in Duchenne dystrophy is reduced synthesis of muscle protein, inhibiting the protease would make very little difference.

Incurable and untreatable are not synonymous and much can be done to make the life of a patient more comfortable. Sometimes the parents of dystrophic children faced with the problem of illness in their child manifest one of two reactions. They either try to ignore the child or they build things for his aid so that he becomes encased in mechanical contraptions. Physicians, on occasion, have been known to have the same reactions and the two extremes are equally to be avoided. It does not help the family to be told that there is nothing to be done and that they should return home to await the inevitable end. On the other hand, bracing the child too early or recommending major reconstructive surgery inappropriately may salve the physician's hurt, but can do the patient a great deal of harm. The proper management of Duchenne dystrophy depends on a team approach, such as that outlined by Vignos et al. (106). The ideal situation is where the neurologist, the orthopaedic surgeon, the physical and occupational therapist, the social worker and the orthotist all take an active part in the clinic.

In the early stages of the illness, passive stretching of the muscles is all that is required. Early attention should be given to two areas. The Achilles tendon should be stretched once or preferably twice daily in these patients. If practiced regularly, this can do much to impede the equinovarus deformity which otherwise develops. The application of light bivalve casts at night or of "night splints" may further retard the development of the foot deformity (Fig. 4.25) and is an important part of the treatment plan. The iliotibial bands should also be stretched daily. Active exercises are usually unnecessary in the young children since they run around to the best of their ability anyway. There is no solid evidence that exercise either injures the muscle in Duchenne dystrophy or helps the patient. There are changes in CK and myoglobin closely associated with exercise (9), but there is no direct evidence that these changes in any way represent muscle damage. A sensible compromise is perhaps to

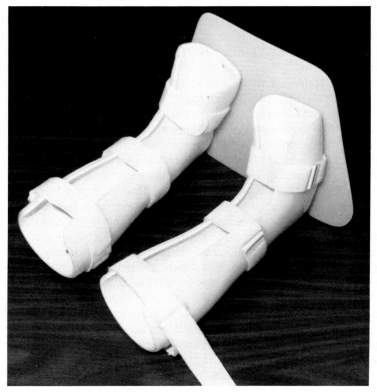

Figure 4.25.   Night splints. These splints are designed to prevent the contractures of the heel cords. They are worn at night and maintain the foot in dorsiflexion. They are fixed in a base plate in a position of slight internal rotation. This prevents the legs from externally rotating during sleep and thus helps to maintain the stretch on the iliotibial bands.

tell the parents that their children can take as much exercise as they wish, but should not exercise to the extent where muscle pains are noted or the child becomes exhausted. While the child is still walking easily, major surgery is inadvisable and surgery is usually unnecessary before the age of 7. The exception is when the tightness of the heel cords is severe enough to make walking difficult. If it is felt that this is the only reason that walking is impeded (and this is an unusual circumstance), a release of the Achilles tendon may be helpful. I used to recommend posterior tibial transposition as a preferable procedure, but over the last 10 years, I have been impressed that the results of the more complicated surgery are no better than a simple percutaneous release in Duchenne dystrophy patients. If surgery is carried out on the Duchenne patient, he should be mobilized as soon as possible and this usually means that the therapy team should stand him up, out of bed, the same day that the surgery is performed. All of us have had the disastrous experience of watching a patient, whose operation was supposed to help him walk, fail to recover his abiity to do so following prolonged bed rest associated with surgery. The phase during which surgery may be usefully recommended is at the point when the patient is about to cease walking. This implies a degree of prescience on the part of the physician, but there are some indications from the patient's history and examination. When the patient can no longer climb stairs, nor step onto a small step, when he is unable to arise from the floor by himself, he is probably 6 months to a year away from using the wheelchair a major part of his day. Furthermore, if he is falling frequently (i.e., daily), it is wise to attempt to stabilize his walking. On physical examination, the quadriceps strength is an important factor to take into account in deciding the treatment. If he can no longer straighten his knee out against gravity in the seated position, the stage is set for bracing and surgery. The parents and the child should have a clear concept of what to expect following the surgery. If they assume that the child will be walking freely, everybody will be in for a severe disappointment. Surgery is almost never done in isolation. It is always accompanied by bracing of the legs. The type of brace may be a matter of personal preference. The whole aim of the procedure is to allow the leg to be as free of contractures as possible so that a long leg brace can be used. The actual procedure will vary, but most of our patients undergo percutaneous release of the hip and knee flexors, iliotibial bands, and heel cords in a manner which has been popularized by Spencer (107) and by Siegel (108). After surgery, the legs are immobilized in lightweight Hexcelite casts to prevent the immediate redevelopment of contractures. This means that the limb is fixed with the foot dorsiflexed as far as practical and the knee straight. Weight bearing in these casts is not only possible but imperative and the patients are made to stand on the day of surgery and at least twice a day thereafter. They usually take their first steps within 2–3 days following surgery and should be able to walk with some facility between parallel bars by the time of discharge a week later. After 1 week, the casts are removed and the long leg braces applied.

Immediately postoperatively, it is important not to allow the legs to go into an external rotation, and so during sleeping hours, the casts are supported laterally by pillows, which prevent the leg from turning outwards. In addition, it is helpful to continue to stretch the hip by having the child lay flat in bed with a support, such as a foam pad or a telephone book, under his buttocks. Often pressure sores develop on the heels following achilles tenotomy. In this situation the heel counter on the boot should be cut away until the skin heals.

As for the braces themselves, there are two basic types (Figs. 4.26 and 4.27). One is the double upright metal brace which fits into the heel of a high top lace up boot and is secured to the leg by knee pads and a thigh band. A "T" strap, which goes around the external malleolus and pulls the ankle medially, may be used to slow the development of further varus deformity. The other type of brace is of light weight plastic which is molded to the child's limb and can be worn inside the child's shoe. The knee lock, which is the functional part of any long leg brace, is the same as in the bilateral upright variety. The advantage of a plastic brace is that it can be worn with any shoe and also that it is lighter. In fact, the weight of the long leg brace seems to make little difference to the patients because they seldom lift the brace against gravity. Most of the time, the brace is used as pendulum, swinging the leg forward. The disadvantage to the plastic brace is that it does not hold the foot in quite

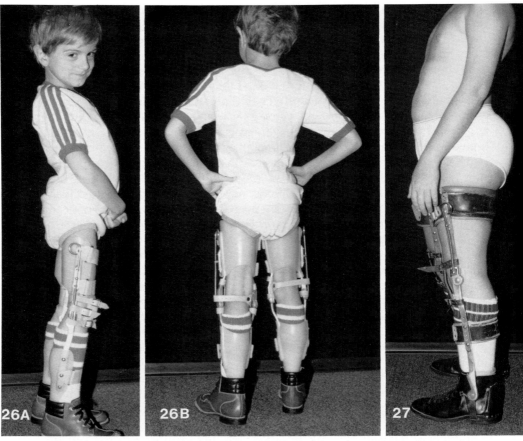

Figures 4.26 and 4.27. Duchenne dystrophy. The use of long leg braces allows the children to stand and walk when their own muscles are no longer strong enough to accomplish this. There are two basic types: the plastic knee foot orthosis (Fig. 4.26, *A* and *B*), which are made of light weight plastic and fit inside the shoe. The second variety is the long leg brace with double upright supports (Fig. 4.27), which are permanently attached to the outside of the shoe.

as secure a position and does not retard the development of a varus deformity as well as the bilateral upright brace.

When surgery is recommended in Duchenne dystrophy, the question of whether any specific precautions should be taken is often raised. The main threat to the child's life is from respiratory failure or the exacerbation of his weakness associated with bed rest of more than a few day's duration. Consequently, respiratory therapy is helpful for a few days before the surgery and also following the procedure. There has been a recent suggestion that malignant hyperthermia may be seen in the patient with Duchenne dystrophy (109–111). Not all of the cases are entirely convincing but because of the possibility of malignant hyperthermia, the use of halothane and succinylcholine should be avoided.

It is important to try to predict which patients will do well with bracing and surgery. One study suggested that the relative preservation of muscle strength, respiratory function, and a more normal creatinine to creatine ratio could be used to select such patients (112). It is curious that these same parameters were independently selected as being characteristic of the boys with Duchenne dystrophy who had a naturally good prognosis and might be expected to walk for a longer period time (5). The other personality trait that was noticed to be associated with successful bracing was the child's determination to continue walking. In a collaborative study, the time taken by boys with Duchenne dystrophy to walk 30 feet was measured. The children whose ambulation was clearly different from their peers would travel the 30 feet remarkably slowly. It was not unusual to watch a child take 4 or 5 min to complete the task. Nevertheless, they continued to the end of the measured distance. Many other children who were equally strong would simply give up after a minute or less and refuse to make any further attempt. These children were less often those in whom bracing successfully prolonged ambulation.

Prolonging walking as an aim in itself would perhaps make little sense. It does give a psychological boost to the patient, but there would be no particular medical importance in keeping the patient out of a wheelchair if it were not for the other complications. When the boy becomes totally confined to a wheelchair, contractures of the legs and arms become worse and may cause the boy some discomfort when he adopts a position other than sitting. Sleeping at night may be a problem. Additionally, the development of a scoliosis is almost always associated with a wheelchair existence. If the child can stand on his feet for as little as 1–2 hours a day, these problems are not as severe. Thus, the aim of prolonging walking is to prevent the complications which formerly made the life of the untreated Duchenne patient so miserable during his last years.

I have no hesitation in recommending a second or third operation for those patients who have already had tendon releases but whose recurrent contractures are once again making it difficult for them to use braces. In addition, in some patients with marked hip weakness, the braces may be extended higher with the addition of a pelvic band which gives the same support to the hip joint as the knee lock provides to the knee joint (Fig. 4.29).

It is important for the physician to recognize when the braces are the wrong size. It is fairly obvious when they are too long, but a brace which is too short may escape the notice of the physician unless he is specifically looks for it. One may suspect that a brace is too short when the patient stands with a lumbar kyphosis with the pelvis rocked back in an attempt to seat the lower part of the gluteal fold on a thigh band which is way too far down the thigh (Fig. 4.28). The proper position for the thigh band of a long leg brace is about 1 inch below the gluteal fold when the patient is in the standing position.

Tightness of the ilio tibial bands may make it impossible for the child to walk in long leg braces even though he has adequate strength. The reason is a mechanical one. The normal way for a child to walk with long leg braces is to stand with the feet fairly close together, one hip is then elevated and the braced leg on that side swings forward rather like a pendulum. The opposite hip is than hiked up and the other leg swings forward. Tightness of the ilio tibial bands makes it impossible for the legs to be adducted and the child

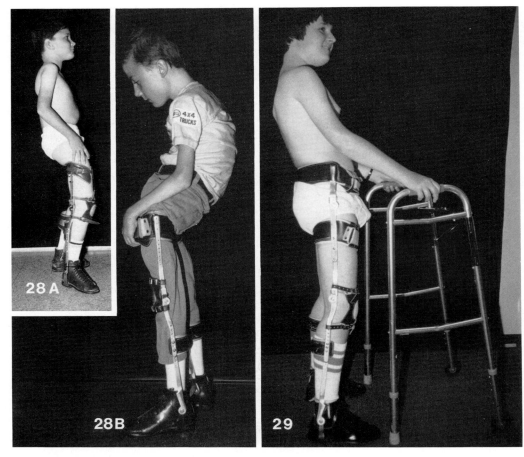

Figures 4.28 and 4.29. Several problems may occur with long leg braces. If they are too short, the patient's pelvis may tilt backwards and eventually a kyphosis occurs (Fig. 4.28, *A* and *B*) this may be corrected in its early stages by adding a pelvic band around the waist which gives the hip joint the same support that the knee obtains from the device (Fig. 4.29).

stands with his feet splayed wide apart (Fig. 4.30). Lifting the hip does nothing and the child's feet remain firmly planted on the ground. If a child who is using long leg braces is noted to be frozen in this position instead of walking normally, the release of the ilio tibal bands and the hip flexors may once again allow him to walk. When evaluating a boy in the braced stage of the illness, one should always check the braces as well as the patient. It is reassuring to see braces with trim that is worn and scuffed. A shiny brace is probably not being helpful, no matter what the family says.

Always inspect the inside of the boot in patients who are wearing double upright braces. The accumulation of fluff at the junction of the sole and the heel inside the boot is an indication of heel cord tightness and that the child is not getting the heel completely down on to the sole of the shoe. Always insist that you see the boy walk in the braces while he is in the clinic. Sometimes the results are informative (Fig. 4.31).

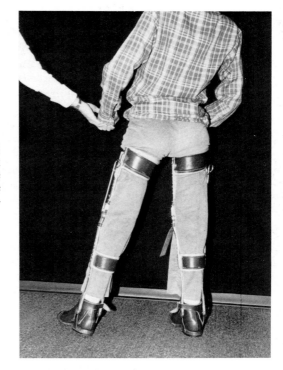

Figure 4.30. If the iliotibial bands are very tight, the patient cannot stand with the feet close together and may then be unable to walk or even maintain his balance without assistance.

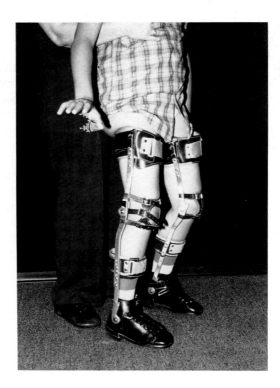

Figure 4.31. These braces are useless, not only are they too short but the knee lock on the left cannot be locked because of knee contractures. The patient was, in fact, being held up by his mother when this photograph was taken.

Eventually, in spite of the best efforts, most patients are confined to a wheelchair and the tendency to develop contractures is accelerated, the arms are now involved and, as previously mentioned, a kyphoscoliosis begins. It is sometimes difficult to prevent these deformities and equally difficult to decide how much energy to put into their correction. Contractures of the hips and knees may make life miserable for the patient since he is unable to sleep in any position except on his side and cannot comfortably be supported in any position other than sitting. Stretching exercises should now be expanded to prevent flexion contractures of the elbows and wrists, as well as the hips and knees. There have been various attempts to impede the development of a kyphoscoliosis, none of them completely succesful. A molded insert which stabilizes the child's position, may be used in the wheelchair. This is of most value before the scoliosis has commenced or when it is very mild. Attempting to correct a severe scoliosis is impossible with such a device. Various accessory pads on the back of the wheelchair have been tried, but are of limited value. I prefer the use of a light plastic body jacket extending from under the armpits to the pelvis (Fig. 4.32). A word of caution is necessary. Some of the treatment failures from the use of a body jacket stem from the fact that the brace spends more time in the closet than it does on the patient. Physicians, however, are the last to be told about this. A child has to get used to a brace. The brace should be used initially for periods of 15 minutes to ½ hour with the time gradually lengthened until the child is able to tolerate the brace all day. In a paretic scoliosis, such as the child with Duchenne dystrophy has, there is no need to wear the body jacket when the child is lying down, but it is imperative that, eventually, the body jacket is worn whenever the child is up out of bed. There are very few occasions when it is justified to recommend a body jacket for a child who is still fully ambulatory. In the first place, any curve that is

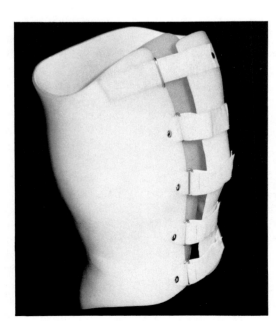

Figure 4.32. A body jacket (thoracolumbosacral orthosis). The body jacket is designed to fit firmly around the trunk and may help prevent further deformity of the spine. This device does not work well in the obese and in order for it to be effective it has to be worn during the entire time except when the boy is in bed.

noticed is usually only a positional one and does not need correction, and in the second place, a body jacket represents an additional burden and a child who is marginally ambulatory will be put completely off his feet.

When the neck muscles become weak, the use of a head support on a wheelchair can increase the boy's comfort. This may take the form of an extension to the back of the wheelchair, or may be a more formal head support such as a self-centering head support attachment. The use of plastic collars and other attachments to the body jacket is not very popular with the patient. Sometimes one sees patients with Duchenne dystrophy who are using a Milwaukee brace. This brace is an "active" brace which requires the patient's strength to straighten the back. Although it is very useful in some forms of scoliosis, it is very difficult for patients with muscle weakness to tolerate this and it should not be used.

The patient whose spine is hyperextended (with an increased lordosis) has less tendency to develop the lateral curvature than those whose spines bow into an early kyphosis (113). It is important, when applying a body jacket, to do so with the spine in extension. Additionally, a wheelchair back which is slightly reclined may be used further to promote the lordosis. Ensuring that the patient's pelvis is level may also help retard the spinal deformity, and a firm board suitably padded should be substituted for the slack seat upholstery of the average wheelchair. Again to be emphasized is that a properly fitting wheelchair is essential. Marked deformities can be produced by wheelchairs which are too big and allow the patient to slump to one side, or those in which the arm rests are too high or too low. Many of us do not have experience in measuring patients for wheelchairs. If this is the case, the patient should be referred to someone who does.

When the curvature is becoming worse in spite of attempts at bracing, surgery should be considered. Surgery of the back has not been a popular method of treatment in the past because of the long hospital stay, the associated discomfort, and the limited lifespan of the patient with Duchenne dystrophy. If present trends continue, though, it is likely to find increasing acceptance in the management of patients (114). With new forms of instrumentation, the postoperative course is made much easier. The patients can be mobilized earlier and leave the hospital earlier. In my own clinic, I am now recommending surgery to most of my patients with Duchenne dystrophy. Since surgery is the only way of permanently stabilizing the spine, it makes a logical choice. An equally logical choice is in orthopaedic surgeon skilled in the management of neuromuscular disease.

Ancillary devices are also of benefit. When the child is having difficulty feeding himself because of weakness of the shoulders, a ballbearing forearm orthosis or ballbearing feeder is helpful. The use of a gel cushion or one of the specialized types of inflatable cushions, such as the Roho, may prevent the development of pressure sores over the buttocks. When the child is no longer able to turn over in bed, the sleep of the entire family is disturbed since family members have to get up and turn him every couple of hours. In this situation, an alternating air mattress (alternating pressure pad) with a pump attached can give the family, as well as the patient, some much needed rest. When the child can no longer walk independently, pulmonary care becomes increasingly important (115) and daily postural drainage should be carried out by the family. Occasionally, nasal administration of oxygen at night can be helpful in giving the patient a comfortable night's rest.

REFERENCES

1. Duchenne de Boulogne. De la paralysie musculaire pseudohypertrophique ou paralysie myosclerosique. (Extrait des Archives generales de Médecine) Asselin, Paris, 1868.
2. Gardner-Medwin. D. Mutation rate in Duchenne type of muscular dystrophy. J. Med. Genet. *7:* 334–337, 1970.
3. Emery A. E. H. Genetic considerations in the x-linked muscular dystrophys. In: *Pathogenesis of Human Muscular Dystrophy*, edited L.P. Rowland. Excerpta Medica, Amsterdam, 1977, pp. 40–52.
4. Roses, A. D., Roses, M. J., Miller, S. E., Hull, K. L., and Appel, S. H. Carrier detection in Duchenne muscular dystrophy. N. Engl. J. Med. *294:* 193–197, 1976.
5. Brooke, M. H., Fenichel, G. M., Griggs, R. C., Mendell, J. R., Moxley, R., Miller, J. P., Province, M. A., and CIDD Group. Clinical investigation in Duchenne dystrophy: 2. Determination of the "power" of therapeutic trials based on the natural history. Muscle Nerve *6:* 91–103, 1983.
6. Scott, O. M., Hyde, S. A., Goddard, C., and Dubowitz, V. Quantitation of muscle function in children: a prospective study in Duchenne muscular dystrophy. Muscle Nerve *5:* 291–301, 1982.
7. Cohen, H. J., Molnar, G. E., and Taft, L. T. The genetic relationship of progressive muscular dystrophy (Duchenne type) and mental retardation. Dev. Med. Child. Neurol. *10:* 754–765, 1968.
8. Leibowitz, D., and Dubowitz, V. Intellect and behavior in Duchenne muscular dystrophy. Dev. Med. Child. Neurol. *23:* 557–590, 1981.
9. Florence, J. M., Fox, P. T., Planer, J., and Brooke, M. H. Activity, creatine kinase and myoglobin in Duchenne muscular dystrophy: a clue to etiology. Neurology *35:* 758–761, 1985.
10. Griggs, R. C., Reeves, W., and Moxley, R. T. The heart in Duchenne dystrophy. In: *Pathogenesis of Human Muscular Dystrophies*, edited L. P. Rowland. Excerpta Medica, Amsterdam 1977, pp. 661–671.
11. Jeliett, A. B., Kennedy, M. C., and Goldblatt, E. Duchenne pseudohypertrophic muscular dystrophy. A clinical and electrocardiographic study of patients and female carriers. Aust. N. Z. J. Med. *4:* 41–47, 1974.
12. Perloff, J. K., Roberts, W. C., de Leon, A. C., and O'Doherty, D. The distinctive electrocardiogram of Duchenne's progressive muscular dystrophy. Am. J. Med. *42:* 179–188, 1967.
13. Skyring, A., and McKusick, V. A. Clinical, genetic and electrocardiographic studies in childhood muscular dystrophy. Am. J. Med. Sci. *242:* 534–547, 1961.
14. Ronan, J. A., Jr., Perloff, J. K., Bowen, P. J., and Mann, O. The vectorcardiogram in Duchenne's progressive muscular dystrophy. Am. Heart. J. *84:* 588–596, 1972.
15. Davis, K. E., Pearson, P. L., Harper, P. S., Murray, J. M., O'Brien, T., Sarfarazi, M., and Williamson, R. Linkage analysis of 2 cloned DNA sequences flanking the Duchenne muscular dystrophy locus on the short arm of the human X-chromosome. Nucleic Acid Res. *11:* 2303–2312, 1983.
16. Monaco, A. P., Bertelson, C. J., Middlesworth, W., Colletti, C., Aldridge, J., Fischbeck, K. H., Bartlett, R., Pericak-Vance, M., Roses, A. D., and Kunkel, L. M. Detection of deletions spanning the Duchenne muscular dystrophy locus using a tightly linked DNA segment. Nature *316:* 842–845, 1985.
17. Demos, J., and Ecoiffier, J. Troubles circulatorie au cours de la myopathie. Etude arteriographique. Rev. Fr. Etud. Clin. Biol. *2:* 489–494, 1957.
18. Hathaway, P. W., Engel, W. K., and Zellweger, H. Experimental myopathy after microarterial embolization. Arch. Neurol. *22:* 365–378, 1970.
19. Mendell, J. R., Engel, W. K., and Darrer, E. C. Duchenne muscular dystrophy: Functional ischemia reproduces its characteristic lesions. Science *172:* 1143–1145, 1971.
20. Parker, J. M., and Mendell, J. R. Proximal myopathy induced by 5-HT-imipramine simulates Duchenne dystrophy. Nature *247:* 103–104, 1974.
21. Silverman, L. M., and Gruemer, H. D. Sarcolemmal membrane changes related to enzyme release in the imipramine/serotonin experimental animal model. Clin. Chem. *22:* 1710–1714, 1976.
22. Murphy, D. L., Mendell, J. R., and Engel, W. K. Serotonin and platelet function in Duchenne's muscular dystrophy. Arch. Neurol. *28:* 239–242, 1973.

23. Paulson, O. F., Engel, A. G., and Gomez, M. R. Muscle blood flow in Duchenne type muscular dystrophy, limb-girdle dystrophy, polymyositis and in normal controls. J. Neurol. Neurosurg. Psychiatry *37:* 685–690, 1974.

24. Jerusalem, F., Engel, A. G., and Gomez, M. R. Duchenne dystrophy: I. Morphometric study of the muscle microvasculature. Brain *97:* 115–122, 1974.

25. Mechler, F., Mastaglia, F. L., Haggith, J., and Gardner-Medwin, D. Adrenergic receptor responses of vascular smooth muscle in Becker dystrophy. A muscle blood flow study using the ^{133}Xe clearance method. J. Neurol. Sci. *46:* 291–302, 1979.

26. McComas, A. J., Sica, R. E. P., and Currie, S. An electrophysiological study of Duchenne dystrophy. J. Neurol. Neurosurg. Psychiatry *34:* 461–468, 1971.

27. Panayiotopoulos, C. P., Scarpalezos, S., and Papapetropoulos, T. Electrophysiological estimation of motor units in Duchenne muscular dystrophy. J. Neurol. Sci. *23:* 89–98, 1974.

28. Ballantyne, J. P., and Hansen, S. New method for the estimation of the number of motor units in a muscle: 2. Duchenne, limb-girdle and facioscapulohumeral, and myotonic muscular dystrophies. J. Neurol. Neurosurg. Psychiatry *37:* 1195–1201, 1974.

29. Nicholson, L. V. Serum myoglobin in muscular dystrophy and carrier detection. J. Neurol. Sci. *51:* 411–426, 1981.

30. Mokri, B., and Engel, A. G. Duchenne dystrophy: electron microscopic findings pointing to a basic or early abnormality in the plasma membrane of the muscle fiber. Neurology *25:* 1111–1120, 1975.

31. Bradley, W. G., and Fulthorpe, J. J. Studies of sarcolemmal integrity in myopathic fibers. Neurology *28:* 670–677, 1978.

32. Bodensteiner, J. B., and Engel, A. G. Intracellular calcium accumulation in Duchenne dystrophy and other myopathies. A study of 567,000 muscle fibers in 114 biopsies. Neurology *28:* 439–446, 1978.

33. Bertorini, T. E., Bhattacharya, S. K., Palmieri, G. M. A., Chesney, C. M., Bifer, D., and Baker, B. Muscle calcium and magnesium content in Duchenne muscular dystrophy. Neurology *32:* 1088–1092, 1982.

34. Bhattacharya, S. K., Palmieri, G. M. A., Bertorini, T. E., and Nutting, D. F. The effect of diltiazem in dystrophic hamsters. Muscle Nerve *5:* 73–78, 1982.

35. Schotland, D. L., Bonilla, E., and Wakayama, Y. Application of the freeze fracture technique to the study of human neuromuscular diseases. Muscle Nerve *3:* 21–27, 1980.

36. Schotland, D. L., Bonilla, E., and Van Meter, M. Duchenne dystrophy: alteration in plasma membrane structure. Science *196:* 1005–1007, 1977.

37. Peluchetti, D., Mora, M., Protti, A., and Cornelio, F. Freeze fracture analysis of the muscle fiber plasma membrane in Duchenne dystrophy. Neurology *35:* 928–930, 1985.

38. Heimann-Patterson, T. D., Bonilla, E., and Schotland, D. L. Concanavalin A binding of the cell surface of Duchenne muscle in vitro. Ann. Neurol. *12:* 305–307, 1982.

39. Mawatari, S., Igisu, H., Kurolwa, Y., and Miyoshino S. Na-K-ATPase of erythrocyte membranes in Duchenne muscular dystrophy. Neurology *31:* 293–297, 1981.

40. Mawatari, S., Takagi, A., and Rowland, L. P. Adenyl cyclase in normal and pathologic human muscle. Arch. Neurol. *30:* 96–102, 1974.

41. Cerri, C. A., Willner, J. H., and Rowland, L. P. Assay of adenylate cyclase in homogenates of control and Duchenne human muscle. Clin. Chim. Acta *111:* 133–146, 1983.

42. Ionasescu, V., Ionasescu, R., Feld, R., Witte, D., Cancilla, P., Kaeding, L., and Stern, L. Z. Alterations in creatine kinase in fresh muscle and cell cultures in Duchenne dystrophy. Ann. Neurol. *9:* 394–399.

43. Thompson, E. J., Yasin, R., Vanbeers, G., Nurse, K., and Al-Ani, S. Myogenic defect in human muscular dystrophy. Nature *268:* 241–243, 1977.

44. Rothman, S. M., and Bischoff, R. Electrophysiology of Duchenne dystrophy myotubes in tissue culture. Ann. Neurol. *13:* 176–179, 1983.

45. Mawatari, S., Miranda, A., and Rowland, L. P. Adenyl cyclase abnormality in Duchenne muscular dystrophy: muscle cells in culture. Neurology *26:* 1021–1026, 1976.

46. Cerri, C. A., Willner, J. H., and Miranda, A. F. Adenylate cyclase in Duchenne fibroblasts. J. Neurol. Sci. *53:* 181–185, 1982.

47. Rowland, L. P. Biochemistry of muscle membranes in Duchenne dystrophy. Muscle Nerve *3:* 3–20, 1980.

48. Falk, R. S., Campion, D., Guthrie, B., Sparkes, R. S., and Fox, C. F. Phosphorylation of the red cell membrane proteins in Duchenne muscular dystrophy. N. Engl. J. Med. *300:* 258–259, 1979.

49. Fischer, S., Tortolero, M., Piau, J. P., Delaunay, J., and Schapira, G. Protein kinase and adenylate kinase of erythrocyte membrane from patients with Duchenne muscular dystrophy. Clin. Chem. Acta *88:* 437–440, 1978.

50. Roses, A. D., Mabry, M. E., Herbstreith, M. H., Shile, E. V., and Balakrishnan, O. V.

152   CLINICIAN'S VIEW OF NEUROMUSCULAR DISEASES

Increased phosphorylation of spectrin peptides in Duchenne muscular dystrophy. In: *Disorders of the Motor Unit*, edited by D. L. Schotland. John Wiley & Sons, New York, 1982, pp. 413–420.

51. Mabry, M. E., and Roses, A. D. Increased ³²P-phosphorylase of triptic peptides of erythrocyte spectrin in Duchenne muscular dystrophy. Muscle Nerve *4:* 489–493, 1981.
52. Roses, A. D., Shile, P. E., Herbstreith, M. H., and Balakrishnan, C. V. Identification of abnormally ³²P-phosphorylated cyanogen bromide cleavage product of erythrocyte membrane spectrin in Duchenne muscular dystrophy. Neurology *31:* 1026–1030, 1981.
53. Shay, J. W., Cook, J., and Fuseler, J. W. Microtubules and Duchenne muscular dystrophy. Ann. Neurol. *6:* 147, 1979.
54. Connolly, J. A., Kalnins, V. I., and Barber, B. H. Microtubular organization in fibroblasts derived from the dystrophic chicken and persons with muscular dystrophy. Nature *282:* 511–513, 1979.
55. Walsh, F. S., Yasin, R., Kundu, K., and Thompson, E. J. Organization of microtubules and microfilaments in fibroblasts and in Duchenne muscular dystrophy muscle cultures. Ann. Neurol. *9:* 202–204, 1981.
56. Ionasescu, V., Zellweger, H., and Conway, T. W. Ribosomal protein synthesis in Duchenne muscular dystrophy. Arch. Biochem. Biophys. *144:* 51–58, 1971.
57. Peter, J. B., Worsfold, M., and Pearson, C. M. Erythrocyte ghost adenosine triphosphatase (ATPase) in Duchenne dystrophy. J. Lab. Clin. Med. *74:* 103–108, 1969.
58. Austin, L., Katz, S., Jeffrey, P. L., Shield, L., Author, H., and Mazzoni, M. Thermodynamic behavior of membrane enzymes in Duchenne muscular dystrophy. J. Neurol. Sci. *58:* 143–151, 1983.
59. Arthur, H., deNiese, M., Jeffrey, P. L., and Austin, L. Plasma lipoproteins in Duchenne muscular dystrophy. Biochem. Int. *6:* 307–313, 1983.
60. Davis, M. H., Cappel, R., Vester, J. W., Samaha, F. J., and Gruenstein, E. Creatine kinase activity in normal and Duchenne muscular dystrophy fibroblasts. Muscle Nerve *5:* 1–6, 1982.
61. Rosenmann, E., Kreis, C., Thompson, R. G., Dobbs, M., Hamerton, J. L., and Wrogeman, K. Analysis of fibroblast proteins from patients with Duchenne muscular dystrophy by two-dimensional electrophoresis. *Nature 298:* 563–565, 1982.
62. Thompson, R. G., Nickel, B., Finlayson, S., Mauser, R., Hamerton, J. L., and Wrogemann, K. 56 K fibroblast protein not specific for Duchenne muscular dystrophy but for skin biopsy site. Nature *304:* 740–741, 1982.
63. Ballard, F. J., Thomas, F. M., and Stern, L. M. Increased turnover of muscle contractile proteins in Duchenne muscular dystrophy as assessed by 3-methylhistidine and creatine excretion. Clin. Sci. *56:* 347–352, 1979.
64. Griggs, R. C., and Rennie, M. J. Muscle wasting in muscular dystrophy decreased protein synthesis or increased degradation. Ann. Neurol. *13:* 125–132, 1983.
65. Rennie, M. J., Edwards, R. H., Millward, D. J., Wolman, S. L., and Halliday, D. Effects of Duchenne muscular dystrophy on muscle protein synthesis. Nature *296:* 165–167, 1982.
66. Bertorini, T. E., Palmieri, G. M. A., Aiorozo, D., Edwards, N. L., and Fox, I. H. Increased adenine nucleotide turnover in Duchenne muscular dystrophy. Pediatr. Res. *15:* 1478–1482, 1981.
67. Carroll, J. E., Norris, B. J., and Brooke, M. H. Defective [*U*-¹⁴C]palmitic acid oxidation in Duchenne muscular dystrophy. Neurology *35:* 96–97, 1985.
68. Wolf, S. (editor). *Genetic Analysis of the X Chromosome.* Plenum Press, New York, 1982.
69. Haldane, J. B. S. The rate of spontaneous mutation of a human gene. J. Genet. *31:* 317–326, 1935.
70. Roses, A. D., Roses, M. J., Metcalf, B. S., Hull, K. L., Nicholson, G. A., Hartwig, G. B., and Rose, C. R. Pedigree testing Duchenne muscular dystrophy. Ann. Neurol. *2:* 271–278, 1977.
71. Lane, R. J. M., Robinow, M., and Roses, A. D. The genetic status of mothers of isolated cases of Duchenne muscular dystrophy. J. Med. Genet. *20:* 1–11, 1983.
72. Lindgren, V., Martinville, B., Horwich, A. L., Rosenberg, L. E., and Francke, U. Human ornithine transcarbamylase locus mapped to band XP21.1 near the Duchenne muscular dystrophy locus. Science *226:* 698–700, 1984.
73. Francke, U., Ochs, H. D., Martinville, B., Giacalone, J., Lindgren, V., Disteche C., Pagon, R. A., Hofker, M. H., VanOmmen, G. J. B., Pearson, P. L., and Wedgewood, R. J. Minor Xp21 chromosome deletion in a male associated with expression of Duchenne muscular dystrophy, chronic granulomatous disease, retinitis pigmentosa, and McLeod's syndrome. Am. J. Hum. Genet. *37:* 250–260, 1985.
74. Lyon, M. F. Evolution of x-chromosome inactivation in mammals. Nature *250:* 651–653, 1974.
75. Roses, M. J., Nicholson, M. T., Kirchner, C. S., et al. Evaluation and detection of

Duchenne's and Becker's dystrophy carriers by manual muscle testing. Neurology *27:* 20–25, 1977.

76. Moser, H., and Emery, A. E. H. The manifesting carrier in Duchenne muscular dystrophy. Med. Genet. *5:* 271–284, 1974.
77. Cavanagh, N. P., and Preece, M. A. Calf hypertrophy and asymmetry in female carriers of X-linked Duchenne muscular dystrophy: an overdiagnosed clinical manifestation. Clin. Genet. *20:* 168–172, 1981.
78. Munsat, T. L., Baloh, R., Pearson, C. M., and Fowler, W. Serum enzyme alterations in neuromuscular disorders. J.A.M.A. *226:* 1536–1543, 1973.
79. Blyth, H., and Hughes, B. P. Pregnancy and serum CPK levels in potential carriers of severe X-linked muscular dystrophy. Lancet *1:* 855–856, 1971.
80. Emery, A. E. H., and King, B. Pregnancy and serum-creatine-kinase levels in potential carriers of Duchenne X-linked muscular dystrophy. Lancet *1:* 1013, 1971.
81. Lane, R. J., and Roses, A. D. Variation of serum creatine kinase levels with age in normal females: implications for genetic counselling in Duchenne muscular dystrophy. Clin. Chem. Acta *113:* 75–86, 1981.
82. Sage, J., Inati, Y., and Samaha, F. The importance of serum pyrurate kinase in neuromuscular disease and carrier states. Muscle Nerve *2:* 390–393, 1979.
83. Percy, M. E., Andrews, D. F., and Thompson, M. W. Duchenne muscular dystrophy carrier detection using logistic discrimination: serum creatine kinase, hemopexin, pyruvate kinase, and lactate dehydrogenase in combination. Am. J. Med. Genet. *13:* 27–38, 1982.
84. Griggs, R. C., Mendell, J. R., Fenichel, G. M., et al. Clinical investigation in Duchenne dystrophy: V. Use of creatine kinase and pyruvate kinase in carrier detection. Muscle Nerve *8:* 60–67, 1985.
85. Pearce, G. W., Pearce, J. M. S., and Walton, J. N. The Duchenne type muscular dystrophy: histopathological studies of the carrier state. Brain *89:* 109–120, 1966.
86. Roy, S., and Dubowitz, V. Carrier detection in Duchenne muscular dystrophy. J. Neurol. Sci. *11:* 65–79, 1970.
87. Emery, A. E. H. Abnormalities in the electrocardiogram in female carriers of Duchenne muscular dystrophy. Br. Med. J. *2:* 418–420, 1969.
88. Gardner-Medwin, D. Studies of the carrier state in the Duchenne type of muscular dystrophy: 2. Quantitative electromyography as a method of carrier detection. J. Neurol. Neurosurg. Psychiatry *31:* 124–134, 1968.
89. Gardner-Medwin, D., Pennington, R. J., and Walton, J. N. The detection of carriers of X-linked muscular dystrophy genes. A review of some methods studied in Newcastle upon Tyne. J. Neurol. Sci. *13:* 459–474, 1971.
90. Moosa, A., Brown, B. H., and Dubowitz, V. Quantitative electromyography carrier detection in Duchenne type muscular dystrophy using a new automatic technique. J. Neurol. Neurosurg. Psychiatry *35:* 841–844, 1972.
91. Hilditch, T. E., Sweetin, J. C., and Thomson, W. H. S. Rubidium and detection of Duchenne carriers. Lancet *2:* 323, 1973.
92. Bonilla, E., Fischbeck, K. H., and Schotland, D. L. Freeze fracture study of muscle plasma membrane in obligate carriers of Duchenne muscular dystrophy. Neurology *33:* 1346–1348, 1983.
93. Ionasescu, V., Zellweger, H., Shirk, P., and Conway, T. W. Identification of carriers of Duchenne muscular dystrophy by muscle protein synthesis. Neurology *23:* 497–501, 1973.
94. Brooke, M. H., and Engel, W. K. The histographic analysis of human muscle biopsies with regard to fiber types: I. Adult male and female. Neurology *19:* 221–233, 1969.
95. Hobbins, J. C., and Mahoney, M. J. In utero diagnosis of hemoglobinopathies. Technic for obtaining fetal blood. N. Engl. J. Med. *290:* 1065–1067, 1974.
96. Ionasescu, V., Zellweger, H., and Cancilla, P. Fetal serum creatine phosphokinase not a valid predictor of Duchenne dystrophy. Lancet *2:* 1251, 1978.
97. Golbus, M. S., Stephens, J. D., Mahoney, M. J., Hobbins, J. C., Haseltine, F. P., Caskey, C. T., and Banker, B. Q. Failure of fetal CK as indicator of Duchenne muscular dystrophy. N. Engl. J. Med. *300:* 860, 1979.
98. Mendell, J.R., and Wiechers, D. O. Lack of benefit of allopurinol in Duchenne dystrophy. Muscle Nerve *2:* 53–56, 1979.
99. Stern, L. M., Fewings, J. D., Bretag, A. H., Ballard, F. J., Tomas, F. M., Cooper, B. M., and Goldbatt, E. The progression of Duchenne muscular dystrophy: clinical trial of allopurinol therapy. Neurology *31:* 422–426, 1981.
100. Stern, L. Z., Ringel, S. P., Ziter, F. A., Menander-Huber, K. B., Ionasescu, V., Pellegrino, R. J., and Snyder, R. D. Drug trial of superoxide dismutase in Duchenne's muscular dystrophy. Arch. Neurol. *39:* 342–346, 1982.
101. Skinner, R., Howden, L. C., and Matthews, M. B. Verapamil in Duchenne muscular dystrophy. Lancet *1:* 559, 1982.

102. Mendell, J. R., Griggs, R. C., Moxley, R. T., Fenichel G. M., Brooke, M. H., Miller, J. P., Province, M. A., and Dodson, W. E. Clinical investigation in Duchenne muscular dystrophy: IV. Double-blind controlled trial of leucine. Muscle Nerve *7:* 535–541, 1984.
103. Moxley, R. T., Brooke, M. H., Fenichel, G. M., Mendell, J. R., Griggs, R. C., Miller, J. P., Province, M. A., Patterson, V., and the CIDD Group. Clinical investigation in Duchenne dystrophy: VI. Double-blind controlled trial of nifedipine. Muscle Nerve (in press).
104. Stracher, A., McGowan, E., and Shafiq, S. Muscular dystrophy; inhibition of degeneration in vivo of protease inhibitors. Science *200:* 50–51, 1978.
105. McGowan, E., Shafiq, S., and Stracher, A. Delayed degeneration of dystrophic and normal muscle cell cultures treated with pepstatin, leupeptin and antipain. Exp. Neurol. *50:* 649–653, 1976.
106. Vignos, P. J., Spencer, G. E., and Archibald, K. C. Management of progressive muscular dystrophy in childhood. J.A.M.A. *184:* 89–96, 1963.
107. Spencer, G. E. Orthopaedic care of progressive muscular dystrophy. J. Bone Joint Surg. *49:* 1201–1204, 1971.
108. Siegel, I. M. *The Clinical Management of Muscle Disease.* William Heineman, London, 1977.
109. Karpati, G., and Watters, G. V. Adverse anesthetic reactions in Duchenne dystrophy. In: *Muscular Dystrophy Research. Advances and New Trends,* edited by C. Angelini, G. A. Danielli, and D. Fontanari. Excerpta Medica, Amsterdam, 1980.
110. Kelfer, H. M., Singer, W. D., and Reynolds, R. N. Malignant hyperthermia in a child with Duchenne muscular dystrophy. Pediatrics *71:* 118–119, 1983.
111. Brownell, A. K., Paasuke, R. T., Elash, A., Fowlow, S. B. Seagram, C. G., Diewold, R. J., and Friesen, C. Malignant hyperthermia in Duchenne muscular dystrophy. Anesthesiology *58:* 180–182, 1983.
112. Vignos, P. J., Wagner, M. B., Kaplan, J. S., and Spencer, G. E. Predicting the success of reambulation in patients with Duchenne muscular dystrophy. J. Bone Joint Surg. *65A:* 719–728, 1983.
113. Wilkins, K. E., and Gibson, D. A. The patterns of spinal deformity in Duchenne muscular dystrophy. J. Bone Joint Surg. *58A:* 24–32, 1976.
114. Bonnett, C., Brown, J. C., Perry, J., Nickel, V., Wallinski, T., et al. Evolution of treatment of paralytic scoliosis at Rancho Los Amigos Hospital. J. Bone Joint Surg. *57A:* 206–215, 1975.
115. Inkley, S. R., Oldenburg, F. C., and Vignos, P. J. Pulmonary function in Duchenne's muscular dystrophy related to stage of disease. Am. J. Med. *56:* 297–306, 1974.

SLOWLY PROGRESSIVE (BECKER) VARIETY OF X-LINKED RECESSIVE MUSCULAR DYSTROPHY

A form of X-linked recessive dystrophy bearing a close resemblance to the Duchenne variety was outlined by Becker (1). The patient develops the same proximal weakness of the hips and shoulders with a tendency to walk on the toes and with the characteristic hypertrophy of the calf muscles (Figs. 4.33 and 4.34). The onset of the disease is much later and survival is prolonged until middle adult life. Such patients are almost always walking until at least the age of 16 and this has been used as the differentiating point between the diagnosis of Becker and Duchenne dystrophy (2). Although the number of families reported in the literature is not large, the Becker variety and the Duchenne type only occasionally coexist in the same pedigree (3), suggesting that they do not, in reality, represent the two extremes in the spectrum of progression of a single disorder. The locus of the gene was formerly suggested to be quite different from Duchenne dystrophy. This was based on a possible linkage with Deutan color-blindness which is located on the long arm of the X chromosome (4). This has now been shown to be incorrect. More careful studies using two new probes have shown that the Becker dystrophy gene is located in the Xp21 band on the short arm of the X chromosome. It is in the same region as the Duchenne gene and these two disorders are quite possibly allelic (5).

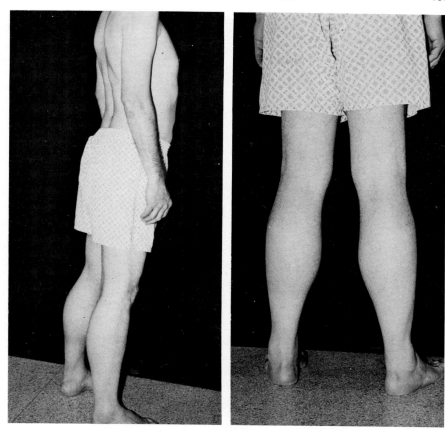

Figures 4.33 and 4.34.   Becker or mild variety of pseudohypertrophic dystrophy. This man was able to walk although he had some difficulty in standing from a low chair. The calf muscles were large and the heel cords tight.

Mental retardation is also less common in Becker dystrophy than in Duchenne. Except for the age of the patient and the degree of weakness, the physical examination in the two diseases is almost identical. There is, perhaps, less tendency for contractures to develop in Becker dystrophy and the skeletal deformities are not as marked, but the gait, the manner of arising from the floor, and other aspects of the disease are similar. Many patients experience cramping pains in the muscles, particularly associated with exercise (6). There is always a problem in confirming the diagnosis in Becker dystrophy since the border between this illness and the other proximal dystrophies in adult life are much less clearly defined than between Duchenne and other causes of childhood weakness. At these boundaries lie the patients whose illnesses belong in the amorphous group of limb girdle dystrophies. It is, therefore, probably unwise to make the diagnosis of Becker dystrophy without a solid family history indicating an X-linked recessive disorder.

Laboratory studies show large increases in the levels of serum CK. The electrocardiogram may also be abnormal, although not as often as in the Duchenne form; probably in the neighborhood of 30–40%. Furthermore, the

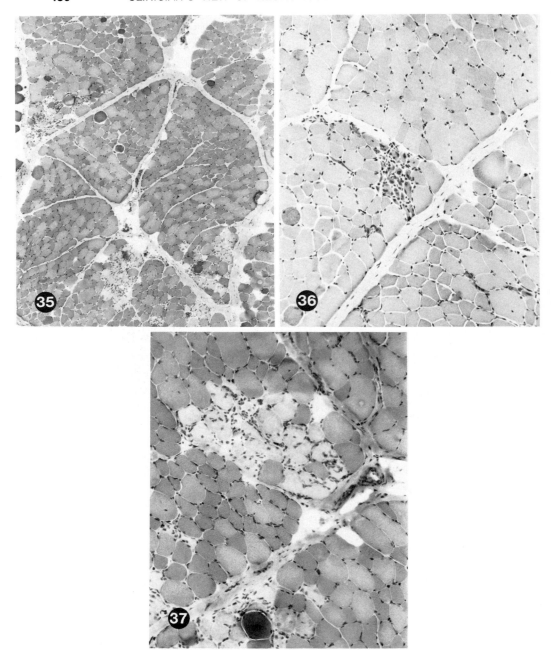

Figure 4.35. Becker dystrophy. In general, the changes in Becker dystrophy resemble those of Duchenne. The degree of fibrosis is perhaps a little less but variation in the size of fibers, the rather rounded fibers, and opaque fibers are noted.

Figure 4.36. Small groups of basophilic fibers are also seen.

Figure 4.37. The routine hematoxylin and eosin stain also shows groups of necrotic fibers which are recognized by their paler stain.

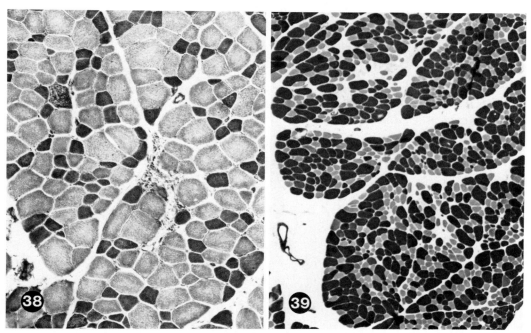

Figure 4.38. Oxidative enzyme reactions again demonstrate the changes which have been noted on the routine stains and do not show any major distortion of the intermyofibrillar network pattern although one "granular fiber" is seen toward the upper part of the left hand side of the photograph.
Figure 4.39. ATPase stains, in general, show a better differentiation of the fiber types into Type 1 and Type 2 than is seen in Duchenne dystrophy.

EKG abnormalities, which are seen, are less specific. The EKG is seldom used to establish the diagnosis, although it may be important in monitoring the disease and some patients may have cardiac involvement (6). The muscle biopsy in Becker dystrophy has been the subject of two reports (2, 7). The changes described in these papers were dissimilar from the biopsy of the typical Duchenne. There is much more in the way of fiber splitting, internal nuclei, and in general, the biopsies resemble those of the "limb-girdle" dystrophy patients. My own experience has been that the biopsy from Becker dystrophy is rather more similar to Duchenne dystrophy with circular fibers embedded in the sea of fibrous tissue and the small groups of basophilic fibers scattered throughout the biopsy (Figs. 4.35–4.39). This may reflect my bias in rejecting the sporadic cases of this type of dystrophy as being unproven, or perhaps, belonging in the "limb-girdle" rubric. I think all of us would feel a good deal more confident about making the diagnosis if we had some pathognomonic clinical, biochemical or pathological abnormality. In the absence of this, the entity remains a little hazy, although the most typical patients are easily recognized.

Carrier detection in Becker dystrophy follows the same lines as that in Duchenne dystrophy; 60% of the carriers are said to have an elevated CK (8). Only the development of appropriate genetic probes will allow us to give accurate advice.

The treatment of the illness follows along the same lines as outlined in the section on Duchenne dystrophy.

The etiology of Becker dystrophy is unknown. Most tacitly assume that the disorder is related to Duchenne muscular dystrophy, but this is by no means certain. The vascular theory has again been invoked as in Duchenne dystrophy, but the muscle blood flow at rest in Becker dystrophy was found to be higher than normal, although the α receptor blockade produced by phentolamine was less than normal (9).

REFERENCES

1. Becker, P. E. Two new familes of benign sex linked recessive muscular dystrophy. Rev. Can. Biol. *21:* 551–566, 1962.
2. Bradley, W. G., Jones, M. Z., Mussine, J. M., and Fawcett, P. R. W. Becker type muscular dystrophy. Muscle Nerve *1:* 111–132, 1978.
3. Furukawa, T., and Peter, J. B. X-linked muscular dystrophy. Ann. Neurol. *2:* 414–416, 1977.
4. Skinner, R., Smith, C., and Emery, A. E. H. Linkage between the loci for benign (Becker type) x-borne muscular dystrophy and Deutan color blindness. J. Med. Genet. *2:* 317–320, 1974.
5. Kingston, H. M., Harper, P. S., Pearson, P. L., Davies, K. E., Williamson, R., and Page, D. Localization of the gene for Becker muscular dystrophy. Lancet *2:* 1200, 1983.
6. Kuhn, E., Fiehn, W., Schroder, J. M., Assmus, H., and Wagner, A. Early myocardial disease and cramping myalgia in Becker type muscular dystrophy: a kindred. Neurology *29:* 1144–1149, 1979.
7. Ringel, S. P., Carroll, J. E., and Schold, S. C. The spectrum of mild x-linked recessive muscular dystrophy. Arch. Neurol. *34:* 408–416, 1977.
8. Skinner, R., Emery, A. E. H., Anderson, A. J. B., and Foxall, C. The detection of carriers of benign (Becker type) X-linked muscular dystrophy. J. Med. Genet. *12:* 131–134, 1975.
9. Mechler, F., Mastaglia, F. L., Harggith, J., and Gardner-Medwin, D. Adrenergic receptor responses of vascular smooth muscle in Becker dystrophy. A muscle blood flow study using the ^{133}Xe clearance method. J. Neurol. Sci. *46:* 291–302, 1980.

FACIOSCAPULOHUMERAL DYSTROPHY

The common concept of facioscapulohumeral dystrophy as a rather benign and slowly progressive weakness of muscles of the face, shoulder, and upper arm is only partially correct. There is marked variability in the severity of symptoms from patient to patient, as there is in the age of onset. This obviously suggests the possibility of genetically distinct entities rather than a continuous spectrum of disease. Research into the illness has progressed very little over the past few years. Indeed the major role of facioscapulohumeral dystrophy in published studies has been as the control population to contrast with Duchenne dystrophy. What follows in the initial paragraphs relates to the classical concepts of facioscapulohumeral dystrophy and will be amplified later to cover the whole gamut of patients with this illness.

Clinical Aspects

The disease is inherited as an autosomal dominant. There is strong penetrance, and the incidence of the illness has been estimated at between 3 and 10 cases per million population (1). As in so many muscle diseases, this incidence is probably erroneously low owing to the large number of undiagnosed cases. Typically, the disease is first noticed towards the end of the first decade or during the second. Facial weakness is present and an inability to whistle is often a symptom, although it may appear to the patient as no more than a mild quirk of nature. During sleep the eyes may remain slightly open and, because the extraocular muscles are unimpaired, a prominent Bell's phenomenon is seen displaying the sclera through partially opened lids. Drinking through a straw or blowing up balloons may be impossible but may again be dismissed by the patient as an idiosyncrasy rather than a true abnormality. The first doubts about muscular strength are often raised in physical education classes where the teenager can neither climb a rope nor perform a push-up successfully. The configuration of the shoulders is often more noticed by schoolmates than by the family and the epithet of "chicken wings" has been applied to not a few of our patients.

The muscles of the upper arm and shoulders are usually involved simultaneously with the facial muscles, and this gives rise to predictable difficulty in handling heavy objects at a level above the shoulders. When the patient sits in a straight backed chair the protruding shoulder blades may catch on the back of the chair. The illness spreads slowly to other muscle groups, including those of the hips. Bilateral foot-drop may be present. Occasionally this is one of the initial symptoms and it is then difficult to know whether to call the disorder facioscapulohumeral dystrophy or scapuloperoneal dystrophy. The overall progression takes place over many decades, interspersed with periods of relatively rapid deterioration.

Although the appearance of the patient with the fully developed illness is characteristic (Figs. 4.40–4.49), the milder varieties may be overlooked. The patient's face is smooth and the forehead usually unlined. The mouth loses the normal contour and appears widened with a more horizontal appearance due to the loss of the normal upward curvature of the lower lip. When viewed from the side, the lips have a pouting appearance ("bouche de tapir"). On either side of the angles of the mouth, a dimple appears, often the only mark on the patient's face. The painting of Mona Lisa illustrates a mild form of this dimpling but it may become pronounced. It also deepens when the patient smiles or attempts to bare the teeth. When the patient is asked to purse his lips, instead of forming the normal "moue," both upper and lower lips move horizontally in opposite directions. The blink is usually slowed and is frequently incomplete.

There is wasting of the neck muscles, and the medial ends of the clavicles jut forwards, forming a distinct step at the base of the neck. Part of this prominence is due to a reorientation of the clavicles. Normally, these bones run slightly upwards and backwards from their medial ends. In facioscapulohumeral dystrophy, there is a droop to the shoulders which causes the clavicles to run horizontally or to slope downwards. When the patient attempts to abduct the arms, the scapulae, having lost their fixation, ride upwards over the back, and the upper borders may be seen rising up into the normal location of the trapezius muscle. Viewed from the side or the back, the scapulae are only loosely apposed to the thorax. The inferior medial angle is the most prominent and juts backwards on attempted movement. Although the term facioscapulohumeral dystrophy would imply that all the muscles of the shoulder and upper arm are atrophic, the deltoid is surprisingly well preserved in many cases. This may be overlooked, however, because poor scapular fixation prevents the deltoid from exerting its maximal effect. Therefore, in testing the muscle it is well to have the patient lying down with the examiner's hand pressing the thorax backwards into the couch in order

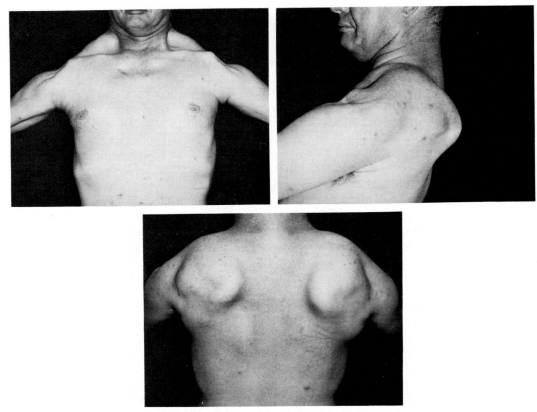

Figures 4.40 through 4.42. Facioscapulohumeral dystrophy. In this disease the shoulders have a characteristic appearance. When the arms are abducted, the trapezius mounds up and a "step" is formed at the point of the shoulder (Fig. 4.40, *left*). The scapulae slide upwards and laterally and the inferomedial corner juts out posteriorly (Figs. 4.41 *right*) and 4.42 (*center below*).

to prevent the scapula from moving. When the deltoid is examined in this fashion, it is often of normal strength or only slightly weak. Both the triceps and biceps are involved early and may waste rapidly. The slender stick-like upper arm is contrasted with the relative bulk of the forearm and a descriptive term for this type of abnormality is the "Popeye" arm. A remarkable discrepancy is seen in the strength of the forearm muscles. In severe cases, particularly the infantile or juvenile variety of facioscapulohumeral dystrophy, there is a marked weakness of the wrist extensors, producing a wrist drop. The wrist flexors, on the other hand, may maintain normal strength even when most of the other muscles of the body, including those of the hips and lower legs, are atrophic. The inability to extend the wrist results in another characteristic posture adopted by patients with this illness, the so-called "praying mantis" position. When asked to extend the arms, the patient holds the arms forward, flexed at the elbows and wrists with the shoulder blades jutting backwards. The pattern of shoulder and arm weakness in facioscapulohumeral dystrophy is different from that of limb-girdle dystrophy. The selective weakness of the biceps and the involvement of the deltoid in limb-girdle dystrophy are helpful in making the differentiation. Facioscapulohumeral dystrophy often affects

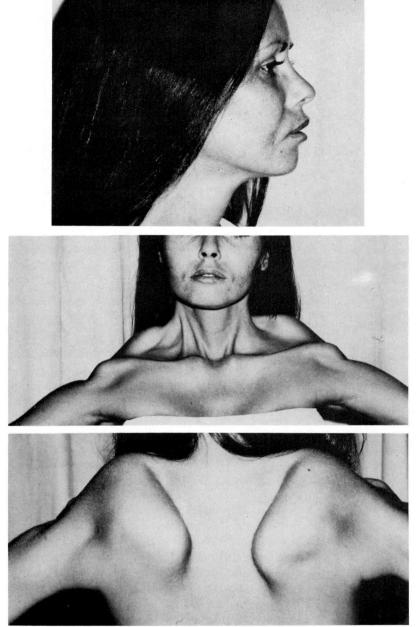

Figures 4.43 through 4.45.   Facioscapulohumeral dystrophy. From the lateral view, the lips have a slight pout (Fig. 4.43, *top*). When seen full face, there is a dimple lateral to the angles of the mouth. The identical appearance of this patients shoulders to those shown in Figure 4.40 should be noted. The posterior view shows the scapulae riding over the lateral part of the thorax (Fig. 4.45, *bottom*).

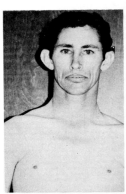 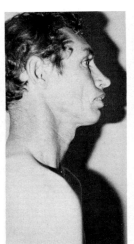 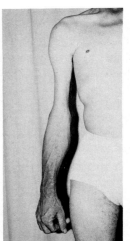 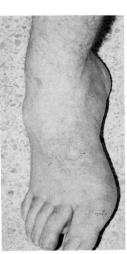

Figures 4.46 through 4.49. Facioscapulohumeral dystrophy. The facial weakness often gives the lips a flattened rectangular appearance when viewed full face (Fig. 4.46, *left*). The lateral view, once again shows the pouting appearance of the mouth (Fig. 4.47, *left center*). Preservation of the deltoid muscle with marked atrophy of the biceps and triceps is seen in Figure 4.48 (*right, center*). The muscles of the forearm are not atrophic and this is given rise to the appelation "Popeye" arm which is well illustrated in this patient. In spite of the fact that this man has a marked foot drop, the extensor digitorum brevis is hypertrophic as shown in this photograph where it appears as a mound on the lateral surface of the foot (Fig. 4.49, *right*).

the limbs in a very asymmetric fashion. It is not unusual to see one arm or leg severely involved while the other maintains reasonable strength.

Weakness of the hips may be found quite early in facioscapulohumeral dystrophy, although it may remain unnoticed by the patient until after he has noticed the weakness of the face and shoulders. There is often a compensatory lordosis, and this differs from other illnesses. Dorsal kyphosis is unusual, and associated scoliosis is also less common. The thoracic spine may remain as straight as a ramrod, but the lordosis which is seen in the lumbar region is much more marked than usual. In extreme cases, the sacrum forms a platform which runs almost horizontally, exaggerating the small of the back into a deep pit. The precarious gait of patients with this form of abnormality is remarkable. In the lower legs the same difference is seen between the plantar flexors and dorsiflexors of the ankle as is noted in the arms. The calf muscles are usually much stronger than the anterior tibial and peroneal group. The extensor digitorum brevis, on the other hand, is often hypertrophied and usually maintains its normal strength. Deep tendon reflexes are decreased early in the disease, more so at the elbows and at the knees than distally.

As was mentioned previously, the preceding refers to the typical and classical disease. The evolution takes place over many decades, and most patients lead a productive and relatively full life, adapting themselves slowly to their illness. There are, however, other clinical pictures, which are in my own experience equally common. They are often neglected in the textbooks.

Infantile Facioscapulohumeral Dystrophy

The first and most characteristic is the infantile variety of facioscapulohumeral dystrophy (2). This is by no means a benign disease and it is noticed within the first 2 years of life. Curiously, it is seldom noted by the parents in their own children, but the babysitter or another friend comments that the child never smiles, or that the eyes are kept open during sleep. This picture is associated with severe weakness. Not only there be total paralysis of the face, including the muscles involved in eye closure (Figs. 4.50 and 4.51), but severe and crippling weakness of the other muscle groups is seen early. Many of these children are using wheelchairs by the time they are 9 or 10 years of age. Even their facial weakness produces serious handicap. They are completely unable to smile and are often ostracized at school because of their total lack of emotional response. Many children develop an audible laugh instead of a smile in order to signify amusement. This produces even more difficulty with acquaintances, whose casual pleasantries are greeted with a harsh chuckle from a mirthless and impassive face. The patient may make constant sucking noises and use the tongue to try and control the drooling of saliva. Such children are frequently far more depressed than those with other disabling childhood diseases, such as Duchenne dystrophy.

The gait of these children may be quite remarkable as the weakness becomes more severe. In order to maintain the balance, the head is often thrown

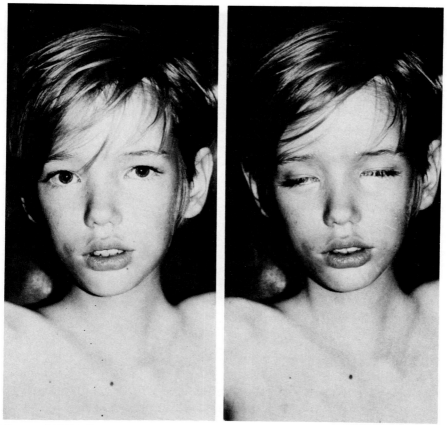

Figures 4.50 (*left*) and 4.51 (*right*). Infantile facioscapulohumeral dystrophy. This boy has had marked weakness of the face since birth. When he attempts to close his eyes tightly and to bare his teeth (Fig. 4.51), the sclera are still showing and he could not move his mouth at all.

backwards. The sacral shelf is horizontal with an extraordinary lumbar lordosis, which causes the buttocks to jut backwards (Figs. 4.52–4.54). The legs are spindly and the knees are locked in hyperextension at each step. The child walks across the room like a flamingo picking its way through shallow water.

Nerve deafness is a common associated finding, although the cause of this and its association with the disease is not clear (3).

The inheritance of this severe form of infantile muscular dystrophy is interesting. In all except one of the patients whom we have seen so far with this illness, there are no overt cases of facioscapulohumeral dystrophy in the parents (3). However, one parent always has mild facial weakness. This may be either the father or mother of the patient, and usually on examination they have the full pouting mouth characteristic of facioscapulohumeral dystrophy. On occasion, such parents have been noted to sleep with their eyes open and have had difficulty with whistling or with drinking through a straw, but again this is often not regarded as an abnormality. In the same family, severe and mild cases are present in both the same and different generations. However, the invarible occurrence of the mild, subclinical variety in a parent

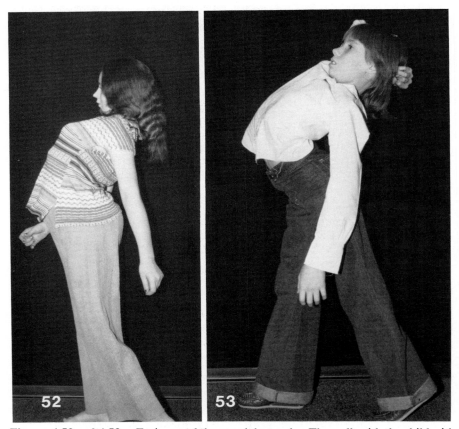

Figures 4.52 and 4.53. Facioscapulohumeral dystrophy. The walk with the child with the infantile variety of facioscapulohumeral dystrophy is rather typical and illustrated by these photographs.

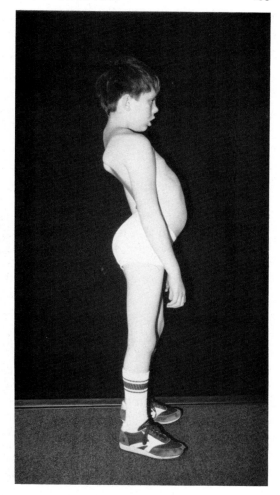

Figure 4.54. The stance of this child is also characteristic, a deep hollow appears in the lower part of the back associated with a pronounced pelvic tilt.

of a child with the severe infantile type requires more explanation and raises the possibility of a modifying gene, perhaps in the other parent.

Coats Syndrome and Facioscapulohumeral Dystrophy

Three reports documented the concurrence of exudative telangiectasia of the retina (Coats syndrome) with facioscapulohumeral dystrophy (4–6). In addition to the muscular weakness, the patients also had sensorineural hearing loss. The hearing loss was severe and bilateral and the patients communicated by lip-reading. Two of the patients reported had a definite family history of the illness and, in one case, this was autosomal dominant although the full syndrome was not always expressed. The telangiectasia is secondary to a loss of the vascular endothelium and the accumulation of PAS positive material in the basement membrane. The weakened vessel then undergoes aneurysmal dilatation and a progressive telangiectasia with fluid accumulation beneath the retina ensues. The importance in recognizing the possibilty of Coats disease is that it may be a treatable condition and the early recognition and photocoagulation of the abnormal vessels may prevent the visual loss. In these patients loss of vision is doubly tragic since the patient is then only able to communicate with the outside world by touch.

Facioscapulohumeral Dystrophy with Late Exacerbation

This variety of facioscapulohumeral dystrophy is more difficult to document. What follows is tentative, and post mortem confirmation is lacking. There are some patients who have a lifelong mild weakness of the face, perhaps with an inability to blow up balloons or difficulty with whistling. At some stage in their life, they may undergo a sudden and rapid deterioration, such that within a matter of 2–3 years they have difficulty walking, and even require the use of a wheelchair. Both the hip and shoulder muscles are involved. Although this sudden deterioration may occur at any time, it is more common in middle life. Obviously, the differential diagnosis includes any of the inflammatory myopathies as well as some of the rapid, progressive varieties of limb girdle dystrophy. The lifelong facial weakness which precedes this worsening, however, suggests that it may be a variety of facioscapulohumeral dystrophy. The picture is complicated by the fact that many such patients have inflammatory changes within their muscles. When treated with steroids they do not show the typical response of patients with polymyositis and the muscle biopsy, although it may reveal an inflammatory response, is different.

Laboratory Studies

Laboratory studies in the investigation of facioscapulohumeral dystrophy usually do no more than confirm the diagnosis. The clinical picture is typical enough and although the serum enzymes are often elevated, the EMG "myopathic," and the muscle biopsy substantiates the diagnosis (Figs. 4.55–4.62), this adds little (other than reassuring the physician) to the management of the patient. However, it is advisable to biopsy all patients with facioscapulohumeral dystrophy, particularly those with a rapidly progressive form of the infantile type. A number of these patients show quite marked inflammatory responses in the biopsy (7, 8) and, when present, a therapeutic trial on steroids is worthwhile. I have never seen any objective improvement from such treatment, but some patients have a symptomatic improvement and claim to be able to walk with more facility, to arise from the floor more easily, and generally feel improved. It is possible that this is a placebo effect, although it is not an effect that we have noted with a placebo, when this has been substituted for the steroids.

Treatment

Treatment of facioscapulohumeral dystrophy follows the usual and general lines for the treatment of neuromuscular diseases. In addition, the possibility of surgical fixation of the scapula should be considered (9). If patients are unable to raise their arms above the horizontal level because of the loss of scapular fixation, they may derive some improvement by surgical attachment of the scapula to the posterior thoracic wall (Figs. 4.63 and 4.64). Unfortunately, such operation is not without complications, and one of the more troublesome is that the scapula may break loose again shortly after the procedure. In many cases, the operation gives considerable benefit. I usually

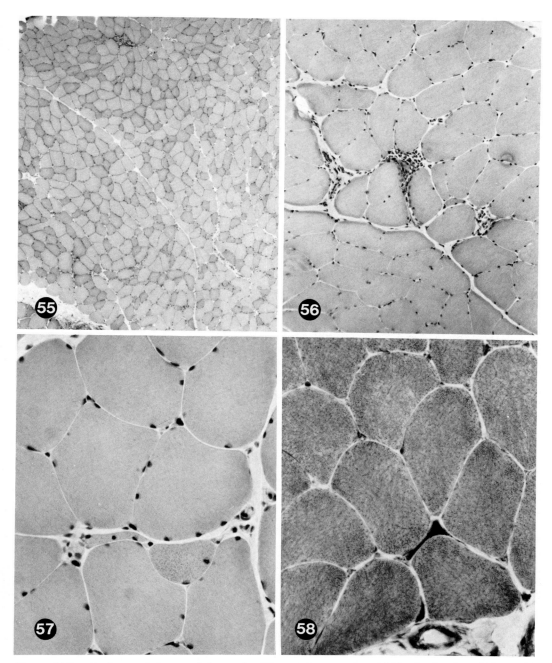

Figure 4.55. Facioscapulohumeral dystrophy. There is increased variability in the size of fibers with small and large fibers being present as shown in the routine hematoxylin and eosin stain. Notice a small cellular response at the extreme top of the photograph.

Figure 4.56. High power view (hematoxylin and eosin stain) illustrates one of the small cellular responses around a necrotic fiber.

Figure 4.57. Notice the presence of some small fibers between more normal sized fibers.

Figure 4.58. These small fibers may be angulated and may be mistaken for denervated fibers. This confusion can be compounded on the oxidative enzyme reaction when they appear to be dark and angulated. Below the obvious angulated fiber is another very small fiber adjacent to a blood vessel. These fibers have a different appearance from ones which are denervated and, for example, are not reactive with the esterase stains. They have been termed "tiny" fibers.

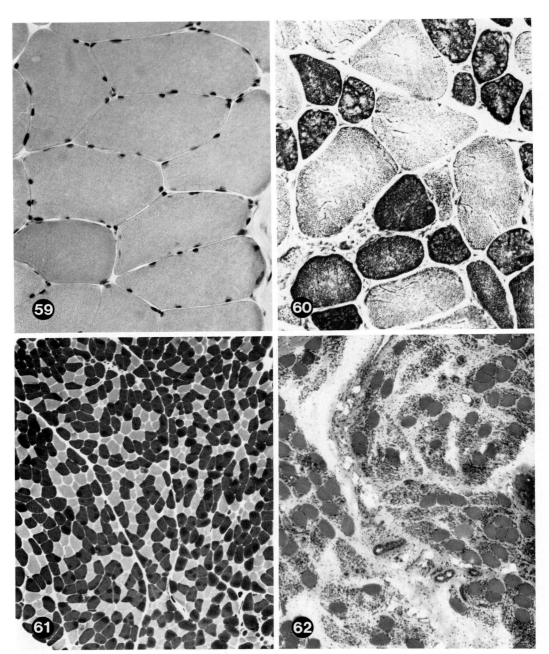

Figure 4.59. In this hematoxylin and eosin stain preparation, there are two nuclei between the two fibers towards the center of the photograph which, on closer inspection, are seen to be associated with two minute fibers. This type of "tiny" fiber is often seen in facioscapulohumeral dystrophy.

Figure 4.60. Another change which is often noted in the illness is the presence of moth-eaten whorled fibers demonstrated by oxidative enzyme reactions. In these fibers the intermyofibrillar network is distorted so that it appears to be whorled after the fashion of an eddying stream. In addition, the enzyme reaction is missing from parts of the fiber.

Figure 4.61. An ATPase stain is illustrated in this preparation and shows the variation in the size of the fibers. Some tiny fibers are visible as small dots with this stain.

Figure 4.62. Facioscapulohumeral dystrophy. In the infantile variety of facioscapulohumeral dystrophy, there is occasionally a pronounced cellular response seen in severely affected muscle.

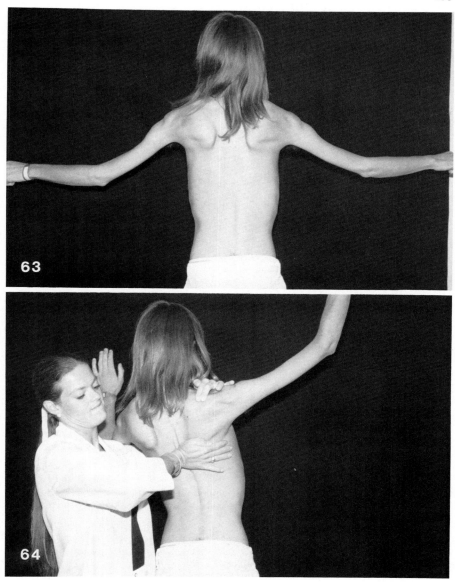

Figures 4.63 and 4.64. One of the functional problems in facioscapulohumeral dystrophy is illustrated in these two photographs. The arm cannot be raised above the level of the shoulder because the scapula floats free from the back and no longer provides a stable base. If the corner of the scapula is pressed firmly on to the thorax and held there by the examiner, the patient can then elevate his hand above the head. This observation provides the basis for recommending surgical fixation in the shoulder in some patients.

recommend surgery on one side only. If it is successful, operation can be considered for the opposite side at some later date. Additionally, useful function of the hand may be restored by providing wrist support when the wrist-drop is marked. If a foot-drop is noticed (Fig. 4.65), ankle supports, either of the shell type or a wire spring brace, should be tried. A review of

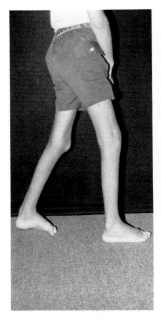

Figure 4.65.   Preservation of strength of the posterior tibal muscle often leads to intorsion of the foot while walking and, eventually, to a permanent equinovarous deformity of the foot.

some of the pertinent clinical literature was published by Kazakov and others (10).

REFERENCES

1. Morton, N. E., and Chung, C. S. Formal genetics of muscular dystrophy. Am. J. Hum. Genet. *11:* 360, 1960.
2. Hanson, P. A., and Rowland, L. P. Moebius syndrome and facioscapulohumeral muscular dystrophy. Arch. Neurol. *24:* 31–39, 1971.
3. Carroll, J. E. and Brooke, M. H. Infantile facioscapulohumeral dystrophy. In: *Peroneal Atrophies and Related Disorders,* edited by G. Serratrice and H. Roux. Masson, New York, 1979.
4. Small, R. E. Coats' disease and muscular dystrophy. Trans. Am. Acad. Opthalmol. Otolaryngol. *72:* 225–231, 1968.
5. Taylor, D. A., Carroll, J. E., Smith, M. E., Johnson, M. O., Johnston, G. P., and Brooke, M. H. Facioscapulohumeral dystrophy associated with hearing loss and Coats' syndrome. Ann. Neurol. *12:* 395–398, 1982.
6. Wulff, J. D., Lin, J. T., and Kepes, J. J. Inflammatory facioscapulohumeral muscular dystrophy and Coats' syndrome. Ann Neurol. *12:* 398–401, 1982.
7. Munsat, T. L., Piper, D., Cancilla, P., and Mednick, J. Inflammatory myopathy with fascioscapulohumeral distribution. Neurology *22:* 335–347, 1972.
8. Dubowitz, V., and Brooke, M. H. *Muscle Biopsy: A Modern Approach.* W. B. Saunders, Philadelphia, 1973.
9. Ketenjiam, A. Y. Scapulocostal stabilization for scapular winging in facioscapulohumeral dystrophy. J. Bone Joint Surg. *60A:* 476–480, 1978.
10. Kazakov, V. M., Bogorodinsky, D. K., Znoyko, Z. V., and Skorometz, A. A. The facioscapulo-limb (or the facioscapulohumeral) type of muscular dystrophy. Eur. Neurol. *11:* 236–260, 1974.

EMERY-DREIFUSS DISEASE
(HUMEROPERONEAL MUSCULAR DYSTROPHY)

This is another of the X-linked recessive disorders, one in which the muscle weakness is associated with other findings and a rather characteristic picture (1–3). Wasting and weakness of a predominantly scapulohumeroperoneal distribution is associated with contractures of the elbows, the posterior part of the neck, and of the Achilles tendon (Figs. 4.66 and 4.67). The muscle weakness seems to be only slowly progressive, but the development of cardiac conduction abnormalities may present a major threat to life. Occasionally a similar clinical picture may be inherited as an autosomal dominant disease (4).

The disease seems to be present during the first decade of life, but is sometimes not apparent to the patient perhaps because the slow progression causes so little change in function. The tendency to walk on the toes and the development of elbow contractures are among the first noticeable manifestations. The weakness is peculiarly of the biceps and triceps and of the peroneal muscles. The deltoids remain relatively strong, as they do in facioscapulohumeral dystrophy. The contractures of the the back of the neck, which prevent more than a few degrees of flexion are often noted only in the doctor's office. Contractures themselves are not unusual in muscle disease. Many of the dystrophies, and particularly the very early onset dystrophies, have marked neck contractures. Contractures of the elbows, however, are less

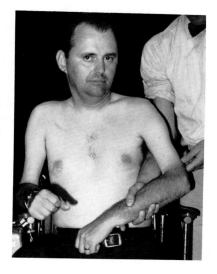

Figure 4.66. Emery-Dreifuss syndrome. This man with a facioscapulohumeral distribution of weakness had associated elbow contractures and heart block. The elbow is shown in maximum extension.

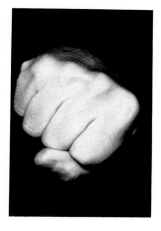

Figure 4.67. Emery-Dreifuss syndrome. Other ligaments may be unusually prominent as illustrated by the tight band joining the second and third metacarpal heads.

common and in the Emery-Dreifuss disease an attempt to straighten the elbows out meets a rock-hard resistance which feels more like an ankylosis (which it isn't) than the firm resistance of contracted tendons. Patients with severe weakness often have contractures of joints which are lying relatively immobile. This cannot be the cause in the patient with Emery-Dreifuss disease since the elbows lock at a time when the patient is still active. Furthermore, there is thickening and contractures of other ligaments in the body which are quite removed from major joints. If the patient is asked to clench the fist, the normally pliable connection between the metacarpal heads stands out like whipcord.

Cardiac abnormalities are so constant that they should be diligently sought for even if the patient shows no evidence of them at the initial visit. Atrioventricular blocks of varying degrees occur, often associated with dropped beats. The installation of a cardiac pacemaker may obviously be essential in such situations. Sudden death, presumably on the basis of acute heart block, has been described in some of the patients.

Other laboratory tests may be of diagnostic value, but perhaps not as much as the typical constellation of clinical findings. The muscle biopsy has been described as myopathic, in association with Type 1 predominance and Type 1 atrophy. This finding generally suggests an illness which occurs early in life. There has been discussion in the literature as to whether the illness may be myogenic or neuropathic, or perhaps consists of both types. The published photographs of the muscle biopsies from these patients, as well as my own experience, would suggest that this is a "myopathic" disease although some of the published changes have been interpreted as neurogenic.

Electromyography has been thought, in some, to demonstrate myopathic and, in others, neurogenic changes, suggesting that there may be two distinct entities giving rise to the same picture. I have learned painfully over the years not to argue with electromyographers about the significance of their findings. Suffice it to say that the EMG in Emery-Dreifuss disease may have some denervating features, but if the student wishes to observe the classic EMG of denervation, he would be better advised to look for a patient with amyotrophic lateral sclerosis or spinal muscular atrophy rather than Emery-Dreifuss disease. It is difficult to know whether the boundaries between Emery-Dreifuss and several of the other early dystrophies will sharpen or blur as time goes by. There are certainly other patients whose posterior cervical contractures and elbow contractures are as severe as those in Emery-Dreifuss disease. Equally, there are other diseases with cardiac conduction defects, nor is the scapulohumeral distribution of weakness particularly unusual. On the other hand, the confluence of these findings in the same patient does, at present, allow the clinician to pop the diagnosis into a neat pigeon hole even though he is no closer to understanding the illness or curing the patient.

REFERENCES

1. Rowland, L. P., Fetell, M., Olarte, M., Hayes, A., Singh, N., and Wanat, F. E. Emery-Dreifuss muscular dystrophy. Ann. Neurol. *5:* 111–117, 1979.
2. Emery, A. E. H., and Dreifuss, F. E. Unusual type of benign x-linked muscular dystrophy. J. Neurol. Neurosurg. Psychiatry *29:* 338–342, 1966.
3. Hopkins, L. C., Jackson, J. A., and Elsas, L. J. Emery-Dreifuss humeralperoneal muscular dystrophy: an x-linked myopathy with unusual contractures and bradycardia. Ann. Neurol *10:* 230–237, 1981.

4. Miller, R. G., Layzer, R. B., Mellenthin, M. A., Golabi, M., Francoz, R. A., Mall, J. C. Emery Dreifuss muscular dystrophy with autosomal dominant transmission. Neurology *35:* 1230–1232, 1985.

SCAPULOPERONEAL DYSTROPHY

Scapuloperoneal dystrophy is probably a variety of facioscapulohumeral dystrophy. In any one case it may be quite difficult to decide which of the two diagnoses is appropriate. In the scapuloperoneal syndrome, the muscles which are involved early are those of the peroneal and anterior tibial group. Foot-drop is among the initial complaints. This is followed shortly by shoulder weakness, which is typically of the type associated with facioscapulohumeral dystrophy (Figs. 4.68 and 4.69). In approximately one-half of the patients there is also associated facial weakness and in this instance the differential diagnosis may not only be difficult but irrelevant. The disease is often inherited as an autosomal dominant, but an X-linked recessive pattern has also been described (1, 2).

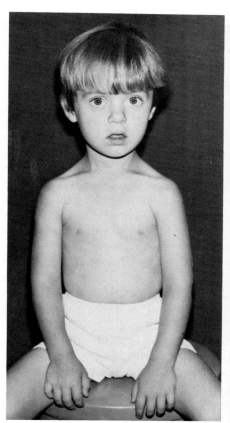 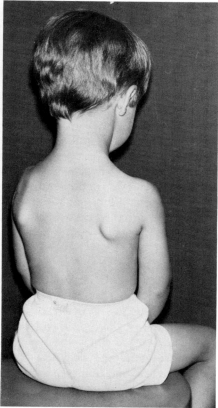

Figures 4.68 (*left*) and 4.69 (*right*). Scapuloperoneal dystrophy. The typical patient with scapuloperoneal dystrophy closely resembles the patient with facioscapulohumeral dystrophy in the apperance of the shoulders. This boy has an abnormal shoulder configuration even though he has little detectable weakness. The clavicles slope downward, the arms are internally rotated with skin creases running upward from the axillae (Fig. 4.68). The inferomedial angles of the scapulae are prominent (Fig. 4.69). His father had classical scapuloperoneal dystrophy.

The importance in the consideration of this diagnosis lies in the fact that other illnesses may mimic scapuloperoneal dystrophy. Perhaps it would be more appropriate to use the term scapuloperoneal syndrome until a definitive diagnosis is made. Nemaline myopathy may present in the adult in this fashion, and perhaps denervating diseases may also cause such a syndrome. It can be quite difficult to distinguish patients whose weakness is limited to the peroneal and anterior tibial muscles from those with hereditary motor neuropathy. Inspection of the extensor digitorum brevis over the dorsum of the foot may be helpful. The muscle is usually atrophic in chronic peripheral neuropathy but is often hypertrophic in the scapuloperoneal syndrome. This is due to the fact that the patient uses the muscle in a futile attempt to dorsiflex the foot. The toes are than drawn upwards, an action which can be seen when the patient walks.

Treatment of the illness is again symptomatic, and ankle supports may be of great help.

REFERENCES

1. Thomas, P. K., Schott, G. D., and Morgan-Hughes, J. A. Adult onset scapuloperoneal myopathy. J. Neurol. Neurosurg. Psychiatry *38:* 1008–1015, 1975.
2. Thomas, P. K., Calne, D. B., and Elliott, C. F. X-linked scapuloperoneal syndrome. J. Neurol Neurosurg. Psychiatry *35:* 208–215, 1972.

HEREDITARY DISTAL MYOPATHY

Of the varieties of muscular dystrophy which affect the distal muscles early, only myotonic dystrophy comes readily to mind. Most of the other forms of neuromuscular disease with predominantly distal involvement are due to denervation. An exception is an illness which was first clearly described by Welander (1). This disease has also been associated with Gowers' name, although his patients may well have had myotonic dystrophy. It is common in Sweden, but is less frequently seen in the rest of the world. Inheritance is as an autosomal dominant with an onset usually between 40 and 60 years of age, when the hand becomes clumsy and fine movements difficult. Once the hand weakness is noticed there is often a slow progression with spread of the illness to the feet and the anterior tibial compartment muscles. Even when no symptoms are noted, examination often shows a mild weakness of the distal muscles of the leg. In Welander's series, the disease was almost completely limited to these muscles, with less than 10% showing weakness of proximal muscles, wrist flexors, or foot plantar flexors. Although there is some disability, the typical case does not progress to total incapacity. Among those few whose illness begins with weakness of the feet, either alone or associated with hand weakness, there is more likelihood that the disease will be progressive and that proximal as well as distal muscles will be involved in this progression. Welander also suggested that there is a homozygous form which commences earlier in life, results in widespread muscle weakness, and has a more rapid course (2).

Reports of the same or a similar entity have appeared from other parts of the world. In general, such reports have stressed that the disease may appear at an earlier age and may produce more generalized weakness even though the distal weakness and late onset pattern remains the more typical presentation. Furthermore in these cases, the initial weakness is often in the feet. The inheritance is not always dominant and autosomal recessive patterns have been noted (12). The literature on this illness has been reviewed (3). Table 4.2 summarizes the findings in the reports of the more typical cases.

Examination of the patient shows wasting of the small muscles of the hand, particularly of thenar eminence. The patient cannot extend the fingers fully, and an attempt to do this produces a posture in which the fingers are held in dissimilar positions (Fig. 4.70). There may be a wrist drop, and the wasting of the wrist extensors produces an oblique groove across the posterior surface of the forearm. Wasting of the intrinsic muscles of the feet and of the anterior tibial and peroneal muscles is less common, as mentioned. The deep tendon reflexes are often preserved early in the disease, diminishing particularly at the ankles and wrists as the diseases progresses. There is usually no sensory abnormality and, if such is found, the possibility of peripheral neuropathy should be entertained. In the younger patients there is often marked atrophy of the gastrocnemius and, when this is combined with anterior tibial weakness, walking may be impossible without ankle stabilization.

Laboratory studies which may be of value include muscle biopsy (4, 5, 10–12), which shows changes suggestive of a myopathy with vacuolar changes. With the acid phosphatase reaction the fibers are often peppered with small punctate reactive areas (Figs. 4.71–4.74). The EMG demonstrates "myopathic" potentials. Motor end point biopsies fail to show any significant abnormality of the distal innervation (6). Serum creatine phosphokinase levels may be normal or slightly elevated. Postmortem studies are rare, but those described by Markesberry et al. (4) show involvement of the cardiac musculature as well as the skeletal musculature. Symptoms of cardiomyopathy are rarely described in the reports. The treatment for this illness is again supportive with recommendation for the appropriate bracing.

REFERENCES

1. Welander, L. Myopathia distalis tarda hereditaria. Acta Med. Scand. Suppl. *265:* 1–124, 1951.
2. Welander, L. Homozygous appearance of distal myopathy. Acta Genet. *7:* 321–324, 1957.
3. Kratz R., and Brooke, M. H. *Distal Myopathy*, edited P. J. Vinken, G. W. Bruyn, and S. P. Ringel. North-Holland, Amsterdam), 1979, pp. 471–483.
4. Markesbery, W. R., Griggs, R. C., Leach, R. P., and Lapham, L. W. Late onset, hereditary distal myopathy, Neurology *24:* 127–134, 1974.
5. Edström, L. Histochemical and histopathological changes in skeletal muscle in late onset hereditary distal myopathy (Welander). J. Neurol. Sci. *26:* 147–157, 1975.
6. Sumner, D., Crawfurd, M. d'A., and Harriman, D. G. F. Distal muscular dystrophy in an English family. Brain *94:* 51–60, 1971.
7. Barrows, M. S., and Duemler, L. P. Late distal myopathy. Report of a case. Neurology *12:* 547–550, 1962.
8. Magee, K. E., and De Jong, R. N. Hereditary distal myopathy with onset in infancy. Arch. Neurol. *13:* 387–390, 1965.
9. Van Der Does de Willebois, A. E. M., Bethlem, J., Meyer, A. E. F. H., and Simons, J. R. Distal myopathy with onset in early infancy. Neurology *18:* 383–390, 1968.
10. Markesbery, W. R., Griggs, R. C., and Herr, B. Distal myopathy; electron microscopic and histochemical studies. Neurology *27:* 727–735, 1977.
11. Kumamoto, T., Fukuhara, N., Nagashima, M., Kanda T., and Wakabayashi, M. Distal myopathy. Histochemical and ultrastructural studies. Arch. Neurol. *39:* 367–371, 1982.
12. Nonaka, I., Sunohara, N., Satoyoshi, E., Terasawa K., and Yonemoto, K. Autosomal recessive distal muscular dystrophy: a comparative study with dystal myopathy with rimmed vacuole formation. Ann. Neurol. *17:* 51–59, 1985.

Table 4.2. Distal Myopathy[a]

Author(s)	Case No.	Sex	Onset Age	Duration in Years	Involvement and Spread	F.H.	EMG	NCV	Muscle Biopsy	Other Findings
Swedish Type										
Welander (1951) (1)	249	M/F = 3/2	20–77	0–44	Hands 192 cases, feet 17 cases, hands and feet 6 cases	244 cases + 5 cases	Myopathic	0	Myopathic	
Barrows and Duemler (1962) (7)	1	M	59	8	Hands→feet	+	Myopathic	0	Myopathic	
Non-Swedish Type										
Magee and De Jong (1965) (8)	1	M	2	38	Feet→hands→thighs	+	Myopathic	N	Myopathic	No progression after age 16
	2	M	2	10	Feet	+	0	0	0	
	3	M	1	26	Feet→hands	+	0	0	0	Possible proximal muscle involvement
Van der Does de Willebois et al. (1968) (9)	1	M	Childhood	35+	Feet→hands	+	Myopathic	N	Myopathic	↑ DH5
	2	M	2	6	Feet	+	Myopathic	0	0	
	3	M	1	4	Feet	+	0	0	0	
Heyck et al. (1968)	1	F	Birth	35	Feet→hands	−	Myopathic	N	Myopathic	
Markesbery et al. (1974) (4)	1	M	51	25	Feet→hands→limb girdles	+	Myopathic	N	Myopathic	No significant CNS findings at autopsy

Reference	No.	Sex	Age	Onset	Distribution	F.H.	EMG	NCV	Biopsy	Enzymes
	2	M	50	18	Feet→hands→thighs and arms	+	Myopathic	N	"End stage" muscle	
Markesbery et al. (1977) (10)	3	M	~40	~6	Feet→lower legs	+	Myopathic	N	Myopathic	
	1	M	20	7	Feet→lower legs→hands	−	Myopathic	N	Myopathic	CPK, LDH + SGOT ↑
	2	M	19	8	Feet→lower legs→biceps	−	Myopathic	N	Myopathic	CPK, LDH + SGOT ↑
Edström (1975) (5)	13	No details				10 cases + 3 cases	Myopathic	0	Myopathic	

[a] F.H. = family history; EMG = electromyography; NCV = nerve conduction velocities; F = female; M = male; 0 = not done; N = normal. (From R. Kratz and M. H. Brooke: *Distal Myopathy*, edited by P. J. Vinken, et al., North-Holland, Amsterdam, 1979.)

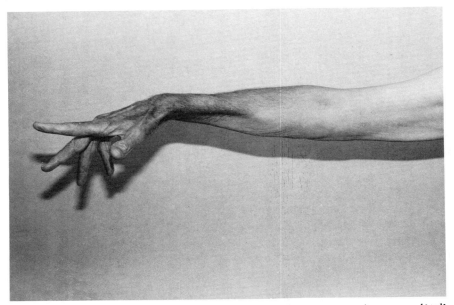

Figure 4.70.   The patient is being asked to extend the fingers and wrist as completely as he can. The finger extensors are variably affected and the fingers adopt different postures. The distal wasting of the muscles is also apparent. (Distal myopathy.)

LIMB-GIRDLE DYSTROPHY

It is difficult to write of limb-girdle dystrophy with much conviction or enthusiasm since the term probably denotes a collection of illnesses with various etiologies. Only the common occurrence of a progressive weakness of the hips and shoulders has resulted in their being considered as a single entity. While it is true that the muscle biopies from such patients are rather similar, this is at best a tenuous connecting thread. In other respects the patients' illnesses differ widely. There is variety in the mode of inheritance, the age of onset, and the progression of the illness, as well as in the distribution of weakness, which seems to underline the need for reappraisal.

Many cases are sporadic, but an autosomal recessive pattern of inheritance is not unusual. When the disease occurs in a family, the various members of the family seem to have the same type of illness, and even the sporadic cases of the disease may conform to one of several general patterns. Perhaps the commonest of these has its onset during the second or third decade. The illness begins with weakness of the hips, and the symptoms are in no way different from other illnesses causing hip weakness. At about the same time, or shortly thereafter, the patient notices shoulder weakness and the illness progresses so that within 20 years after the onset walking will be difficult, if not impossible. Although the patient is confined to a wheelchair, the skeletal deformities so common in some of the other forms of neuromuscular disease are not frequent. Death may occur from cardiopulmonary complications and terminal pneumonia.

In another version of the disease, the weakness is not noted until the fourth decade or even later, but this late onset does not always mean a good prognosis. In some patients there is a rapid progression of the weakness with

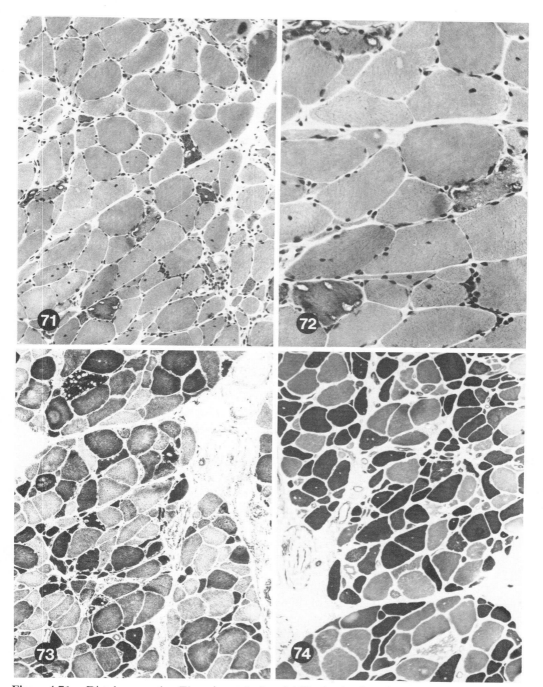

Figure 4.71. Distal myopathy. There is marked variability in the size of the fibers, some fibrosis and a few internal nuclei. Several of the fibers contain characteristic "vacuoles" which are edged with basophilic material. These are termed "rimmed vacuoles" and probably correspond autophagic vacuoles seen with the electron microscope. The biopsy from patients with distal myopathy shows many similarities with those of patients with oculopharyngeal dystrophy and with inclusion body myositis.

Figure 4.72. High power view of the same biopsy to show the rimmed vacuoles in greater detail.

Figure 4.73. The fibers which contain the vacuoles are intensely stained. Otherwise there are only mild changes in the intermyofibrillar network pattern in this oxidative enzyme stain (NADH-tetrazolium reductase).

Figure 4.74. The routine ATPase reaction confirms the variation in the size of fibers. This is neither predominance in one type of fiber nor is there any selective atrophy of a fiber type.

an inability to walk within 3 years of the onset of the disease. The majority of such patients exhibit an autosomal recessive inheritance of the disease. In yet other patients, the disease seems to be predominantly of the hips and thighs or of the shoulders and arms, leading to the term pelvifemoral dystrophy for the one and scapulohumeral dystrophy for the other. These varieties are usually associated with a better prognosis. As in some other neuromuscular diseases, the illness is named for the muscle groups in which the weakness commences. This does not imply that the muscles outside of these groups are uninvolved, and in the terminal stages of the illness the muscles of the lower legs, forearms, and hands are weak, too.

Rarely, families with an autosomal dominant pattern of inheritance have been found and, equally unusually, limb-girdle dystrophy may present in the first decade. Occasionally mild weakness of the face is seen; if facial weakness is severe, consideration should be given to the diagnosis of facioscapulohumeral dystrophy. Involvement of the tongue or pharynx is not part of the illness. Sensory symptoms are absent, and other muscular symptoms such as myoglobinuria or muscle pain are also lacking. Many patients with limb-girdle dystrophy suffer from severe and intractable low back pain. Unless there are associated signs of nerve compression, surgical intervention is usually inadvisable and may indeed exacerbate the pain. The weakness of the lumbar muscles which predisposes to the development of low back pain is not reversed by operation and the instability of the lumbar spine may well be worsened by any surgical maneuver.

Examination of the patient shows the usual abnormalities of gait associated with either hip or shoulder weakness. There may be weakness of the neck muscles, both flexors and extensors. The set of the shoulders may be abnormal. The tips are depressed, giving a webbed appearance to the neck, and the clavicles slope downwards. There is often a crease running from the axilla diagonally toward the neck. This is produced by the shoulders folding forward as scapular fixation is lost; the crease is accentuated by the atrophy of the underlying pectoral muscles. The pattern of weakness is different from that seen in facioscapulohumeral dystrophy (q.v.) since in the latter the strength of the deltoid muscle may be relatively preserved. Similarly, winging of the scapula may be seen, but the tendency of the scapula to ride up over the back and appear as a prominence in the trapezius when viewed from in front is not marked in limb-girdle dystrophy. Preferential weakness and atrophy of the biceps is a useful diagnostic sign (Fig. 4.75). Although not pathognomonic of limb-girdle dystrophy, it is noted frequently in even mild cases. The degree of wasting may be so pronounced that a concavity appears in the upper arm where the biceps should normally be.

The pattern of weakness in the hips is not so characteristic. Both hip flexors and extensors as well as the paravertebral muscles are involved, and the quadriceps and hamstrings share this involvement. Deep tendon reflexes are usually depressed at the elbows and knees early in the illness. Intellectual difficulty is not present and other complications, such as cardiac conduction defects, are rare.

The differential diagnosis includes any of the causes of proximal weakness and it is axiomatic that, if the diagnosis of limb girdle dystrophy can be made,

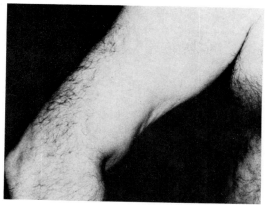

Figure 4.75. Severe wasting of the biceps is not infrequently seen in limb girdle dystrophy. Instead of the normal muscle belly a concavity is noted.

juvenile spinal muscular atrophy should also be considered. The selective absence of the biceps may be helpful in making the diagnosis of limb-girdle dystrophy, whereas the occurrence of more than an occasional fasciculation would suggest spinal muscular atrophy.

Laboratory studies that may be helpful include the usual abnormalities of serum creatine phosphokinase and lactic dehydrogenase. The elevation of these enzymes is seldom spectacular, but it may occasionally be increased by a factor of 10. Electromyography reveals the presence of small, short poly-phasic potentials. There may be bizarre high frequency discharges, but in general the pattern is a "myopathic" one. Muscle biopsy shows considerable variation in the size of fibers, coupled with numerous internal nuclei and fiber splitting. Moth-eaten, whorled fibers are usually profuse (Figs. 4.76–4.81).

There are probably many conditions causing a proximal myopathy and, as more sophisticated methods of evaluation become possible, it is likely that we will discover more and more conditions of known etiology which we can split off from the heterogeneous collection called limb girdle dystrophy. A measure of my open hostility to this whole entity can be deduced from the lack of bibliographic references for this particular section.

OCULAR MYOPATHIES

There are three types of neuromuscular disease in which the eye muscles are involved and which share many features in common. These are ocular dystrophy, oculopharyngeal dystrophy, and oculocraniosomatic neuromuscular disease with ragged red fibers. As to the first of these, I have not knowingly seen a case and I shall only parrot what has appeared in the literature. My experience with the second entity involves a number of patients, but since they are probably all derived from a common genetic background in a Spanish-American population in the United States, it may not be readily applicable to other areas. The third entity seems to be the subject of great controversy. It is not that the clinical picture remains unclear, but uncertainty remains as to the name by which the disease should be known. A further

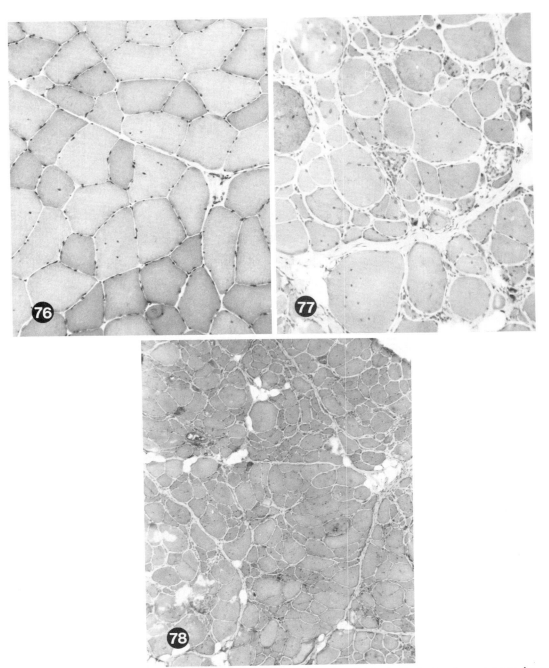

Figure 4.76. Limb-girdle dystrophy. In spite of the fact that limb-girdle dystrophy seems to be a collection of heterogeneous diseases there is one particular type of biopsy which is often associated with these patients and this is illustrated in the following figures. In the early stages of limb-girdle dystrophy there is the same increased variability in the size of fibers that characterizes many of the dystrophies. In addition, a slightly increased amount of fibrous tissue is present between the fibers. The sarcolemmal nuclei have moved from their normal position at the periphery of the fiber to become centralized.

Figure 4.77. Internal nuclei are readily seen. Splitting of fibers is often associated with this change.

Figure 4.78. An advanced stage of the illness. There is more variation in the size of the fibers, internal nuclei are profuse, and careful inspection shows many of the fibers to be developing lines across them which indicate fiber splitting.

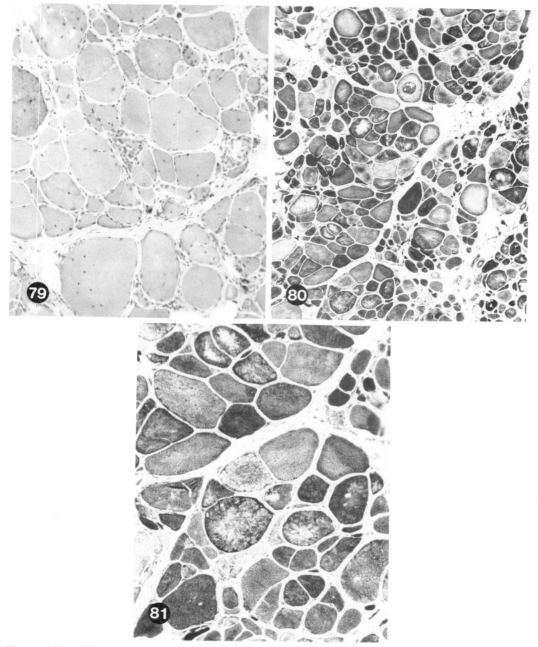

Figure 4.79. Higher power view of the biopsy shown in Figure 4.78 to illustrate some of these features in more detail.
Figures 4.80 and 4.81. Profound change in the intermyofibrillar network is seen, with moth-eaten and whorled fibers in profusion. (NADH-tetrazolium reductase).

description of this last illness is given in the section on metabolic diseases, where it belongs by virtue of the striking abnormalities seen in the mitochondria. Clinically, though, it is often considered in the differential diagnosis of the two preceding illnesses. Although they are called "myopathies," in some instances the proof remains a little shaky. Since the changes of myopathy and denervation are even harder to distinguish in the extraocular muscles than elsewhere, most of the evidence that the ocular diseases are indeed "myopathic" is based on a few postmortem studies showing normal brainstem neurons. In view of these circumstances, this section is undertaken with temerity since it is guaranteed to please no one and irritate many.

Ocular Dystrophy

The existence of a form of dystrophy causing ptosis and weakness of the extraocular muscles has been recognized for many years. Although there are several previous reports, the paper of Kiloh and Nevin (1) was the first of the modern papers delineating this entity. The ptosis usually precedes the weakness of the eye muscles and, although it may occur at any age, the onset is much more common the first 20–30 years of life (2). The symptoms are caused by drooping of the eyelids which interferes with vision. It is rare for diplopia to be a complaint. The disease is slowly progressive over many years and, although it may be limited to the eye muscles in some stage of the disease, there is always evidence of involvement of other muscle groups later on. Facial weakness is probably most common; a number of patients also have weakness in the limbs. Even those without overt weakness may have areflexia or an abnormal muscle biopsy. An unusual aspect of ocular myopathy is the curare sensitivity reported by Ross (3) and by Matthew et al. (4). Some patients with ocular myopathy have developed profound ptosis, extraocular palsies, and weakness of the neck and limbs with small doses of curare. This raises a difficult diagnostic problem. Patients with myasthenia who have extraocular weakness also have an extreme sensitivity to curare. If weakness of the eye muscle is the only major expression of the myasthenia, the diagnosis may be quite difficult to prove since the extraocular palsies may not respond to the administration of edrophonium or neostigmine. Differentiating a patient with ocular dystrophy from one with a congenital myasthenic syndrome may be a real clinical conundrum and on more than one occasion has proved impossible. Ross (3) felt that the entity, ocular myopathy, was nevertheless a real one. It differed from myasthenia since there was a long and slowly progressive history of eye findings which did not wax and wane and which was succeeded by an equally unvarying weakness of the limbs without any of the bulbar signs of myasthenia. Whatever the solution to this diagnostic dilemma, if surgery is to be considered in patients with ocular myopathy, the possibility of abnormal sensitivity to curare should be emphasized.

The disease is often inherited as an autosomal dominant. Occasional sporadic cases and cases with autosomal recessive inheritance have also been described. On examination, the weakness is commonly severe enough to produce a total paralysis of the eye muscles. The marked ptosis causes the patient to retroflex the head. The pupillary responses are normal. Treatment is symptomatic and is aimed at the relief of the ptosis. This may involve surgery or the use of eyelid crutches.

A significant number of the patients who have been diagnosed as having ocular myopathy may complain of dysphagia, thus the entity merges with the following one, oculopharyngeal dystrophy. The only case I have seen which could have been classified clinically as a relatively pure ocular myopathy (ptosis, extraocular palsies, and mild facial weakness beginning in the 20s) was in fact a member of a large family with many members suffering from classical oculopharyngeal dystrophy.

Oculopharyngeal Dystrophy

An illness which is perhaps similar but which causes more widespread abnormalities is oculopharyngeal dystrophy (5). This illness, which is usually inherited as an autosomal dominant, is rare in most parts of the world but occurs in circumscribed geographical areas. It is quite common in French Canadian families in Quebec, and the disease has been traced to a common ancestor who landed in Quebec from France in 1634 (2, 6). A similar large focus is found among Spanish American families in southern Colorado, northern New Mexico, and Arizona.

The illness begins later than the pure ocular dystrophy, with its onset in the third or fourth decade. It has always surprised me that patients with oculopharyngeal dystrophy seem to survive to a great age even in the face of their severe disability. The weakness is frequently asymmetrical: a marked ptosis may develop on one side while the other eyelid is only minimally involved (Figs. 4.82–4.84). Eventually, however, both lids are extremely ptotic, and all extraocular movement is lost, although pupillary responses remain normal. Usually the dysphagia follows the weakness of the eye muscles although in the French Canadian families difficulty with swallowing occurs at the same time as, or even precedes, weakness of the eyes. Most of the patients have some degree of facial weakness and, as the disease slowly worsens, weakness of the hips and shoulders is common. In one report distal weakness of the limbs was associated with ocular myopathy and dysphagia (7). With increasing age the dysphagia becomes incapacitating. Saliva pools in the pharynx and it may be impossible for the patient to swallow any solid foods; even liquid foods present some difficulty. In the face of this, there is considerable weight loss and the patient becomes emaciated. In one patient this emaciation did not respond to the administration of a daily diet of 3500 calories by a nasogastric tube over a period of 4 weeks. The patient still continued to lose weight even though caloric intake should have been sufficient to prevent this.

Examination of the patient will be abnormal, the extent of the abnormality depending upon the stage of the disease. Ptosis, extraocular palsies, and facial weakness are almost always apparent. Weakness and wasting of the masseter muscles may be seen. The tongue may be atrophic, and the pharynx moves poorly. Proximal weakness of the limbs with areflexia is not uncommon. Usually there is no problem in making the diagnosis in view of the strong family history seen in many of these patients. Myotonic dystrophy and myasthenia gravis can give rise to some confusion with this entity, but there are obvious significant differences between oculopharyngeal dystrophy and these two common diseases. Other neuromuscular diseases can present with ptosis and ophthalmoplegia; these vary from myotubular myopathy to oculocraniosomatic neuromuscular disease.

Laboratory studies may be of help. The EMG shows small amplitude

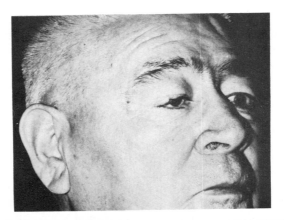

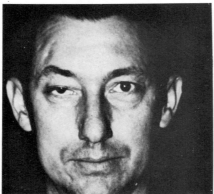

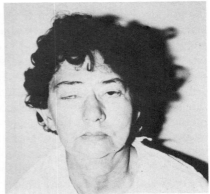

Figures 4.82 through 4.84.   These patients with ocular pharyngeal dystrophy have paralysis of extraocular movement and ptosis. Although the ptosis is bilateral, it is very often assymmetrical as shown here.

polyphasic potentials with short duration. Although electrical evidence of denervation is not customary in oculopharyngeal dystrophy, it has been described and, in one of these cases, was associated with severe axon loss in the peripheral nerves (8, 9).

The serum "muscle" enzymes may be elevated but are seldom more than 3–4 times normal and more usually are within normal limits. EKG abnormalities may be found and vary from conduction deficits to changes suggesting old infarction. Since this population is older than the usual group of patients with neuromuscular disease, the causes should not always be ascribed to the illness.

Microscopic abnormalities of the muscle have been described and include variability in the size of fibers, fibrosis and the presence of rimmed vacuoles which are probably autophagic (Figs. 4.85–4.89) (10). An interesting finding which appears to be pathognomonic of the disease is the appearance of intranuclear filamentous inclusions. These occur only in muscle nuclei and are noted in between 3% and 5% of the nuclei. They are tubular and extend up to 0.25 μm. Their significance is unclear, but they have not been seen in any other illness (11, 12). Radiological studies of swallowing show a hypotonic

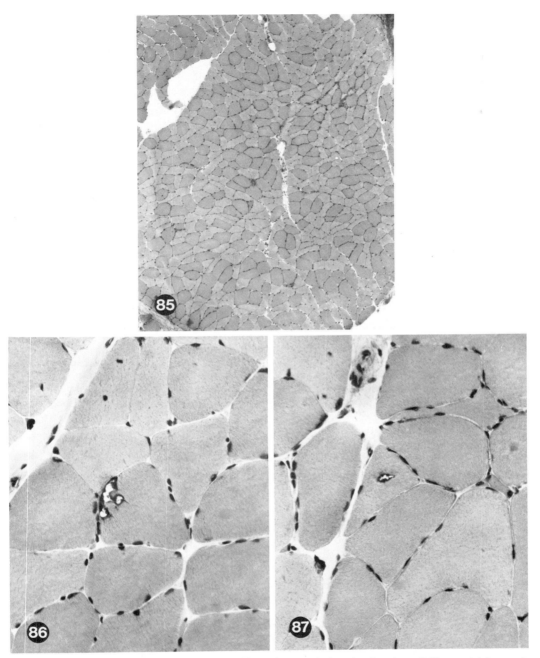

Figure 4.85. Oculopharyngeal dystrophy. There is a variation in the size of fibers which can be readily seen with a routine hematoxylin and eosin stain. Internal nuclei, fibrosis, and fiber splitting are not noted.

Figures 4.86 and 4.87. Many of the fibers contain "rimmed" vacuoles. These are probably autophagic vacuoles and are illustrated here in higher power in Figure 4.87.

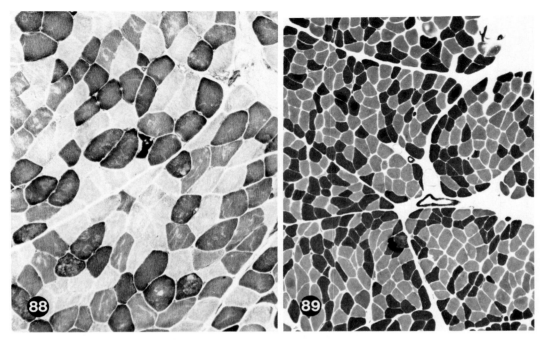

Figure 4.88.   Oxidative enzyme reaction shows occasional moth-eaten changes in the fibers. Fibers containing rimmed vacuoles often stain intensely as illustrated by the slightly small and somewhat angulated fiber in the center of the photograph.

Figure 4.89.   ATPase stains show good fiber type differentiation into Type 1 and Type 2 and show no tendency for one particular fiber type to be affected more then any other.

pharynx with pooling and more importantly, some incoordination of the pharyngoesophageal sphincter (13). The dysphagia caused by the illness has responded in a few patients to cricopharyngeal myotomy (13, 14). Autopsy studies confirm the abnormality in the pharynx where there are severe pathological abnormalities of the striated muscle. There is also evidence that the striated muscle does not extend as far down the esophagus as in the normal patient (15). Abnormalities of smooth muscle were not demonstrated pathologically (16, 17), but investigation of esophageal motility showed abnormalities throughout the length of the esophagus with decreased peristalsis and incoordinate muscle contraction from the pharynx to the lower part of the esophagus, implying that smooth muscle was involved as well as striated muscle.

REFERENCES

1. Kiloh, L. G., and Nevin, S. Progressive dystrophy of the external ocular muscles (ocular myopathy). Brain *74:* 115–143, 1951
2. Bray, G. M., Kaarsoo, N., and Ross, T. Ocular myopathy with dysphagia. Neurology *15:* 678–684, 1965.
3. Ross, R. T. Ocular myopathy sensitive to curare. Brain *86:* 67–76, 1963.
4. Matthew, N. T., Jacob, J. C., and Chandy, J. Familial ocular myopathy with curare sensitivity. Arch. Neurol *22:* 68–74, 1970.
5. Victor, M., Hayes, R., and Adams, R. D. Oculopharyngeal muscular dystrophy: a familial disease of late life characterized by dysphagia and progressive ptosis of the eyelids. New Engl. J. Med. *267:* 1267–1272, 1962.

6. Barbeau, A. The syndrome of hereditary late onset ptosis and dysphagia in French Canada. In: *Progressive Muskeldystrophie Myotonie Myasthenie*, edited by E. Kuhn. Springer, Berlin, 1966, pp. 102–109.
7. Schotland, D. L., and Rowland, L. P. Muscular dystrophy: Features of ocular myopathy, distal myopathy and myotonic dystrophy. Arch. Neurol. *10:* 433–445, 1964.
8. Probst A., Tackmann, W., Stoeckli, H. R., Jerusalem, F., and Ulrich, J. Evidence for a chronic axonal atrophy in oculopharyngeal "muscular dystrophy." Acta Neuropathol. *57:* 209–216, 1982.
9. Schmitt, H. P., and Krause, K. H. An autopsy study of a familial oculopharyngeal muscular dystrophy (OPMD) with distal spread and neurogenic involvement. Muscle Nerve *4:* 296–305, 1981.
10. Brooke, M. H. The differentiation of oculopharyngeal dystrophy from oculocraniosomatic neuromuscular disease: A clinical, pathological correlation. In: *Third Symposium on Neuromuscular Disorders*, edited by Nesvadba. Balnea, Prague, 1973, pp. 107–112.
11. Tome, F. M. and Fardeau, M. Nuclear inclusions in oculopharyngeal dystrophy. Acta Neuropathol. *49:* 85–87, 1980.
12. Coquet, M., Vallat, J. M., Vital, C., Fournier, M., Barat, M., Orgogozo, J. M., Julien, J., and Loiseau, P. Nuclear inclusions in oculopharyngeal dystrophy. An ultrastructural study of six cases. J. Neurol. Sci. *60:* 151–156, 1983.
13. Bender, M. D. Esophageal manometry in oculopharyngeal dystrophy. Am. J. Gastroenterol. *65:* 215–221, 1976.
14. Dayal, V. S., and Freeman, J. Cricopharyngeal myotomy for dysphagia in oculopharyngeal muscular dystrophy. Report of a case. Arch. Otolaryngol. *102:* 115–116, 1976.
15. Little, B. W., and Perl, D. P. Oculopharyngeal muscular dystrophy. An autopsy case from the French-Canadian kindred. J. Neurol Sci. *53:* 145–158, 1982.
16. Roberts, A. H., and Bamforth, J. The pharynx and esophagus in ocular muscular dystrophy. Neurology *18:* 645–652, 1968.
17. Weitzner, S. The histopathology of the pharynx and esophagus in oculopharyngeal muscular dystrophy: case report and literature review. Am. J. Gastroenterol. *56:* 378–382, 1971.

QUADRICEPS MYOPATHY

Occasionally patients are seen who are experiencing moderately severe weakness of the quadriceps group, but who do not demonstrate any other weakness. Electrophysiological and biopsy evidence of myopathy are found and the disease may remain limited to the thigh muscles for many years. This entity has been termed quadriceps myopathy (1, 2). Even though the clinical findings are limited to the quadriceps muscle, there is often pathological evidence of myopathy in other clinically unvolved muscles. Over long periods of time, most of these patients develop weakness in other muscle groups and the illness is almost certainly a variant of the limb-girdle dystrophy group.

REFERENCES

1. Swash, M., and Heathfield, W. Quadriceps myopathy. A variant of the limb girdle dystrophy syndrome. J. Neurol. Neurosurg. Psychiatry *46:* 355–357, 1983.
2. vanWijngaarden, G. K., Hagan, C. J., Bethlem, J., and Meyer, A. E. F. H. Myopathies of the quadriceps muscle. J. Neurol. Sci. *7:* 201–206, 1968.

BRANCHIAL MYOPATHY

Branchial myopathy, causing enlargement of the masseter and temporalis muscles, is something of a medical curiosity. It has been reviewed by Mancall et al. (1). The disorder described was a slightly tender enlargement of the masseter and temporalis muscles, which was sufficient to interfere with the patient's use of glasses and which caused some difficulty in chewing because of the lump inside the cheek. The masses were resected several times and it is difficult to know what to make of the muscle pathology. A subsequent case showed a very asymmetric hypertrophy of the masseter, as well as symmetrical enlargement of the temporalis muscles. Again, the patient's difficulty seemed to be simply that associated with an increased mass in the face. No weakness was noted. It was significant that this patient had an adverse reaction to anesthetic, perhaps reminiscent of the patient with malignant hyperthermia, the stiffness of whose jaw muscles often betrays the onset of an attack during anesthesia. It is totally unclear where this entity should be classified.

REFERENCE

1. Mancall, E. L., Patel, A. N., and Hirschhorn, A. M. Hypertrophic branchial myopathy. Neurology *24:* 1166–1170, 1974.

5 myotonia

Myotonia is found in several illness. In some it plays a dominant part; in others it is overshadowed by different aspects of the disease. Myotonia is a phenomenon in which the relaxation of the muscle, after it contracts, is delayed. Ther period of gradual relaxation may be prolonged over several seconds. Contraction of a myotonic muscle may be produced by mechanical stimulation (e.g., percussion) as well as voluntarily. Electromyography shows repetitive action potentials of the muscle fibers associated with the phase of contraction and relaxation. These trains of potentials may wax and wane in both amplitude and frequency. The phenomenon seems to arise at the sarcolemmal membrane since curare, although obviously preventing the development of myotonia following voluntary activity, does nothing to diminish the myotonia generated by percussion. In addition to human disease, myotonia has also been noted in goats, mice and horses. Experimentally, myotonia has been produced by the administration of 20,25-diazacholesterol, by monocarboxylic aromatic acids, such as the insecticide 2,4-D and 9AC, and by other compounds (1,2).

In many varieties of myotonia, there seems to be a generalized abnormality of membranes, those of the muscle and red blood cells being the most extensively investigated. Not all myotonia arises from the same physiological error. Myotonia congenita, hereditary myotonia in goats, and that produced by the aromatic carboxylic acids are all associated with a decreased ability of the cell membrane to conduct chloride (3–5). The action potential in a normal muscle cell is conducted inward by the transverse tubules. Such a potential is associated with an outflow of potassium which would easily diffuse away from the site if the membrane were a flat open surface. The transverse tubule is not, however, such a structure. It is a narrow tube and accumulation of potassium presents a real problem in disposal. A succession of action potentials might well raise the potassium in the tubules to levels which result in membrane depolarization. Ordinarily this does not present a problem because the chloride conductance is so large and the relatively free passage of chloride ions will negate the effect of any small change in potassium in the extra cellular fluids (6). If chloride conductance is impeded the increased potassium concentration might well lead to a depolarization sufficient to activate the sodium channels again and lead to repetitive electrical discharge of the membrane or myotonia (7). The exact cause of the decreased permeability to chloride is not known, although the fault must lie in the membrane. Several theoretical possibilities are obvious. It could result from a change in the structure of the membrane, such that the chloride channel is altered, or from some compound which blocks the chloride channel.

In light of all this, it is not surprising that the hunt for the cause of myotonia is centered around the membrane. The myotonia associated with 20,25-diazacholesterol is not associated with abnormal chloride conductance. This compound interferes with cholesterol biosynthesis by inhibition of one of the terminal steps in the pathway. Desmosterol is formed instead and this is incorporated into the membrane causing an alteration in the properties of the membrane (8). This may result in failure in inactivation of the sodium channel, leading to repetitive electrical activity (1).

Patients with myotonic dystrophy also seem to demonstrate abnormalities in membrane function, although not the same ones as in the experimental models. The chloride conductance is normal and the specific defect is unknown.

The illnesses which are outlined in this section are myotonic dystrophy, myotonia congenita, and paramyotonia.

MYOTONIC DYSTROPHY

Clinical Aspects

The adult with advanced myotonic dystrophy has an appearance so characteristic that it is hard to mistake it for any of the other neuromuscular illnesses (Figs. 5.1–5.7). The face is drawn and lugubrious, with hollowing of

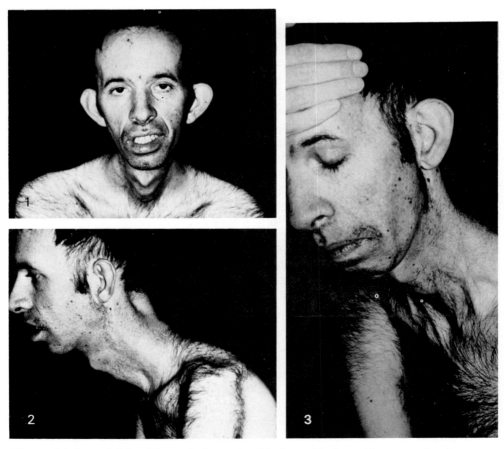

Figures 5.1 through 5.3. Myotonic dystrophy. The long, thin face with temporal and masseter wasting and frontal balding is characteristic (Fig. 5.1). Weakness and wasting of the sternocleidomastoids and other muscles in the neck gives a "swan neck" appearance (Fig. 5.2). When the patient attempts to flex his neck against the examiner's hand, atrophy of the sternocleidomastoid is seen (Fig. 5.3).

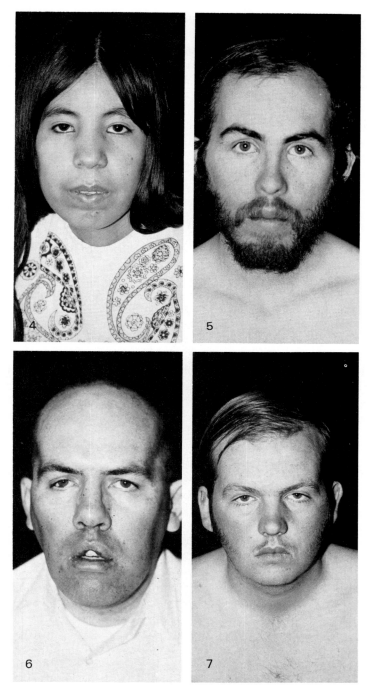

Figures 5.4 through 5.7. Myotonic dystrophy. Various features are to be noted including the elongated face (Figs. 5.4–5.6), the temporal and masseter wasting (Figs. 5.5 and 5.6), and the ptosis (Figs. 5.4, 5.6, and 5.7). Also notice the shape of the patient's mouth in Figure 5.6 and compare it with Figure 5.8.

the muscles around the temples and jaws. The eyes are hooded, the lower lip droops, and the facial weakness imparts a curious sag to the lower part of the face. The wasting of the neck muscles, particularly the neck flexors, gives a slender appearance, and the patient balances his head precariously rather like trying to balance a cherry on top of its stalk. Descriptive terms such as "hatchet-faced" and "swan-necked" have been given to the myotonic patient. It is perhaps the very typical appearance of the fully developed disease which has caused so many of us to miss the diagnosis in its milder forms. Such diagnostic errors are aided and abetted by the patients themselves, who exhibit an unusual degree of denial towards their illness and towards the existence of the same illness in their families. Indeed, I would suspect that almost half of the patients with myotonic dystrophy present with complaints which have nothing to do with their neuromuscular disease. Neither is it unusual to hear a patient with myotonic dystrophy insist that his disease began only 2–3 years ago when the hospital charts document the presence of the illness for decades.

Myotonic dystrophy is inherited as an autosomal dominant condition with a prevalence estimated at between 3 and 5 per 100,000 population and an incidence of 13 per 100,000 live births (5). This makes it one of the commoner neuromuscular disorders. Some have suggested genetic heterogeneity of the illness, with one type occurring early and another later in life (3). In one, the patients are thought to have more severe weakness of the limbs which is often irregularly distributed and facial weakness in proportion to that of the rest of the body. Another variety was characterized by more severe facial weakness and milder limb weakness. The second type is more often associated with mental retardation, male infertility, and neonatally affected children (9). It has also been suggested that neonatal myotonia occurring in the child of a myotonic mother indicates a high risk of subsequent infants having the neonatal form of the disease (10). The contrary view, that the disease is extremely variable and does not represent two genetic populations, has also been expressed (5). My own view is that the unreliability of the clinical and family history obtained from patients with myotonic dystrophy often precludes any hard and fast conclusions being drawn on this basis. I believe that the disease is extremely variable, and I do not see a clear division into different clinical entities in my own practice.

The illness may show some "anticipation" when, with each succeeding generation, the illness appears earlier and is more severe. Part of this reflects the inaccuracy of the myotonic's memory. If an adolescent is seen to suffer from the disease, his parent may very often claim that his own illness lasted but a short while. When this history is taken at face value, then anticipation is surely the rule. On the other hand, there is usually evidence for the parent's illness having lasted much longer than he believes, and in my own experience, the phenomenon of anticipation has been less common than in other series.

Typically, the symptoms of the disease are not noticed until adolescence or early adult life. However, examination of the patient even in the first decade may reveal the presence of myotonia and the characteristic long-faced child with a slightly nasal voice. Although myotonia is noted quite early, it is seldom presented as a complaint by the patient. They may be troubled by some muscle stiffness, cramping pains, or, on occasion, difficulty with relaxing the grasp, but more commonly it is the onset of weakness of the feet and hands which the patient first notices. The weakness increases slowly but steadily and eventually spreads to involve all the muscle groups. Weakness of the flexor muscles of the neck is an early finding, and atrophy of the sternocleidomastoid muscles, which may disappear totally or be present as a thin band, has often been used as a diagnostic clue.

The presence of myotonia upon direct percussion of the muscle is a striking finding in more ways than one. In evaluating myotonia, two aspects should be borne in mind. The first is the tendency for the myotonia to disappear as the weakness progresses. Thus, in patients with severe wasting and weakness of the hands it is preferable to search for myotonia in muscles of the forearm or shoulders. Second, myotonia should never be confused with the normal contraction response which may be produced by percussion of a muscle. This normal response is usually a brief flickering movement of the muscle but may be pronounced enough to cause the joint to move. The delay in relaxation so characteristic of the myotonic is not seen. The symptoms may be accentuated by cold, even through there is no evidence that exposure to cold worsens the electrical activity.

With the passage of time, the voice becomes increasingly dysarthric and nasal and there may be difficulty in swallowing food. It is interesting that the earlier the illness begins, the more severe is the involvement of the bulbar musculature. With increasing handicap the patient is eventually confined to a wheelchair. Death often occurs during the fifth or sixth decade from cardiorespiratory failure. Recurrent dislocation of the jaw may occur. In the typical situation, the patient opens the mouth widely either in yawning or biting an apple, and the jaw remains stuck in this position. This dislocation can often be reduced by the patient and seldom needs further treatment.

In addition to the neuromuscular symptoms, involvement of other organs reflects the fact that myotonic dystrophy is a diffuse disorder. Mild mental retardation is not uncommon and, as already mentioned, there is an odd form of denial in these patients. This is frequently reflected in a suspicious and mildly hostile attitude toward the physician. Further, the multifarious symptoms which are presented by the myotonic patient during a succession of clinic visits can be so baffling and elusive that the physician may be tempted into a similar attitude on occasions. I am ashamed to admit that in my own clinic, any symptom which is not easily explained, has to be presented on two successive occasions before it receives the attention which it probably deserves. This slightly reprehensible suggestion would never have appeared in print were it not that other clinicians with large myotonic practices have expressed similar views to me in private (they, personal communication).

Cataracts are common in myotonic dystrophy. A careful search with the slit lamp will reveal them is almost all cases. Commonly, multihued specks are found in the anterior and posterior subcapsular zones. Other forms of cataracts are also seen and surgical extractions may be necessary.

Endocrine abnormalities include disturbances of hypothalamic, thyroid, pancreatic and gonadal function (11–15). Testicular atrophy is common, with disappearance of the seminiferous tubules. A secondary rise in gonadotrophic hormone occurs in males as a reaction to this. In the female, infertility, habitual abortion, and menstrual irregularities are noted, but no definite hormonal cause has been found. Abnormalities in growth hormone and prolactin secretion have been implicated, but the results of different studies or even different patients within the same study have been so variable it is not clear what the abnormality is.

The incidence of diabetes in patients with myotonic dystrophy is probably only slightly higher than in the general population, if indeed it is at all different. On the other hand, abnormalities of the glucose tolerance test with abnormally high glucose levels, particularly in the late phases of the test, and an overproduction of insulin have been recorded repeatedly (16–18). There are several possible explanations for this, but the choice seems to have narrowed down to abnormalities in the insulin receptor. This has been investigated in several different systems. Glucose uptake into muscle is normally stimulated by insulin. This response is decreased in the forearm muscle of myotonics (19). Increasing the amount of insulin given did not return the response to normal, which implies that it is not merely a matter of an insufficient number of receptors being available to insulin, but that somehow the receptor function is altered. This would, of course, be consistent with an alteration in the cell membrane.

Skin fibroblasts cultured from patients with myotonic dystrophy have also been shown to have decreased insulin binding to the high affinity sites (20). The receptors on circulating mononuclear cells also have an overall decreased affinity for insulin. Unfortunately, the monocytes seem to behave as badly as most of the cells in the blood, and other than the overall impression of an abnormality in insulin binding, the results are inconsistent and often contradictory (16, 21).

Involvement of smooth muscle may be responsible, perhaps, for the increased incidence of gallbladder problems. Patients also complain of mild difficulty with swallowing and radiological studies often show abnormalities even in the absence of syptoms (22). Peristalsis in the hypopharynx, proximal esophagus and, in some patients, in the distal esophagus, is decreased. The upper esophageal sphincter relaxes normally, but again the pressure is decreased. The normal relaxation would indicate an absence of the myotronic phenomenon in the pharynx. The abnormality in esophageal motility probably accounts for the feeling that patients often express of food being caught behind the sternum and is due to weakness and not to myotonia. Although patients frequently complain of chronic constipation and urinary symptoms, these are less clearly associated with abnormalities of smooth muscle function.

Cardiac muscle is also affected in the illness. One of the commoner abnormalities is a conduction defect, such as first degree heart block (PR interval > 0.2 second) and cardiac arrhythmias, which are seen in over half the patients (7). Mitral valve prolapse has been noted in up to 17% of the patients (23). A much more ominous cardiac problem was suggested following radionucleide studies of myocardial function in myotonic muscular dystrophy (24). The normal effect of exercise in men is to increase the excursion in the left ventricular wall and to increase the left ventricular ejection fraction. Patients with myotonic dystrophy had an abnormal response with exercise, with a tendency to balloon out the ventricular wall and decrease the ventricular ejection fraction. This has important implications in recommending exercise to patients with myotonic dystrophy. It will be interesting to see if the finding is confirmed when larger numbers of patients are studied.

Many patients, particularly those who are more severely affected, have a disturbance in their sleep. They tend to doze off frequently during the day time and may sleep for 10–12 hours at night. This may be related to pulmonary hypoventilation. Some have shown a decrease in the central ventilatory response with an absence of the anticipated increase in respiration following increasing carbon dioxide concentrations (25). Others have stressed that the central mechanisms are intact, but that the respiratory muscles are weak to a degree not usually suspected by the clinician and only revealed by more specific testing of respiratory function, such as maximum expiratory pressure (26). When the resting breathing pattern of myotonics is evaluated without the patient being conscious of his breathing, the pattern is often a chaotic one. Perhaps related to the respiratory abnormalities is the increased risk which has been reported with general anesthesia. Patients with myotonic dystrophy may be unduly susceptible to barbiturates and to other medications such as morphine, which may depress the ventilatory drive (27–30).

In infancy, myotonia presents a different clinical picture. When myotonic dystrophy manifests itself in the neonatal period, it may do so without any evidence of myotonia. Indeed, the only clinical findings may be extreme hypotonia and facial paralysis. These children have an oddly shaped mouth with the upper lip, forming an inverted "V," an appearance which has been called the "shark-mouth" (Figs. 5.8 and 5.9). Club feet are also common (Fig. 5.10). The prior pregnancy is often complicated by hydramnios and poor fetal movements. As the children grow older, mental retardation is discovered as a prominent part of the picture, more so than in those whose disease commences later. In one series, the mean IQ of children with neonatal myotonic dystrophy was 66 (31). Frequent respiratory infections are seen at an early age. Clinical myotonia eventually makes it appearance, but may be delayed even until the fifth year or later. One of the unusual aspects is that such children are almost always born to myotonic mothers rather than inheriting the disease from the father (32). Out of 118 patients with congenital myotonic dystrophy, paternal transmission was shown in only 2 cases. This has two implications. The first is that the diagnosis of neonatal myotonic dystrophy is relatively simple to confirm by examination of the child's mother. The second is that, since there is no genetic explanation for this maternal transmission, it must be due to some influence, perhaps intrauterine, of the mother's disease upon the child. Deoxycholic acid has been proposed as a candidate for such a role. Bile acids with side chains longer than usual were detected in the serum of patients with myotonic dystrophy. One is deoxycholic acid (33), the synthesis of which has been demonstrated in human liver through an alternative pathway of cholesterol metabolism. The suggestion of such an abnormality is intriguing in a disease in which the cell membrane has been implicated, since cholesterol plays such an important part in the function of membranes. A second paper confirmed the findings to some extent, but weakened the association between deoxycholic acid and the birth of children with neonatal myotonia (34). Two of three mothers with children

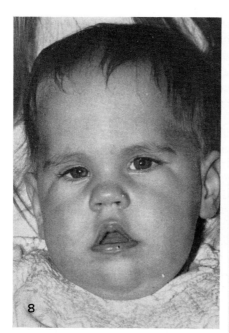

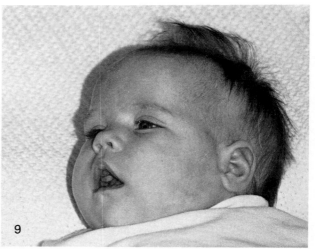

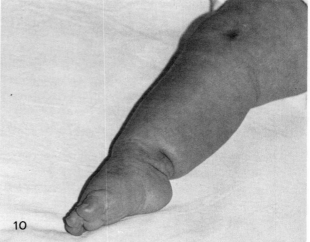

Figures 5.8 through 5.10. Infantile myotonic dystrophy may present a facial diplegia with hypotonia at birth. This is associated with an abnormality of the appearance of the mouth in which the upper lid forms an inverted V (Figs. 5.8 and 5.9). Skeletal abnormalities such as club foot (Fig. 5.10) are also seen.

expressing the neonatal form of myotonia had increased levels of deoxycholic acid. The third, however, had normal levels, and two other women, one of whom had a child with the later onset disease, had slightly increased levels.

Laboratory Studies

The diagnosis of myotonic dystrophy is usually a clinical one and diagnostic laboratory tests are seldom necessary in the advanced case. In the early stages when the weakness is still slight, it may be reassuring to obtain the appropriate studies. Fortunately, in the situation where the patient's disease is mildest, the muscle biopsy is usually the most diagnostic with a combination of internal nuclei and Type 1 fiber atrophy (35) (Figs. 5.11–5.19). This is also

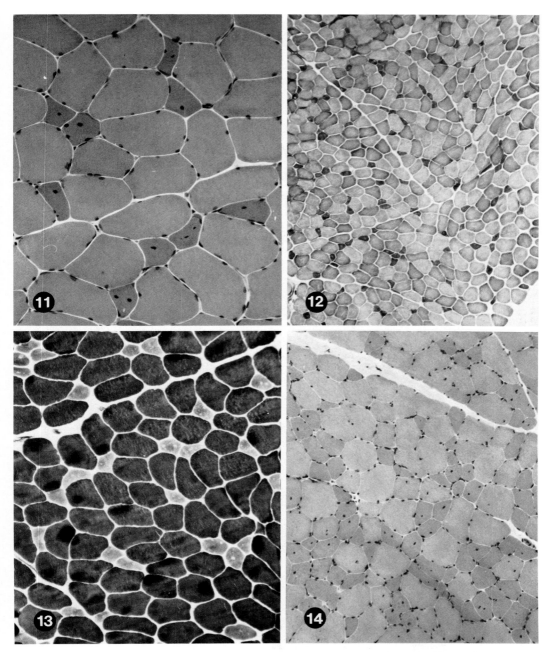

Figure 5.11. Myotonic dystrophy. This is a hematoxylin and eosin stain of the biopsy from a young adult in the early stages of the disease. A population of atrophic fibers with internal nuclei is noted.

Figure 5.12. These small fibers are often dark with the oxidative enzyme reactions (NADH-tetrozolium reductase).

Figure 5.13. Routine ATPase stains (pH 9.4) confirm that they are Type 1 fibers. Type 1 fiber atrophy and internal nuclei are thus characteristic of the early stages.

Figure 5.14. As the disease progresses the internal nuclei become more numerous.

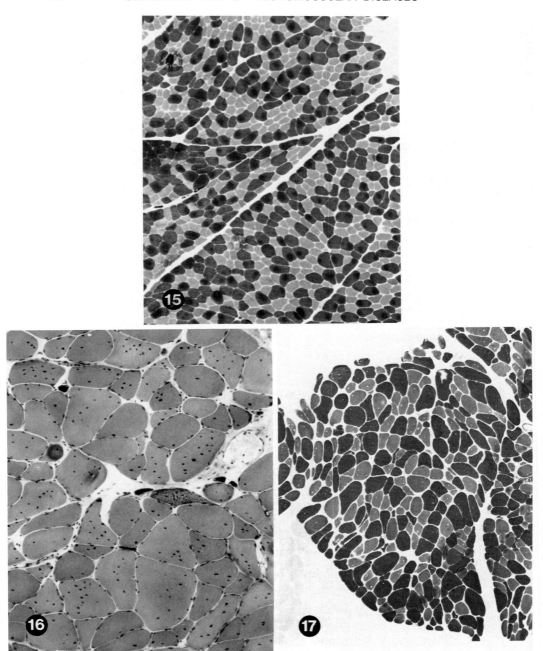

Figure 5.15. The Type 1 fiber atrophy although still present becomes less clear as illustrated in this routine ATPase (pH 9.4) reaction. In addition to the small Type 1 fibers, some of the Type 2 (dark) fibers are also becoming atrophic.

Figure 5.16. In the later stages of the disease there is variation in the size of the fibers, myriads of internal nuclei and clumps of pyknotic nuclei scattered between the fibers.

Figure 5.17. Selective Type 1 fiber atrophy is not now distinguishable (ATPase, pH 9.4).

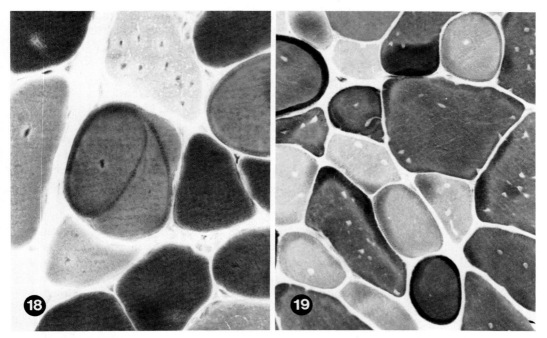

Figures 5.18 and 5.19.   In addition, there is often a bizarre distortion of the fiber architecture; the so called ring fiber. In these ATPase reactons of cross sections of muscle fibers, the majority of the myofibrils are cut end on. Some bundles of myofibrils are oriented in the same plane as the paper and are cut longitudinally rather than transversely. Because myofibrils in longitudinal sections demonstrate a definite striation, they are easily seen. Often they form a ring around the outside of the muscle fiber. The striated appearance of this small bundle gives the ring fiber its other name: the striated annulet.

true in the neonatal disease. The biceps muscle is more prone to this change than other commonly biopsied muscles such as the gastrocnemius and the vastus lateralis (36). As the muscle involvement progresses, the number of muscle nuclei within the muscle fibers increases and the severity of the Type 1 atrophy decreases. This is partly due to changes in the other fiber types with random variation in the size of fibers, fibrosis, and fiber splitting. There are often signs which would traditionally indicate denervation, such as pyknotic nuclear clumps and small atrophic fibers. Such changes may be interpreted as "neurogenic," but it is probably more logical to consider them part of the illness and not to make inferences about the integrity of the motor nerves. Abnormalities in the muscle spindle have been described with fragmentation of the fibers and hypertrophic changes in the axon supplying the muscle spindle (36, 37).

Electromyography demonstrates the classical findings of myotonia with waxing and waning of the amplitude and frequency of the motor units. When this activity is heard over a loudspeaker, it has been likened to the sound of a dive-bomber. As World War II recedes, it is more appropriate to compare it to a motorbike being revved up. True myotonia should not be confused with pseudomyotonia or bizarre high frequency potentials in which the amplitude does not wane so markedly and the frequency is more regular, perhaps producing the sound of a motorboat. Associated with the electrical myotonia, small short polyphasic potentials are also found. Although this has been advanced as evidence for the myogenic origin of myotonic dystrophy, evaluation of the motor units of the illness has suggested that the nerve may also be abnormal. Careful measurement of the cutaneous branches of the common peroneal nerve did not reveal any significant morphological abnormality (39).

Serum "muscle" enzymes are often abnormal, but are of little help in establishing the diagnosis. Abnormal catabolism of IgG and hypogammaglobulinemia are seen in some patients (40). Bony abnormalities have been described with thickening of the cranial vault and a small pituitary fossa. These changes do not seem to be of any particular significance.

Other findings point to widespread abnormalities in the function and structure of cell membranes. Abnormalities in the behavior of the insulin receptors has already been mentioned. Whenever the cell membrane is implicated in an illness, one may expect to find a large number of studies on blood cells. In addition to its role in oxygen transport, the red blood cell seems to have a second major role of provoking arguments among clinical scientists. It does this by a whimsical alteration of its properties as it travels from laboratory to laboratory. The literature is not much less confusing in myotonic dystrophy than it is in Duchenne dystrophy in this regard and protestation, recantantion and, what sometimes sound suspiciously like, incantations have appeared with regard to the fluidity of the membranes, phosphorylation of membrane protein, sodium flux, adenylcyclase, calcium dependent phosphatidic acid synthesis, sodium potassium ATPase and calcium magnesium ATPase, total phosphate concentration, abnormalities in cholesterol esters, and platelet aggregation. Eventually, all of this will settle down into some consistent abnormality, but at the time of writing, it is difficult to know what to make of all of these abnormalities (41–57).

Genetics

Genetic counseling is an important, although often unsuccessful, part of the management. The gene for myotonic dystrophy is on chromosome 19 and linked with ABH receptor genes, Lutheran and Lewis blood groups, C_3 complement, and a peptidase (58, 59). Since an autosomal dominant gene is involved, any myotonic parent must be warned that there is an even chance of any of his children developing the disease. The genes for ABH blood group secretion (which determine whether these ABH substances are secreted into the body fluids such as saliva) are closely linked to that for myotonic dystrophy. The Lutheran blood group antigens are also linked but less closely than the secretor antigens. In some families in which the secretor genotype can be evaluated the determination of whether the fetus is a secretor or nonsecretor can be used to predict the likelihood of its suffering from myotonic dystrophy (60, 61). Since the secretor type of the fetus can be determined from amniocentesis, prenatal diagnosis of myotonic dystrophy may be possible. In any individual case, this will depend upon whether the myotonic dystrophy gene can be shown to be traveling with either the secretor gene or the nonsecretor gene. In some families, this may prove to be impossible. A myotonic who is a nonsecretor is homozygous for the nonsecretor gene. If a myotonic is secretor positive, the secretor gene could be either on the same chromosome as the myotonic gene or on the other chromosome. By knowing that other members of the family who are secretor negative cannot transmit the secretor positive gene to their offspring and that relatives who do not have myotonic dystrophy cannot pass on the gene for myotonic dystrophy on either of their chromosomes, it is often possible to work out whether the myotonic dystrophy gene is associated with the secretor positive or secretor negative status in the individual family. If this can be done, than prenatal diagnosis is possible. There will always be an error of approximately 10% because of the possibility of recombination.

Treatment

The treatment of myotonic dystrophy follows the general principles laid down for other illnesses. Mechanical devices such as ankle supports may be helpful to patients as they develop distal weakness, if they can be persuaded to wear them. Breathing exercises and postural drainage should probably be carried out in the advanced stages of the illness. The sensitivity of patients to drugs such as sedatives and narcotics which depress the respiratory center should be borne in mind. Drugs such as quinine, quinidine, dilantin, carbamazepine, procainamide, and Diamox have all been recommended for the treatment of patients with myotonic dystrophy. All these drugs are aimed at alleviating the myotonia. Therapy is not universally successful, because the patient with myotonic dystrophy is seldom aware of the myotonia and is more troubled by weakness. A therapeutic trial of one of the medications is worthwile if the patient's stiffness is a significant part of his complaint. It is difficult to know which of the drugs to recommend for initial therapeutic trial. Procainamide and quinine prolong the PR interval of the electrocardiogram. Since this interval is abnormally prolonged in many patients with myotonic dystrophy, there are theoretical reasons for starting with dilantin, a drug which shortens the PR interval (7). The other side effects of dilantin, however, can be troublesome to the patient, especially since myotonics are occasionally erratic in their dosage schedules. Carbamazepine has been held to be as effective as dilantin. Dantrolene sodium has not only been of no help, but patients feel markedly worse on this medication with an increase in their weakness. As a rule, the patient derives greater benefit from an ankle support than from any of the pills.

REFERENCES

1. Barchi, R. L. A mechanistic approach to the myotonic syndromes. Muscle Nerve 5: S60–S63, 1982.
2. Palade, P. T., and Barchi, R. L. On the inhibition of muscle membrane chloride conductants by aromatic carboxylic acids. J. Gen. Physiol. 69: 875–896, 1977.
3. Bundey, S., and Carter, C. O. Genetic heterogeneity for dystrophia myotonica. J. Med. Genet. 9: 311–315, 1972.
4. Shore, R. N., and Maclachlan, T. B. Pregnancy with myotonic dystrophy: course complications and management. Obstet. Gynecol. 38: 448–454, 1971.
5. Harper, P. S. *Myotonic Dystrophy.* W. B. Saunders, London, 1979.
6. Bird, M., and Tzagournis, M. Insulin secretion in myotonic dystrophy. Am. J. Med. Sci. 260: 351–358, 1970.

7. Griggs, R. C., Davis, R. J., Anderson, D. C., and Dove, J. T. Cardiac conduction in myotonic dystrophy. Am. J. Med. *59:* 37–42, 1975.
8. Chalikian, D., and Barchi, R. Sarcolemmal desmosterol accumulation in membrane physical properties in 20,25-diazacholesterol myotonia. Muscle Nerve *5:* 118–124, 1982.
9. Bundey, S. Clinical evidence for heterogeneity in myotonic dystrophy. J. Med. Genet. *19:* 341–348, 1982.
10. Pearse, R. C., and Howeler, C. J. Neonatal form of dystrophia myotonica. Arch. Dis. Child. *54:* 331–338, 1979.
11. Steinbeck, K. S., and Carter, J. N. Thyroid abnormalities in patients with myotonic dystrophy. Clin. Endocrinol. *17:* 449–456, 1982.
12. Canal, N., Smirne, S., Comi, G., Guidobono, F., Pecile, A., and Caviezel, F. Study on growth hormone and prolactin secretion in myotonic dystrophy. Acta Neurol. Belg. *82:* 178–184, 1982.
13. Rudman, D., Chyatte, S. B., Patterson, J. H., Ahmann, P., and Gordan, A. Observations on the responsiveness of human subjects to human growth hormones: effects of endogenous growth hormone deficiency in myotonic dystrophy. J. Clin. Invest. *50:* 1941–1949, 1971.
14. Henriksen, O. A., Sundsfjord, J. A., and Nyberg-Hansen, R. Evaluation of the endocrine functions in dystrophia myotonica. Acta Neurol. Scand. *58:* 178–189, 1978.
15. Culebras, A., Podolsky, S., and Leopold, N. A. Absence of sleep related growth hormone elevations in myotonic dystrophy. Neurology *27:* 165–177, 1977.
16. Stuart, C. A., Armstrong, R. M., Provow, S. A., and Plishker, G. A. Insulin resistance in patients with myotonic dystrophy. Neurology *33:* 679–685, 1983.
17. Moxley, R. T., Griggs, R. C., Forbes, G. B., Goldblatt, D., and Donohoe, K. Influence of muscle wasting on oral glucose tolerance testing. Clin. Sci. *64:* 601–609, 1983.
18. Moxley, R. T., Livingston, J. N., Lockwood, D. H., Griggs, R. C., and Hill, R. L. Abnormal regulation of monocyte insulin binding affinity after glucose injection in patients with myotonic dystrophy. Proc. Natl. Acad. Sci. U.S.A. *18:* 2567–2571, 1981.
19. Moxley, R. T., Griggs, R. C., and Goldblatt, D. Decreased insulin sensitivity of the forearm muscle in myotonic dystrophy. J. Clin. Invest. *62:* 857–867, 1978.
20. Lam, L., Huston, A. J., Strickland, K. P., and Tevaarwerk, G. J. Insulin binding to myotonic dystrophy fibroblasts. J. Neurol. Sci. *58:* 289–295, 1983.
21. Festoff, B. W., and Moore, W. V. Evaluation of the insulin receptor in myotonic dystrophy. Ann. Neurol. *6:* 60–65, 1979.
22. Swick, H. M., Werlin, S. L., Dodds, W. J., and Hogan W. J. Pharyngo-esophageal motor function in patients with myotonic dystrophy. Ann. Neurol. *10:* 454–457, 1981.
23. Reeves, W. C., Griggs, R. C., Nanda, N. C., Thomson, K., and Gramiak, R. Echocardiographic evaluation of cardiac abnormalities in Duchenne dystrophy and myotonic muscular dystrophy. Arch. Neurol. *37:* 273–277, 1980.
24. Hartwig, G. B., Rao, K. R., Radoff, F. M., Coleman, E., Jones, R. H., and Roses, A. D. Radionucleide angiocardiographic analysis of myocardial function in myotonic muscular dystrophy. Neurology *33:* 657–660, 1983.
25. Carroll, J. E., Zwillich, C. W.., and Weil, J. V. Ventilatory response in myotonic dystrophy. Neurology *27:* 1125–1128, 1977.
26. Serisier, D. E., Mastaglia, F. L., and Gibson, G. J. Respiratory muscle function and ventilatory control. I. In patients with motor neuron disease: II. In patients with myotonic dystrophy. Q. J. Med. *51:* 205–226, 1982.
27. Ravin, M., Newmark, Z., and Saviello, G. Myotonia dystrophica: an anesthetic hazard: two case reports. Anest. Analg. *54:* 216–218, 1975.
28. Dundee, J. W. Thiopentone in dystrophica myotonica. Anesth. Analg. *31:* 257–262, 1952.
29. Kaufman, L. Anesthesia in dystrophia myotonica. Proc. R. Soc. Med. *53:* 183–188, 1960.
30. Bourke, T. D., and Zuck, D. Thiopentone in dystrophia myotonica. Br. J. Anesth. *29:* 35–38, 1957.
31. Harper, P. S. Congenital myotonic dystrophy in Britain: I. Clinical aspects. Arch. Dis. Child. *50:* 505–513, 1975.
32. Harper, P. S. Congenital myotonic dystrophy in Britain: II. Genetics basis. Arch. Dis. Child. *50:* 514–521, 1975.
33. Tanaka, K., Takeschita, K., and Takita, M. Abnormalities of bile acids in serum and bile from patients with myotonic muscular dystrophy. Clin. Sci. *62:* 627–642, 1982.
34. Soderhall, S., Gustafsson, J., and Bjorkhem, I. Deoxycholic acid in myotonic dystrophy. Lancet *I:* 1068–1069, 1982.
35. Engel, W. K., and Brooke, M. H. Histochemistry of the myotonic disorders. In: *Progressive Muskeldystrophie, Myotonie, Myasthenie*, edited by E. Kuhn. Springer-Verlag, New York, 1966, pp. 203–222.

36. Carroll, J. E., Brooke, M. H., and Kaiser, K. Diagnosis of infantile myotonic dystrophy. Lancet 2: 608, 1975.
37. Daniel, P. M., and Strich, S. J. Abnormalities in the muscle spindles in dystrophia myotonica. Neurology *14:* 310–316, 1964.
38. Swash, M., and Fox, K. P. Abnormal intrafusal muscle fibers in myotonic dystrophy: a study using serial sections. J. Neurol. Neurosurg. Pscyhiatry *38:* 71–99, 1975.
39. Pollock, M., and Dyck, P. J. Peripheral nerve morphometry in myotonic dystrophy. Arch. Neurol. *33:* 33–39, 1976.
40. Wochner, R. D., Drews, G., Strober, W., and Engel, W. K. Accelerated breakdown of immunoglobulin G (IgG) in myotonic dystrophy: a hereditary error of immunoglobulin catabolism. J. Clin. Invest. *45:* 321–329, 1966.
41. Roses, A. D., Butterfield, A., Appel, S. H., and Chestnut, D. B. Phenytoin and membrane fluidity in myotonic dystrophy. Arch. Neurol. *32:* 535–538, 1975.
42. Hull, K. L., and Roses, A. D. Stoichiometry of sodium and potassium transport in erythrocytes from patients with myotonic muscular dystrophy. J. Physiol. *254:* 169–178, 1976.
43. Bousser, M. G., Conard, J., Lecrubier, C., and Samama, M. Increased sensitivity of platelets to adrenalin in human myotonic dystrophy. Lancet 2: 307–309, 1975.
44. Mawatari, S., Takagi, A., and Rowland, L. P. Adenyl cyclase in normal and pathologic human muscle. Arch. Neurol. *30:* 96–102, 1974.
45. Kuhn, E. Myotonia: A lecture. In: *Clinical Studies in Myology: Proceedings of the 2nd International Congress on Muscle Diseases*, edited by B. A. Kakulas. Excerpta Medica. New York, 1973, pp. 471–479.
46. Omachi, A., Sarpel, G., Podolski, J. L., Barr, A. N., and Lazowski, E. Lysophosphatidylcholine induced lysis of erythrocytes in Duchenne and myotonic dystrophies and in Huntington's disease. J. Neurol. Sci. *56:* 249–258, 1982.
47. Yamaoka, L. H., Vance, J. M., and Roses, A. D. Myotonic muscular dystrophy, calcium dependent phosphatidate metabolism in the erythrocyte membrane. J. Neurol. Sci. *54:* 173–179, 1982.
48. Meredith, A. L., Harper, P. S., and Bradley, D. M. In vitro studies on calcium activated phosphatidylinositol phosphodiesterase of erythrocyte ghosts from normal individuals and those with myotonic muscular dystrophy. Clin. Chem. Acta. *120:* 201–206, 1982.
49. Moore, R. B., Appel, S. H., and Plishker, G. A. Myotonic dystrophy calcium dependent phosphatidylic acid synthesis in erythrocytes. Ann. Neurol. *10:* 491–493, 1981.
50. Butterfield, D. A. Myotonic muscular dystrophy. Time dependent alterations in erythrocyte membrane fluidity. J. Neurol. Sci. *52:* 61–67, 1981.
51. Sarpel, G., Lubansky, H. J., Danon, M. J., and Omachi, A. Erythrocytes in muscular dystrophy. Investigation with 31P nuclear magnetic resonance spectroscopy. Arch. Neurol. *38:* 271–274, 1981.
52. Nagano, Y., and Roses, A. D. Abnormalities or erythrocyte membranes in myotonic muscular dystrophy manifested in lipid vesicles. Neurology *30:* 989–991, 1980.
53. Muller, M. M., Kuzmits, R., Frass, M., and Mamoli, B. Purine metabolism of erythrocytes in myotonic dystrophy. J. Neurol. *223:* 59–66, 1980.
54. Chalikian, D. M., and Barchi, R. L. Fluorescent probe analysis of erythrocyte membranes in myotonic dystrophy. Neurology *30:* 227–285, 1980.
55. Gaffney, B. J., Drachman, D. B., Lin, D. C., and Tennekoon, G. Spin label studies of erythrocytes in myotonic dystrophy. No increase in membrane fluidity. Neurology *30:* 272–276, 1980.
56. Podolski, J. L., Lubansky, H. J., Sarpel, G., Danon, M. J., Lazowski, E., and Omachi, A. Erythrocyte membrane lysophospholipase activity in muscular dystrophy. J. Neurol. Sci. *59:* 423–429, 1983.
57. Johnsson, R., Somer, H., Carli, P., and Saris, N. E. Erythrocyte flexibility, ATPase activities, and calcium efflux in patients with Duchenne muscular dystrophy, myotonic muscular dystrophy and congenital myotonia. J. Neurol. Sci. *58:* 399–407, 1983.
58. Harper, P. S., Rivas, M. L., Bias, W. B., Hutchinson, J. R., Dyken, P. R., and McKusick, V. A. Genetic linkage confirm between the locus for myotonic dystrophy and the ABH secretion and Lutheran blood group loci. Am. J. Med. Genet. *24:* 310–316, 1972.
59. Davies, K. E., Jackson, J., Williamson, R., Harper, P. S., Ball, S., Sarfarazi, M., Meredith, L., and Fey, G. Linkage analysis of myotonic dystrophy and sequence of chromosome 19 using a cloned complement 3 gene probe. J. Med. Genet. *20:* 259–263.
60. Schrott, H. G., and Omenn, G. S. Myotonic dystrophy: opportunities for prenatal prediction. Neurology *25:* 789–791, 1975.
61. Insley, J., Bird, G. W. G., Harper, P. S., and Pearce, G. W. Prenatal prediction of myotonic dystrophy. Lancet 2: 806, 1976.

MYOTONIA CONGENITA (THOMSEN'S DISEASE)

Clinical Aspects

In myotonia congenita the muscle stiffness is the predominant if not the only complaint from which the patient suffers. There are two varieties: one with an autosomal dominant inheritance, which Dr. Thomsen first recognized in his own family; the second, and probably the commoner form, is an autosomal recessive well reviewed by Becker (1). In the autosomal dominant variety, the myotonia is noticed in earliest childhood, but it may be rather mild and shows no progression. Both sexes are equally affected and there are no associated findings such as the cataracts or testicular atrophy which are found in patients with myotonic dystrophy. In the recessive variety, the disease is noticed in the middle of the first decade and the myotonia is more severe than in the dominant type. Two-thirds of the patients with the recessive variety are male.

The patient describes his symptoms in a rather steretoyped way. After resting, the muscles are stiff and difficult to move. With continued exercise, the muscles loosen and the patient's movement becomes almost normal. This is seen very typically when the patient arises from a chair. He moves clumsily and starts to walk with a stiff and wooden appearance almost as if he had no joints in his body. As he continues, he can first walk freely and finally can run with ease. A muscle which is stiff from myotonia cannot exert normal power, and this may give a spurious impression of weakness. As the myotonia disappears, the strength returns. All the striated muscles of the body seem to share this abnormality and, although it is most noticeable in the limbs, evidence of myotonia can also be found in the face and tongue. In addition to the presence of myotonia, muscular hypertrophy may be noted (Fig. 5.20). This is not always present and seems to be more pronounced in the recessive form than in the autosomal dominant and in men more than women. It is so striking on occasion as to give the appearance of the Farnese Hercules, but the majority of patients, although well muscled, do not demonstrate this degree of hypertrophy and it is certainly not as common as one would anticipate from the various dramatic pictures to be found in the literature. True muscle weakness may be noted in some patients with the recessive form but when it is marked, the clinician should be suspicious that the diagnosis lies elsewhere.

Laboratory Tests

Electromyography can be helpful in establishing the diagnosis. Well marked myotonia is found with none of the associated dystrophic potentials. The muscle biopsy reveals an absence of Type 2B fibers in some patients (2). This is a subtype of muscle fiber and is characterized by its histochemical properties (Figs. 5.21–5.23). Increase in the size of fibers, internal nuclei and various other changes may also be seen in the muscle biospy but these changes are less specific. Evidence for abnormalities of the membrane is also found in myotonia congenita. These abnormalities are different from those present in myotonic dystrophy. The phosphorylation of membrane proteins (protein kinase activity) is normal, chloride conductance is reduced and the membrane resistance is greater than normal. Electron spin resonance shows increased

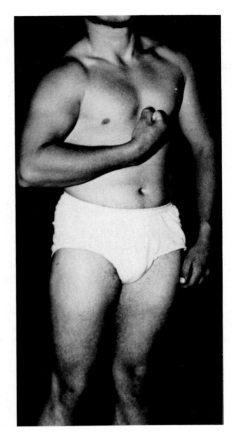

Figure 5.20. Myotonia congenita is often, although not always, associated with a well developed musculature.

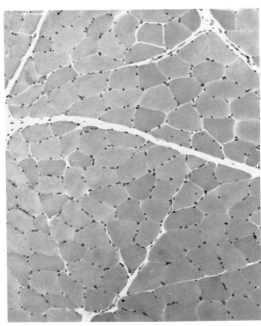

Figure 5.21. Myotonia congenita. The hematoxylin and eosin stains may be completely normal. In the photograph of this patient's biopsy, the only abnormalities are a few small fibers and one or two internal nuclei.

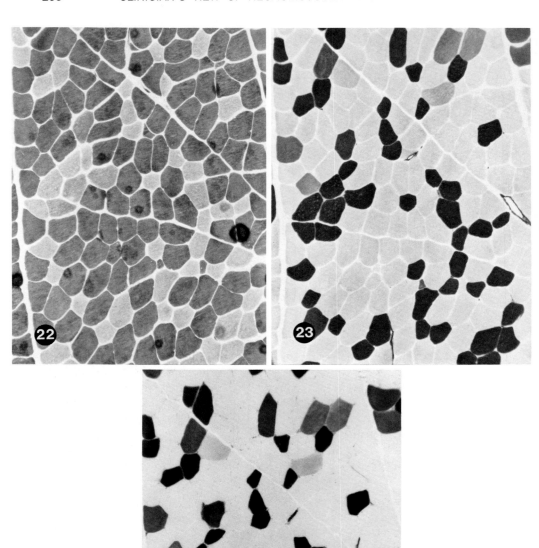

Figs. 5.22–5.24

fluidity of the erythrocyte membrane as in myotonic dystrophy although not necessarily from the same cause (3).

In the autosomal dominant form of the illness, the fatty acid content of the muscle phospholipids is different from that seen in control muscle. Linoleic acid (an 18 carbon fatty acid) is decreased and some of the 20 carbon fatty acids are increased (4).

Treatment

Unlike patients with myotonia dystrophy, the patient with myotonia congenita suffers the effects of the myotonia. A therapeutic trial of one of the medications aimed at preventing this is thus worthwhile. In a double-blind comparison of diphenylhydantoin and procainamide, the former drug was found to be more effective (5). The side effects of procainamide were said to be more troublesome than those of dilantin. Quinine is also well tolerated by some patients and seems to be quite effective in the management of myotonia. All of these drugs have side effects. Quinine may cause gastrointestinal upsets, tinnitus, visual disturbances, and headache. More seriously, it may be associated with vasculitis, bone marrow depression and renal disease. Procainamide, in addition to several minor side effects, may produce bone marrow depression and a lupus-like syndrome. Dilantin does have the advantage of being used in large quantities in patients with epilepsy and, therefore, the side effects are better known. It is relatively well tolerated, but even the minor side effects, such as gastrointestinal upsets and gingival hyperplasia, are seldom tolerated by the patient whose only symptom is myotonia.

In my own experience, the beneficial effects of medications is rather short-lived and tends to disappear after 2 or 3 months. For this reason, patients have usually taken such medication at times when they may be particularly under stress, such as when an undue amount of activity has to be undertaken. As in myotonic dystropy, Diamox, ACTH, and corticosteroids have also been tried, with varying results.

Figures 5.22 through 5.24. These are serial sections of a muscle biopsy from a patient with myotonia congenita demonstrating the absence of Type 2B fibers. Each photograph is of the same corresponding area in three different sections: Routine ATPase (pH 9.4) (Fig. 5.22), ATPase following perincubation at pH 4.6 (Fig. 5.23), and ATPase following preincubation at pH 4.3 (Fig. 5.24). With the routine ATPase (pH 9.4) stains (Fig. 5.22), the Type 2 fibers are dark and the Type 1 fibers light. Following preincubation at pH 4.6 (Fig. 5.23) the darkest fibers are Type 1 and the lightest fibers are Type 2A. Ordinarily Type 2B fibers demonstrate an intensity of staining intermediate between Type 1 and 2A. Superficially it appears that scattered Type 2B fibers are present in the biopsy as indicated by those with an intermediate staining intensity. However, comparison between this photograph and the ATPase following preincubation at pH 4.3 (Fig. 5.24) shows that these are Type 2C fibers, a characteristic of which is that they retain their stain even following preincubation at pH 4.3. There is, in fact, one Type 2B fiber which is best identified in Figure 5.23 as the very small intermediate staining fiber in the middle of the lower third of the photograph. Notice in Figure 5.24 that this fiber has completely lost its stain. Why the Type 2B fibers disappear is not known.

REFERENCES

1. Becker, P. E. Zur Genetik der Myotonien. In: *Progressive Muskeldystrophie, Myotonie, Myasthenie,* edited by E. Kuhn. Springer-Verlag, New York, 1966, pp. 247–255.
2. Crews, J., Kaiser, K. K., and Brooke, M. H. The pathology of myotonia congenita. J. Neurol. Sci. *28:* 449–457, 1976.
3. Butterfield, D. A., Chestnut, D. B., Appel, S. H., and Roses, A. D. Spin label study of erythrocyte membrane fluidity in myotonic and Duchenne muscular dystrophy and congenital myotonia. Nature *263:* 159–161, 1976.
4. Kuhn, E., Fiehn, W., Seiler, D., and Schroder, J. M. The autosomal recessive (Becker) form of myotonia congenita. Muscle Nerve *2:* 109–117, 1979.
5. Munsat, T. L. Therapy of myotonia. Neurology *17:* 359–367, 1967.

PARAMYOTONIA CONGENITA

Clinical Aspects

Paramyotonia congenita was described by Eulenburg in 1886. It is a rare disorder whose existence has occasionally been denied because of some resemblances to hyperkalemic periodic paralysis. It is a disease of autosomal dominant inheritance, and its hallmark is that the muscle symptoms are worsened by exposure to the cold and by exercise (1). Paramyotonia is similar to myotonia and the muscle refuses to relax properly. It differs from myotonia because repetitive use of the muscle, far from easing the problem, causes an increased delay in relaxation. Thus, when the patient is asked to squeeze his eyelids tightly shut, he may initially be able to open them again, but after repeated attempts, the eyelids remain firmly closed and may open again only after a minute or two of inactivity. The facial muscles and the muscles of the forearms and hands are predominantly involved. Paramyotonia of the face may be noticed by stiffness of the expression, narrowing of the palperbral fissures or dimpling of the chin owing to the contraction of the mentalis muscle. A patient who steps outside into winter weather may find that his smile freezes on his face in the literal sense. A similar stiffness is noted in the tongue. Often the patient prefers not to eat cold foods because of this. When paramyotonia occurs in the hand, a peculiar posture may be seen, with the middle three fingers slightly flexed, particularly at the metacarpal phalangeal joint and the thumb and little finger held abducted.

Exposure to the cold also causes weakness of the muscle and when the muscle is sufficiently chilled, the paramyotonia disappears and the muscle is flaccid and paralyzed. This weakness may far outlast the exposure to cold and it is common for the muscle not to regain its full use for hours after returning to room temperature. Strong voluntary contraction may also be associated with a long lasting decrease in strength, not clearly due to an increase in myotonia (2). These symptoms are manifest from birth and do not improve as the patient gets older.

Some patients with a different variety of the illness also have true myotonia, noted both on voluntary activity and following percussion, which is present when the muscle is at a normal temperature. There are often mild attacks of weakness which the patient finds difficult to describe. These may occur several times a day and are similar to the type of spells seen in hyperkalemic periodic paralysis.

Laboratory Studies

The EMG of the resting muscles at room temperature shows myotonia, which is present on percussion or with movement of the needle. The most remarkable findng is the appearance of spontaneous activity on cooling (3). As the muscle is cooled, low amplitude fibrillary activity makes its appearance. This is present at rest and initially disappears following voluntary contraction. It is most intense when the muscle temperature is 30°C. As cooling continues, this spontaneous activity completely disappears. In contrast to myotonia, during the delayed muscle relaxation of paramyotonia electrical activity of the muscle is not prominent, which may indicate that the stiffness is due to a change in the contractile apparatus in the muscle.

The muscle biospy is abnormal and demonstrates marked variability in the size of fibers with internal nuclei and some vacuoles (4).

The pathophysiology was studied in relatively intact muscle fibers obtained from an intercostal biopsy (5). Cooling these fibers reduced the resting membrane potential from approximately −80 mv to −40 mv, at which point they were inexcitable. As the muscle cooled, it passed through a phase of hyperexcitability, presumably equivalent to the changes seen on EMG. Since this depolarization was prevented by tetrodotoxin which blocks sodium channels, it is probable that the illness is due to an abnormality in the membrane associated with increased sodium conductance.

Treatment

On an experimental basis, the drug tocainide has been used in oral doses of 400 mg, 3 times a day. This drug, which is a derivative of lidocaine, is an antiarrhythmic agent which blocks the sodium conductance of the cell membrane. Out of eight patients treated, all improved both with regard to the stiffness and to episodes of weakness. Whether it will be possible to treat patients with a lifelong illness such as paramyotonia with chronic administration of this drug remains to be seen (6). In view of the possible association of paramyotonia congenita with hyperkalemic periodic paralysis, treatment has been attempted with acetazolamide. Although this reduced the myotonia, use of the drug was associated with profound weakness. It use is, therefore, to be avoided in this illness (4).

REFERENCES

1. Thrush, D. C., Morris, C. J., and Salmon, M. V. Paramyotonia congenita: a clinical histochemical and pathological study. Brain 95: 537–552, 1977.
2. Riggs, J. E., Gutmann, L., and Brick, J. F. Exercise induced membrane failure in paramyotonia congenita. Neurology 34: (Suppl. 1): 131, 1984.
3. Haass, A., Ricker, K., Rudel, R., Leman-Horn, F., Bohlen, R., Dengler, R., and Mertens, H. G. Clinical study of paramyotonia congenita with and without myotonia in a warm environment. Muscle Nerve 4: 388–395, 1981.
4. Riggs, J. E., Griggs, R. C., and Moxley, R. T. Acetazolamide induced weakness in paramyotonia congenita. Ann. Intern. Med. 86: 169–173, 1977.
5. Lehmann-Horn, F., Rudel, R., Dengler, R., Lorkovic, H., Haass, A., and Ricker, K. Membrane defects in paramyotonia congenita with and without myotonia in a warm environment. Muscle Nerve 4: 396–406, 1981.
6. Ricker, K., Haass, A., Rudel, R., Bohlen, R., and Mertens, H. G. Successful treatment of paramyotonia congenita (Eulenburg): muscle stiffness and weakness prevented by tocainide. J. Neruosurg. Psychiatry 43: 268–271, 1980.

OTHER FORMS OF MYOTONIA

I suspect that I share with other clinicians the experience of having seen patients with definite voluntary and percussion myotonia whose diagnosis baffles me. Sometimes one tries to fit them into the pattern of myotonic dystrophy or perhaps an unusual recessive form of myotonia congenita, but they really do not look like the other patients. I have, for example, seen a young man with marked myotonia, who also has total ophthalmoplegia and elbow contractures, such that his arms are locked 45° short of full extension. A "new" syndrome worthy of publication, perhaps, except for the fact that his uncle has very typical myotonic dystrophy with cataracts and all the rest. There are other unusual reports in the literature (1), but until more cases are collected and they coalesce into recognizable clinical patterns, it is difficult to make any sense out of them.

"Myotonia acquisita" is probably a mythical entity. The sudden acquisition of myotonia has been described following trauma, electric shock, and other disasters. However, the usual association is of a sudden traumatic episode which brings to light hither to undiagnosed myotonic dystrophy or myotonia congenita. Poisoning with 2,4-diazacholesterol, or some of the other compounds discussed in the introduction to this section, may give rise to myotonia and perhaps should be considered as true myotonia acquisita.

REFERENCE

1. Sun, S. F., Streib, E. W. Autosomal recessive generalized myotonia. Muscle Nerve 6: 143–148, 1983.

6

inflammatory myopathies

POLYMYOSITIS AND DERMATOMYOSITIS

Clinical Aspects

Muscle, no less than other tissues in the body, is at the mercy of various inflammatory processes. The range and diversity of these conditions are impressive: bacterial, viral, and parasitic infections have all been described, as well as the granulomatous conditions due to tuberculosis and sarcoidosis. Yet it is remarkable how seldom one sees any of these diseases and their importance fades, at least in the nontropical countries, when compared to the prevalence of inflammatory diseases of muscle of unknown cause, often associated with disturbances of the immune system. Dermatomyositis and polymyositis are common diseases in any muscle clinic. The combination of a typical skin rash with the signs and symptoms of muscular weakness makes the diagnosis of dermatomyositis not only probable but, on occasions, inescapable. However, the diagnosis of polymyositis in the absence of the rash may indeed be difficult, and provides a variety of traps for the unwary. There are other illnesses in which inflammatory changes are seen in the muscle; nor does the lack of such pathology exclude the diagnosis of polymyositis. These and other problems in the diagnostic criteria for polymyositis have bedeviled the literature and clouded the evaluation of therapy. It is also hard to know whether to consider polymyositis and dermatomyositis as one entity or whether the two diseases are discrete as to cause, prognosis, and treatment. Before treading this particular clinical morass it would be perhaps better to set down some of the typical features of the illness.

Dermatomyositis is an acquired illness with an acute or subacute course. It may occur at any age, but it is slightly more common in childhood and again in the 5th and 6th decades. It is unusual to see a case between the ages of 15 and 25 (1). Some have suggested that women are more prone to the disease than men (2). This is not supported by later studies, except in patients with associated collagen vascular disease. As with many other muscle diseases, the true incidence is hard to discover but lies somewhere between 5 and 10 patients per million annually. This disease often begins with a variety of systemic symptoms, including fever, malaise, or mild and nonspecific gastrointestinal symptoms. Sometimes there is a preceding illness or event which causes the patient and even the physician to suspect that it might be related to the onset of the inflammatory myopathy. Such episodes have included upper respiratory infections, immunizations, and drug reactions. Prolonged exposure to sunlight can precede the development of the rash in dermatomyositis.

The rash may appear before, after, or concomitant with the weakness and may take several forms. There may be a blotchy flush over the cheekbone which blanches on pressure, with a rather slow return of color when the pressure is released. The eyelids, particularly the upper eyelid, may assume a purple color which has been likened to lavender, lilac, or heliotrope. In the black races the rash is neither lavender nor red, but rather a dusky, deep purple shadow on the skin. In severe involvement, the rash is accompanied by marked edema which can cause a puffiness around the eyes. The skin may also break down and present a scaly or weeping appearance. An erythematous rash of the chest and neck often develops in the area that would be exposed by an open shirt or scoop neck dress. The associated telangiectasia makes the rash reminiscent of that associated with irradiation. The skin over the elbows and knees becomes not only discolored but also thickened. Frequently nodules develop which may become necrotic and extrude calcinous material. The rash is equally characteristic on the hands. It varies from a slight puffiness and discoloration around the nail beds to marked edema with telangiectasia. Changes in the blood vessels, around the nail bed may be noted. It is advisable to use a hand lens to detect these. The initial change is often one of hemorrhage and thrombosis. With progression of the illness, giant dilated capillaries may be noted combined with avascular areas. The cuticle is often stained a muddy orange color (3). There may be areas of erythema and thickening over the knuckles and the interphalangeal joints. When the skin changes are severe there is a shiny atrophic appearance to the skin over all the fingers and back of the hand. At other times the rash may be diffuse, covering almost the whole body, though there is usually sparing of the skin in the axilla. The end result of such diffuse changes can be disastrous, with the patient's skin reduced to a chitinous, atrophic shell which cracks at every attempted manipulation, although I have seen this only in the childhood variety.

The ancient tenet that inflammation is accompanied by "calor, dolor, turgor, et rubor" is nowhere more misleading than in polymyositis. Fully half of the patients with the disease have no symptoms of muscle pain whatsoever. The all too often noted comment that a patient could not have polymyositis because of the absence of muscle pain is extremely ill-advised. Not only is its absence no bar to the diagnosis of polymyositis but the majority of patients who do complain of muscle pain have some other illness such as polymyalgia or the ubiquitous "aches, cramps, and pains" syndrome. When pain is present it is usually described as a deep aching within the muscles, a soreness which is helped to some extent by rest and made worse with continued activity. The muscles may be swollen, particularly the proximal muscles of the leg, and palpation of the muscle belly may accentuate the tenderness. In chronic and long standing disease, the muscles may not only become firmly indurated but may be the site of contractures. Rarely, widespread calcification of the soft tissues follows severe poly- or dermatomyositis (Fig. 6.1). Although this calcification is occasionally disabling, it is usually found only when the disease itself is inactive. Soft tissue x-ray studies often reveal a diffuse calcification of the subcutaneous tissue to a degree which is not suspected clinically.

The symptoms of weakness may begin with surprising suddenness and may render a patient bedfast within several days, but usually the measure of the progression is not in days but in weeks. The symptoms differ in no way from those of patients with other forms of proximal weakness; difficulties in arising from a chair, climbing stairs, and lifting objects onto shelves are common.

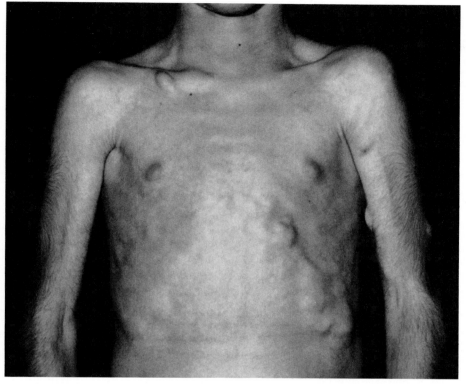

Figure 6.1. Dermatomyositis. In the late stages of the disease, calcified nodules may appear under the skin.

Polymyositis may have a predilection for the neck muscles. The anterior neck muscles are often involved in which respect it differs from myasthenia gravis where weakness of the posterior muscles is more usual. Weakness of the facial muscles, although recorded, should suggest the possibility of some other diagnosis. Bulbar symptoms of dysphonia or dysarthria are unusual, but dysphagia is a more common feature and may be so severe as to necessitate nasogastric tube feeding. The limb weakness is initially proximal and spreads to involve more distal muscles as the disease progresses. Whether or not polymyositis is a different disease from dermatomyositis, those patients without the rash have a similar story. They experience the same initial systemic complaints followed by an acute or subacute bout of weakness. It is unusual for a child to have polymyositis (without the rash) so the disease is chiefly seen in adults.

The incidence of Raynaud's phenomenon has been estimated to be as high as 28%. Most of us have encountered this symptom less frequently in uncomplicated polymyositis and a subsequent series set the incidence at less than 20% unless one includes those patients with the "overlap" syndrome. Cardiac abnormalities with heart block and pathologically proven involvement of the heart have been noted (4, 5). Abnormalities of the lung with interstitial fibrosis and pneumonitis may also occur as a rare complication

(6, 7). This type of illness links patients with idiopathic polymyositis whose symptoms chiefly reflect the muscle disease to other patients in whom the muscle disease is clearly complicated by (or perhaps a complication of) some diffuse collagen vascular disease.

It is difficult to be sure of the natural history although attempts have been made to characterize it (1, 2, 8, 9). Some studies have been plagued by the shifting miasmic quality of the criteria used to diagnose polymyositis. The typical case of dermatomyositis is easy to document, but when cases are adjudged on the basis of the clinical picture alone or of mild inflammatory responses in the muscle biopsy, it is hard to be certain that dystrophies or metabolic myopathies of various types are excluded (10, 11).

The disease may run a variable course. There may be subsequent complete recovery even in the untreated patient. Other patients suffer a remitting, relapsing illness, usually with imperfect recovery between bouts of myositis. A third variety, and one which may evolve from the previous type, is a chronic indolent form. The best that can be hoped for if this happens (although this is perhaps a physician's viewpoint, not that of a patient) is that the disease burns out before the patient's pulmonary functions are compromised. Death, when it takes place, is usually from inanition, intercurrent infection, or respiratory failure. The mortality rate as reported in the literature varies from 15 to 30%. Many of the patients followed in these studies were not observed over long periods of time and it is difficult to be certain of the real mortality (8, 9). One study also suggested that the more acute the disease the better the prognosis (8). Of those patients whose disease had lasted less than 6 months, almost half went into remission, whereas of those whose illness was of longer duration, barely a quarter achieved remission. Perhaps the axiomatic corollary of this should be noted: namely, the longer one suffers a disease the more likely it is to be severe.

It is quite probable that the natural history of polymyositis will never be established. We are long into an age when steroid therapy and immunosuppressive drugs have become commonplace, and it is difficult to stand by and watch a patient become enfeebled from polymyositis without at least attempting treatment. The only certain statement which can be made is that patients with dermato- and polymyositis do poorly enough in general that some therapy should be sought.

To have arrived thus far in the discussion of inflammatory myopathies without attempting their classification would be regarded in some circles as a tour de force and in others as a lapse in judgment. The ways in which the various forms of polymyositis may be classified are not yet settled, nor even the question as to whether there really are different forms of myositis. In any group of diseases the advantage of a good system of classification is that it simplifies matters, whereas the disadvantage of a bad one is that it only complicates the subject. Although the classification which has been proposed for the inflammatory myopathies is not based upon the certainty of different etiologies, it does serve as a reminder that the several varieties are not necessarily identical. If this function is to be served it is better to maintain rather wide and general categories. If and when the details are filled in at a later time a new classification will assuredly come into being. For this reason the system suggested by Bohan and Peter (10, 11) approaches a reasonable compromise. It is as follows:

Group 1. Primary idiopathic polymyositis.
Group 2. Primary idiopathic dermatomyositis.
Group 3. Dermatomyositis (or polymyositis) associated with neoplasia.
Group 4. Childhood dermatomyositis (or polymyositis) associated with vasculitis.
Group 5. Polymyositis or dermatomyositis associated with connective tissue disorder (overlap syndromes).

The first two groups are separated on the basis of information which is already available. There is enough difference between polymyositis and dermatomyositis at least to give rise to doubt as to their common identity.

Childhood dermatomyositis seems to be a slightly different disease. It begins with a change in behavior. The children become fretful and irritable and a normally good child may become impossible and unruly. Although the usual course is of relapse and remission, the illness may be monophasic with a relatively acute decline in strength and then a more prolonged recovery to normal strength in the absence of any therapy. Calcinosis is more prone to occur in the childhood variety and may be very severe. There is more evidence of an acute vasculitis in the illness as is discussed below. A category of cases associated with cancer gives tacit recognition to the fact that these patients need to be managed differently while that associated with collagen vascular disease admits the thin end of a very large wedge to the classification.

Polymyositis and Dermatomyositis Associated with Neoplasms

There is a relationship between dermatomyositis (less often polymyositis) and neoplasm. This is chiefly seen in the adult form of dermatomyositis. The underlying neoplasm is usually a carcinoma. The breast, lung, ovary and stomach have been commonly implicated. The true incidence of this relationship is difficult to extract from the literature but is probably in the neighborhood of 10–20%. Whatever the exact figure, it is high enough that the possibility of a neoplasm should be entertained in an adult presenting with dermatomyositis (12). The usual clinical situation is that of a patient with known malignancy who presents with the typical rash and weakness. It is only rarely that laboratory tests reveal the presence of an unsuspected cancer in a patient with dermatomyositis. One review of the relationship between dermatomyositis and malignancy concluded that elaborate or invasive tests for malignancy were unrevealing unless a careful history or examination suggested signs and symptoms of cancer (13). A practical approach might be to obtain a chest x-ray, to refrain from the temptation to bypass the rectal and pelvic examination, and to test the stool for occult blood in any patient with dermatomyositis. Obviously, if the patient's symptoms warrant a complete investigation this would be advisable. When I reviewed our own series of patients, I found that we had detected only four neoplasms, two of the lung, one of the stomach and one of the thyroid (the last was discovered incidentally postmortem), in an unselected series of 75 patients with poly- or dermatomyositis. The mortality rate in the group associated with malignancy is higher than in the other groups. Most patients die from the effects of the disseminated cancer rather than from the muscle weakness, but the reverse is occasionally seen.

Polymyositis in Association with Other Collagen Vascular Disease (Overlap Syndrome)

Lupus erythematosus, polyarteritis nodosa, and scleroderma may all have weakness as a facet of the disease complex. The prognosis in such a situation is not as good as with uncomplicated polymyositis. This may again imply that the more widespread a disease, the more likely it is to have serious consequences. The "overlap syndromes" are those in which features of several types of collagen vascular disease coexist. Fifteen percent of the patients with polymyositis had associated collagen vascular disease (14). In this situation myositis is seen in association with arthritis, fibrosing alveolitis, features of scleroderma, nephritis and keratoconjunctivitis sicca. One particular combination, in which polymyositis coexists with Raynaud's phenomenon, sclerodactyly, arthritis and pulmonary fibrosis, was termed mixed connective tissue disorder. It was suggested that the disease could be identified by the presence of an extractable nuclear antibody which was sensitive to digestion by ribonuclease (15, 16). The illness had a benign cause and was responsive to steroids. Recent studies have expressed some doubt as to whether this exists as a real entity. In one study exploring the presence of this antibody in patients with the overlap syndrome, 72% of the patients had the antiribonucleoprotein antibody, but not all of them had mixed connective tissue disorder (17). Although occasional patients with positive titers may have polymyositis alone, the presence of any significant levels of antinuclear antibody in polymyositis suggests the presence of an associated collagen vascular disease (18). Predictably, the incidence of arthritis, myalgia and Raynaud's phenomenon is higher in patients with overlap syndromes, averaging around 50%.

Laboratory Studies

If clinical criteria are difficult and therapeutic response uncertain, How may one essay the diagnosis of poly- or dermatomyositis? There are abnormalities in laboratory tests which are often helpful. The serum "muscle" enzymes are elevated and the serum creatine kinase (CK) and myoglobin are almost always increased during the acute phase. This has been disputed (2), but it is true in the great majority of cases. The CK tends to be higher when the disease is active than when it is inactive, but a relatively normal enzyme level is seen in a few patients in whom the disease is in exacerbation, particularly if these patients are taking steroids. The serum CK should therefore be used only as one of the criteria to judge the progress of the disease and a change in muscle strength would take precedence over any change in the level of CK for determining the activity of the illness. Nevertheless, on occasion, the CK may be a reliable predictor of changes to come and when interpreted in this fashion may provide useful information. In other patients the sedimentation rate may reflect the activity of the illness but this finding is nonspecific and cannot be used to establish the diagnosis.

An electromyograph (EMG) can be helpful since the typical finding in polymyositis is of a so called myopathic EMG with short low amplitude polyphasic potentials with which are associated marked signs of muscle irritability. Bizarre high frequency repetitive discharges, fibrillations, and positive denervation potentials may all be seen.

The muscle biopsy is often strikingly abnormal (Figs. 6.2–6.9) and may differ in the two forms of the illness. In dermatomyositis there tends to be a characteristic atrophy which involves the fibers around the periphery of the muscle fascicles (perifascicular atrophy), whereas in polymyositis this change is often lacking. Inflammatory changes are obviously part and parcel of the disease, but they again may be absent in up to one-third of the patients. Another rather characteristic finding is the "ghost fiber" illustrated in Figures 6.8 and 6.9.

Abnormalities in the esophagus are often detected by cineradiography. In one study of 16 patients who were incompletely responsive to steroid therapy, there were abnormalities in the distal esophagus in 14. This part of the esophagus, of course, contains smooth muscles, suggesting that the disorder is more wide spread than usually thought. There was diminished peristalsis, dilation of the lumen, and a reduction of the lower esophageal spincter pressure. Reflux into the esophagus is also noted. Only three of the patients had symptoms associated with this difficulty. These changes were noted in patients with relatively chronic disease (19).

Etiology

Although much is known about the underlying pathology of the disease, the precise etiology is still elusive. It has been suggested that the perifascicular distribution of the atrophic muscle fibers indicates vascular insufficiency with selective atrophy of those fibers furthest "downstream" (20). Paulson et al. (21) employed xenon-131 to measure the blood flow in a limb at rest and during hyperemia induced by ischemic exercise and histamine. They showed decreased muscle blood flow in patients with polymositis that was present neither in Duchenne dystrophy nor in limb-girdle dystrophy. Morphometric analysis of the skeletal muscle capillaries reveals hypertrophy of the capillary endothelial cells and also basement membrane reduplication, suggesting repeated capillary degeneration as the primary event in the disease (22). Subtle differences are also found between the changes in polymyositis and in dermatomyositis.

An experimental animal model of myositis was attempted by the injection of muscle extracts in conjunction with complete Freund's adjuvant (23). Inflammatory lesions were produced, the worst involvement being noted in those animals injected with a myofibrillar fraction (24). Circulating antibodies to muscle were detected in this animal model. The disease was transferred to other animals by an infusion of washed lymphocytes from an affected animal. Anti-muscle antibodies have also been detected in patients with polymyositis, but the force of this evidence is weakened by their detection in normal controls as well (25). The possibility of an altered immune state raises the question of whether the damage is produced by humoral factors or by cellular means. As is so often the case there are major differences between the animal model and the human disease, and it is not at all clear whether justifiable inferences can be drawn from these experiments.

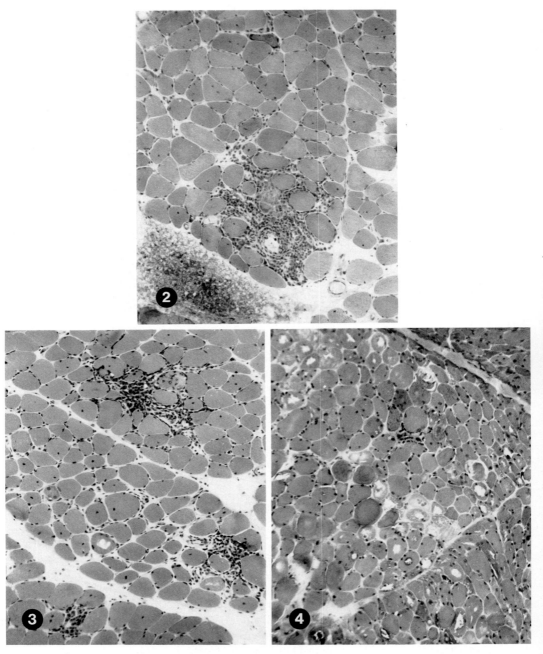

Figure 6.2. Polymyositis. The best known change in the biopsy of patients with polymyositis is the inflammatory response. The routine hematoxylin and eosin stain demonstrates a perivascular inflammatory response in which the cells are gathered around a medium size blood vessel. This is a typical feature and strongly suggests the diagnosis.

Figure 6.3. In this patient the cellular response was apparently associated with necrotic fibers rather than with the blood vessels. Although this patient did indeed have polymyositis, interpretation of such a biopsy should be more cautious since other genetic dystrophies may give rise to cellular responses associated with the fibers.

Figure 6.4. Another biopsy shows a vacuolar change in many of the fibers.

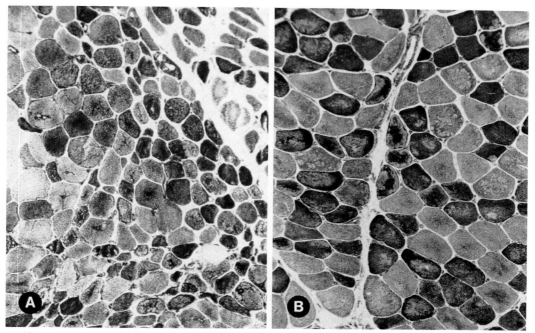

Figure 6.5. (*A* and *B*) The oxidative enzyme reactions may show changes in the intermyofibrillar network of almost any type. There are small dark staining fibers seen in the lower right of *A*, while in the center of both photographs fibers with an increased central stain are noted. These "dark centered fibers" are often seen in polymyositis and other illness in which there is degeneration and regeneration, such as in the myoglobinurias.

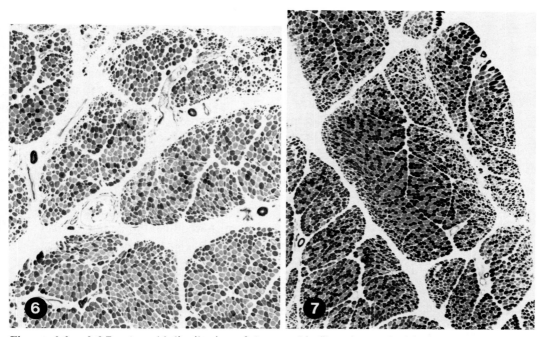

Figures 6.6 and 6.7. An odd distribution of the atrophic fibers is noted with the ATPase reactions in dermatomyositis and less often polymyositis. These atrophic fibers tend to cluster around the outside of the fascicles. This change is known descriptively as "perifascicular atrophy."

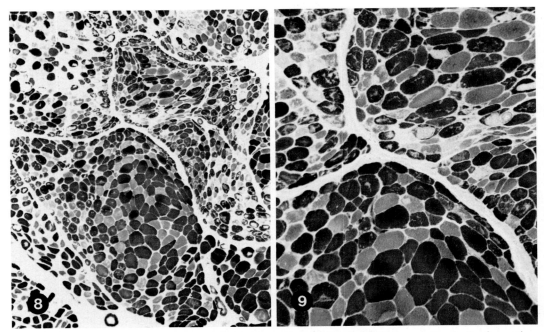

Figures 6.8 and 6.9. Another characteristic change noted with the ATPase reaction is the formation of "ghost fibers." These begin as a central pale area in which the enzyme reaction is lost and this area of altered reaction ultimately extends until the fiber becomes invisible; only the shadow of where it used to be is detectable.

The background to the autoimmune theory in the etiology of polymyositis has been well reviewed (26). It is well accepted that autoimmunity must play some part in the production of this illness, a supposition which has turned the attention of investigators to the complicated system which governs the immune response. On chromosome 6 in the human, there is a region, the HLA gene complex, which determines the human leukocyte antigens whose activity is instrumental in determining whether foreign substances shall be rejected or not. This is the major histocompatibility complex. Since these antigens determine whether a graft shall be rejected by the host animal, they have been known as the transplant antigens. The genes encode four types of antigens, the HLA-A, B, and C antigens and the D/DR antigens. This genetic region is very unusual because instead of the usual 1–2 alleles, HLA, A, B, C, and D have as many as 20 or 30 alleles. This creates the possibility of extreme variability in the HLA makeup of any individual. In practice, certain combinations occur more commonly than others. The genes in the A, B, and C loci produce a glycoprotein of about 45,000 molecular weight which is tethered to the surface of the cell by means of a β_2-microglobulin. These antigens are on the surfaces of all cells. The D region, on the other hand, encodes for glycopeptides of molecular weight 34,000 and 29,000 which form a two-chain molecule and are found on the surface, not of all cells, but only of B lymphocytes and some T cells. It seems that a prime function of the HLA, A, B and C gene products is to determine the number and specificity of the killer T cells. Additionally, the killer cell and its victim must share at least one HLA-A or B allele in common. The HLA-D gene products determine whether an immune response will take place and probably determine its magnitude. Because these genes are so polymorphic, there has been an active search in many laboratories to determine whether certain combinations of HLA types are particularly associated with a response when a particular antigen is presented. Even if the antigen cannot be identified, the finding that patients with the same illness all share the same HLA antigens would reinforce the need to search for a given precipitating cause and underline its autoimmune basis. HLA-A, B and C antigens are identified by numerals as in HLA-A1, A2, A3, etc. D specificity is indicated by Dw1, Dw2, Dw3, etc., indicating a tentative designation (27, 28). The HLA-D gene products are determined in two ways. DR antigens are defined by serological typing of B cells and monocytes. Dw typing is accomplished with the mixed lymphocyte response. There is fairly close correlation between DR typing and Dw typing and they are probably just different ways of identifying the same product.

As mentioned above, certain combinations occur commonly. Thus, the combination of HLA-A1, B8, and Dw3 occurs in 5% of the European white population. A3, B7, and Dw2 occurs in 3%. The largest category of HLA associated diseases are associated with the HLA-D type. Since the HLA-D antigens are preferentially associated with certain of the HLA-A and B antigens, this may give rise to a secondary association of autoimmune diseases with the HLA-A and B type. Myasthenia gravis and lupus erythematosus seem to be preferentially associated with HLA-B8 and DR3. Multiple sclerosis is more associated with HLA-B7 and DR2. An increase in HLA-B8 and HLA-DR3 has been reported in Caucasian patients with polymyositis, and HLA-B7 and HLA-Dw6 in black patients with the illness (29). Other studies have reported HLA-B8 in up to 72% of white patients with childhood dermatomyositis, compared to 21% of normal controls (30).

At present, HLA typing gives no further information with regard to the pathogenic mechanisms, even though it does suggest an altered immune state of the basis of the disease.

The immune response in the body is under the regulation of the now familiar T and B lymphocytes. T cells fall into subcategories whose function is designated by a variety of picturesque names such as helper, amplifier, suppressor and killer cells. Cytotoxic T cells recognize the major histocompatibility complex gene products (HLA antigens) in the tissues and are responsible for cell-mediated immunity. Killer cells destroy antibody-coated target tissue, whereas "natural killer" cells recognize alterations in a cell's surface composition without the need for the antibody. The B cells may be transformed into plasma cells and produce a specific antibody. Macrophages, B cells, and activated T cells can be identified by an antibody (Ia) which recognizes the HLA-DR antigen displayed on their surface. The systems are interrelated and the subsets of the T cells regulate B cell activity. It is therefore understandable that studies designed to show that polymyositis is due to either a cellular or a humoral cause are often confusing. Some evidence supporting the proponents of cellular immunity was found from experiments in which lymphocytes from patients with polymyositis were incubated with muscle. These lymphocytes were activated and released a lymphotoxin which was demonstrated using human fetal muscle as the target organ (31). A quantitation was attempted by assaying the incorporation of ^{14}C-labeled amino acid into the target cells. The lymphocytes which had been incubated with muscle produced a 50% decrease, which was not quite as complete as the 95% decrease in amino acid incorporation when the lymphocytes were nonspecifically stimulated with phytohemagglutinin. It was nevertheless clearly different from normal. Others have failed to demonstrate any abnormal response of lymphocytes from patients with polymyositis to stimulation by muscle extract or other agents and have concluded that cell mediated immunity does not play a part in the illness (32). A more direct demonstration of cytotoxicity was possible by incorporating ^{51}Cr into cultured chick muscle cells (33). These cells were then incubated with either the serum or lymphocytes from patients with polymyositis and the release of labeled chromium into the supernatant was measured. Only lymphocytes from patients with active disease produced an increased release of chromium into the medium, an indirect indication of damage to muscle cells. The greatest release of chromium, and therefore the most damage, was seen in the untreated patients, or patients being treated with low dose or alternate day steroids. A similar experiment compared the effect of mononuclear cells from the blood of 10 patients with polymyositis to those from control patients, when incubated with rat muscle cultures. In this experiment, no chromium was released (34). A possible explanation for the discrepancy might be that in the first experiment chick muscle was used and in the second, muscle from the rat.

Using monoclonal antibodies to type lymphocytes, Behan et al. (35) showed a decrease in the number of suppressor/cytotoxic T cells in polymyositis. Studies of the cellular response in a muscle biopsy showed an increase in the number of helper cells. Another attempt to identify the type of cell in the cellular infiltrate in the muscle demonstrated an abnormally large number of T cells in those patients who had a marked inflammatory component (36).

In a careful study comparing dermatomyositis with polymyositis, Duchenne muscular dystrophy and inclusion body myositis, the cells of the inflammatory response were identified not only by cell type but by location in the muscle biopsy (37).

In dermatomyositis there were more B cells than in the other illnesses. When the cellular responses around the muscle fibers were compared with those situated around the blood vessels, the percentage of cells which were T cells was highest around the muscle fibers and least around the blood vessels. T helper cells were found in close proximity to the macrophages at all sites, supporting the hypothesis that the helper cells were triggered by an antigen on the surface of the other cells. Killer and natural killer cells were rare. This would suggest that the major responsibility for dermatomyositis lies with humoral factors, although a T cell response against vascular or connective tissue components could not be completely ruled out.

In polymyositis the inflammatory reaction was predominantly associated with muscle fibers or was around the fascicles. The distribution of cells was similar to that seen in dermatomyositis. B cells were more numerous around the blood vessel than around muscle fibers. The reverse was true of T cells.

The proportion of T cells displaying the Ia antigen (i.e., activated T cells) was twice as high around the muscle fibers as at perivascular sites. About 1% of the cells around the muscle fibers were killer cells.

The problem was explored further by an analysis of the cells which were surrounding non-necrotic muscle fibers (38). Such cells are likely to reflect a primary response rather than being a secondary infiltration provoked by a necrotic fiber damaged by some other factor. The surface antigen T8 identifies cytotoxic T cells and it was these cells which were found to be the most abundant among those which were actually invading the muscle fibers. About half of these cells were activated as indicated by the presence of the Ia antigen. These results would suggest that polymyositis is due to T cells which have become sensitized to a muscle surface antigen and that the mechanism is cell mediated.

Immune complexes, which represent the combination of an antibody with its antigen, may be deposited in tissues in diseases which have an autoimmune basis. Immune complexes have been detected in the perimysial veins in muscle biopsies from children with dermatomyositis (39, 40). Similar deposits were found in adults with dermatomyositis, but not in polymyositis. This may support the suggestion made on pathological grounds that dermatomyositis in children is more associated with vasculitis than the disease in the adult. In a search for circulating antigen-antibody complexes, 33 patients with polymyositis were studied and such complexes found in 70%. The controls for this study were patients with amyotrophic lateral sclerosis and myasthenia gravis, two diseases which are characterized either by no destruction of the muscle or a rather passive atrophy rather than the acute destruction seen in polymyositis. It is, therefore, possible that these complexes might be found in other necrotizing myopathies (41).

Several investigators have attempted to identify specific antibodies which not only might be used diagnostically but might give some clue as to the etiology of the disease. Antibodies to myosin have been detected in serum (25, 42), but this is nonspecific. Of more interest is the antibody which has been termed Jo-1. This is an antibody to soluble cellular constituents which is detected by immunodiffusion studies in 60% of patients with polymyositis. Independently, the same antibody was labeled Pl-1 although the term Jo-1 has precedence. Further studies of this system showed the antigen to be a polypeptide which appears to be a subunit of histidyl transfer RNA synthetase with a molecular weight of 50,000 (43). The authors pointed out that antibodies against tRNA seems to be a hallmark of myositis in contrast to the finding in lupus erythematosus in which DNA antibodies are abundant. They believed the difference might reflect the high ratio of cytoplasm to nuclei in muscle. It was suggested that the anti-Jo-1 response was due to the binding of tRNA-hist to a viral RNA, which might allow the viral RNA to be carried past the body's immune defenses with subsequent cell damage and the release of viral RNA complexed with histidyl tRNA.

The last observation raises the possibility of a triggering mechanism in the disease. Since the illness often comes on in adult life after previous good health, it is difficult to imagine that the immune system would spontaneously embark on a course of tissue destruction and it seems reasonable that some mechanism is responsible for triggering it. Viral infections have often been suspected as a cause for the illness. Coxsackie B virus was implicated in one study. This myotropic virus is known to be associated with muscle symptoms in Bornholm's disease and has also been implicated in a cardiomyopathy. In a small study, the serum from four patients with polymyositis neutralized coxsackie B virus (44). Serial blood samples from patients effected this neutralization in increasingly high dilutions suggesting rising titers of the antibody. The time from the onset of symptoms to peak levels of the neutralizing antibody ranged from 2 to 7 months. Another infectious agent which has been implicated in the illness is toxoplasma. Toxoplasma itself may cause a marked myositis when the organism is detected in the muscle. However, one case of dermatomyositis was reported in which toxoplasma was also found in the muscle (45). Whether this was coincidental is uncertain, but treatment of the toxoplasmosis was associated with improvement in the patient's dermatomyositis. In another report, IgM antibodies against toxoplasma were detected in 24% of patients with polymyositis/dermatomyositis (46). Serologic evidence of old toxoplasma infection is found in up to 50% of the population, but the presence of increased levels of IgM antibodies is supposedly associated with a recent infection. Thus, their existence in patients with polymyositis/dermatomyositis is suspicious. However, it will be of interest to see whether additional confirmation of this is obtained in subse·quent studies.

Treatment

The treatment of dermato- and polymyositis is simpler to describe than it is to justify (47). Controlled trials of steroids or other immunosuppressants are few and far between. One large study concluded that the same number of patients achieved remission with no steroids as with a high dose of steroids (8). A low dose of steroids seemed to be ineffective and only one patient on low dose steroid therapy did well. A hopeful sign for those who believe in the use of these drugs was that twice as many patients were "better" with a high dose of steroids than with no steroids at all. Two seemingly contradictory studies on the results of high dose steroid therapy in polymyositis demonstrated in one series that 7 of 18 patients died and only 3 maintained any improvement (48). In the other larger series (118 patients), two-thirds of the patients improved to the point where they had no functional disability (49). In an analysis of 100 cases of patients with polymyositis and dermatomyositis, Henriksson and Sandstedt (50) found that about half of the patients improved on steroid therapy, the other half did not. They also suggested that those treated with steroids within the first 24 months of the illness did better than those who were treated during later phases. If one subtracts from this study the patients with accompanying malignancy the overall mortality rate is around 15%. The authors also felt that the degree of improvement was related to the dose of steroids. There may be, however, a fallacy in this reasoning. The potential degree of improvement in patients who are severely affected is much greater than those in whom only slight disability exists. Physicians are likely to use the larger dose of steroids in the patient with the more severe disease and this might lead to a false correlation. However, the finding does echo the study previously mentioned in which low dose steroid therapy seemed to be ineffective as compared to high dose steroids. The only prospective control trial in the literature was not a trial of steroids vs. placebo but of a combination of prednisone and azathioprine evaluated against patients treated with prednisone alone. The study was a small one, the initial period of follow-up short, and the conclusion was that there was no difference (51). A subsequent paper following these patients in an uncontrolled fashion suggested that the group of patients who were given both prednisone and azathioprine were slightly better than those treated with prednisone alone (52). However, the statistical underpinnings of this opinion were not impressive (47).

There is now increasing interest in using azathioprine in neuromuscular diseases. Although the drug has its share of side effects, including potential fatal leukopenia, and is hepatotoxic, it is often much more easily tolerated by the patient than prednisone. It is used in doses of 1.5–2 mg per kilogram or even higher. Therapy is instituted by using a low dose (for example, 50 mg a day in an adult) and then gradually increasing the dosage while monitoring the blood count. In the early stages, the white cell count evaluation should be carried out every 2 or 3 days. As the dosage is increased the white cell count will start to fall and it is advisable to keep the leukocyte count above 3,000–4,000. In some patients an unusual systemic reaction occurs early in the treatment characterized by fever, abdominal pain, nausea, vomiting and anorexia (53).

Other forms of immunosuppression have included low dose total body radiation (54, 55). A total dose of 150 R was given over a period of several weeks. Individual treatments consisted of a dose of 15 R and was given twice a week. One patient had a dramatic improvement in his condition and the second patient also improved, but relapsed shortly afterwards. One patient has been treated in our clinic with total body irradiation. He was an elderly man with dermatomyositis of long standing which was severely disabling and which was refractory to all other forms of therapy. No response was seen to irradiation. An additional patient who did not respond to the therapy was reported by Schon et al. (56).

Plasmapheresis has been reported to be of benefit on occasions but has been popular only in a few centers (57, 58).

It is possible that the popularity of one form of treatment over another may depend on which one is tried first in any given clinic. The illness seems to be much more responsive to therapy in its early stages than when it has become chronic and indolent. Perhaps any of the several forms of treatment are likely to be impressive when used early, whereas used late in the illness all may tend to fail. Those of us who use total body irradiation or plasmapheresis late in the illness may therefore develop an unnecessarily gloomy impression of their lack of efficacy. This simply underlines the need for controlled trials; an almost impossible demand in a situation in which the patient is sick and the clinician is committed by faith to his favorite medicine. In spite of the dismal state of our knowledge, few of us can observe the worsening of a patient with acute dermato- or polymyositis without prescribing prednisone or some other agent.

What follows is a distillation of my own prejudices, based on no firm scientific principles. It seems to me that there are three errors which are prevalent in the treatment of patients with steroids. The first occurs when the medication is started too late, the second is the administration of steroids in doses which are too small, and the third is the termination of the therapy too soon. If steroids have an effect on the disease, they should be used as soon as the diagnosis is made. It seems, in general, that patients who are treated earlier do better (49, 59). If steroids are to be used they should be used in adequate suppressive doses of between 50 and 80 mg of prednisone daily (1–2 mg per kilogram of body weight in children). Using smaller doses of prednisone early in the disease in the hope of sparing the patient the untoward side effects is an unhappy compromise at best and may even result in the appearance of side effects in the absence of the possible benefit of suppressive doses. Physician's insecurity over the value of prednisone also leads to an early withdrawal of the drug, which may sometimes be not only unnecessary but harmful. A typical situation is the patient with moderately severe polymyositis and an elevated CK whose diagnosis is well substantiated. The patient is placed on suppressive doses of steroids and, instead of the expected immediate improvement, no change in the patient's condition is seen for a week to 10 days. At this point the physician is either given to doubts about the diagnosis or concludes that steroids are ineffective. Consequently the medication is withdrawn. Very frequently the serum CK will fall during the first week. The clinical improvement, however, may be quite delayed, a matter of 4–6 weeks after the decline in the CK. The return of the enzyme to more normal levels is not only an encouraging finding but is an indication to persevere with the use of steroids for at least 2–3 months before assuming the patient is steroid resistant. The length of time during which patients should be maintained on suppressive doses of steroids is another question with no proven answer. If the disease is acute and the patient has been started on 80 mg of prednisone daily, or higher, the dose can be reduced to levels of 60 mg daily after 2 months or when the enzyme returns to normal. Tapering the steroids below this level depends upon the clinical situation. I do not like to taper steroids while the patient's strength is still improving. The only exception to this is in the situation when the side effects of the medicine are insupportable. Once the improvement in muscle strength has leveled off, I usually further reduce the prednisone dosage. In practical terms this will mean that most patients will be taking suppressive doses of prednisone for a year or more. By appropriately reducing the alternate daily dose the patient may be converted to an alternate day regimen of steroids. Some patients do quite well on such a schedule; others do not. Once the dosage is below the equivalent of 25 mg daily the reduction may be even slower, 2.5 mg at a time. Sometimes an exacerbation of the polymyositis during steroid withdrawal is heralded by a gradual increase in the serum muscle enzyme levels. Such an increase should be treated with respect and, if there is a consistent and progressive elevation of the enzyme, an increase in the dose of steroids may be indicated even in the absence of clinical change.

Ancillary therapy includes the administration of potassium supplement and an antacid regimen in those with a history of gastric discomfort. A high protein, low carbohydrate diet with decreased salt intake is also recommended. The commonest side effect which has been noted in patients in our clinic has been the occurrence of cataracts. These were usually seen in patients who had been taking steroids for 2 months or more and occurred in about 30% of such patients. On one occasion surgical extraction was necessary. One patient had a hypertensive crisis with an encephalopathy but there have been no serious problems with diabetes or gastrointestinal disturbance. Osteoporosis was seen in several patients and compression fracture of the thoracic vertebra was seen in one. During this time there have been 12 deaths in over 100 patients seen over the last 15 years, 3 in childhood and 9 in middle to late age. Valid statistics cannot be derived from our results because many patients were followed for a brief time. A different view on the management of juvenile dermatomyositis has been proposed by Dubowitz (60). Based on the results of steroid therapy in eight cases he suggested using smaller doses of prednisone and tapering the dosage as soon as clinical improvement begins. Dubowitz also suggested that serum enzyme levels are less reliable than the patient's clinical response. In a subsequent paper from Hammersmith (61), children with dermatomyositis were treated with prednisone 1–1.5 mg/kg daily for 2 weeks and then the dose was reduced at the rate of 2.5 mg/week. When the dosage reached a level of 10 mg daily it was reduced by 1 mg/week. The author believed that a group of children treated in this manner alone and without any prior treatment fared better than another group of children who had also received prior and more prolonged treatment with steroids. The problem with using this second group of children as controls is that it will naturally select out those who have "failed" treatment before being referred to a tertiary referral center. It is not justified to compare them with a group of children who have never been treated.

In addition to steroids and azathioprine, various immunosuppressant agents have been used (62–68). Patients reported in the literature have responded to methotrexate and cytoxan. There are good theoretical grounds for trying these medications. My own experience has been limited to azathioprine and, in only two patients, methotrexate. The results obtained were not as good as those in the literature, but it is quite possible that the medications were used too late. Presumably, if they are to be effective, they will be more effective early in the disease. Various dosage schedules have been recommended for the various drugs. Methotrexate has been given both intravenously and orally. The least toxic and most effective regimen seems to be to give the drug orally in increasing doses until 0.8 mg per kilogram of body weight is given per week. The side effects of the medication have been pronounced in some series and relatively absent in others. Among those mentioned were buccal ulcers, hepatitis, pleuritis, and pneumonitis. With methotrexate therapy the maximal response occurred after about 13 weeks of treatment (67). It is important to prevent the joint contractures which may develop during the illness, and a program of "range of motion" passive exercises should be carried out during the acute stages of the disease.

REFERENCES

1. Medsger, T. A., Dawson, W. N., and Masi, A. T. The epidemiology of polymyositis. Am. J. Med. *48:* 715–723, 1970.

2. Pearson, C. M. Polymyositis. Annu Rev. Med. *17:* 63–82, 1966.
3. Nussbaum, A. I., Silver, R. M., and Maricq. H. R. Serial changes in nailfold capillary morphology in childhood dermatomyositis. Arthritis Rheum. *26:* 1169–1172, 1983.
4. Schaumburg, H. H., Nielsen, S. L., and Yurchak, P. M. Heartblock in polymyositis: case with proven involvement of heart. N. Engl. J. Med. *284:* 480–481, 1971.
5. Singsen, B., Goldreyer, B., Stanton, R., and Hanson, V. Childhood polymyositis with cardiac conduction defects. Am. J. Dis. Child. *130:* 72–74, 1976.
6. Duncan, P. E., Griffin, J. P., Garcia, A., and Kaplan, S. B. Fibrosing alveolitis and polymyositis. Am. J. Med. *57:* 621–626, 1974.
7. Schwartz, M. I., Matthay, R. A., Sahn, S. A., et al. Interstitial lung disease in polymyositis and dermatomyositis; analysis of six cases and review of the literature. Medicine *55:* 89–104, 1976.
8. Winkelmann, R. K., Mulder, D. W., Lambert, E. H., Howard, F. M., and Diessner, G. R. Dermatomyositis-polymyositis: comparison of untreated and cortisone treated patients. Mayo Clin. Proc. *43:* 545–556, 1968.
9. Bohan, A., Peter, J. B., Bowman, R. L., and Pearson, C. M. A computer assisted analysis of 153 patients with polymyositis and dermatomyositis. Medicine *56:* 255–286, 1977.
10. Bohan, A., and Peter, J. B. Polymyositis and dermatomyositis. N. Engl. J. Med. *292:* 344–347, 1975.
11. Bohan, A., and Peter, J. B. Polymyositis and dermatomyositis. N. Engl. J. Med. *292:* 403–407, 1975.
12. Barnes, B. E. Dermatomyositis and malignancy, a review of the literature. Ann. Intern. Med. *84:* 68–76, 1976.
13. Callen, J. P., Hyla, J. F., Bole, G. G., and Kay, D. R. The relationship of dermatomyositis and polymyositis to internal malignancy. Arch. Dermatol. *116:* 295–298, 1980.
14. Henriksson, K. G. Recent advances in investigation of polymyositis. Acta Neurol. Scand. Suppl. *78:* 60–67, 1980.
15. Sharp, G. C., Irvin, W. S., Tan, E. M., Gould, R. G., and Holman, H. R. Mixed connective tissue diseases. Am. J. Med. *52:* 148–159, 1972.
16. Levitin, P. M., Weary, P. E., and Ginliano, V. J. The immunofluorescent "band" test in mixed connective tissue disorders. Ann. Intern. Med. *83:* 53–55, 1975.
17. Venables, P. J., Mumford, P. A., and Maini, R. M. Antibodies to nuclear antigens in polymyositis; relationship to autoimmune "overlap syndrome" and carcinoma. Ann. Rheum. Dis. *40:* 217–223, 1981.
18. Bradley, W. G. Polymyositis. Br. J. Hosp. Med. *17:* 351–355, 1977.
19. de Merieux, P., Verity, M. A., Clements, P. J., and Paulus, H. E. Esophageal abnormalities and dysphagia in polymyositis and dermatomyositis. Arthritis Rheum. *26:* 961–963, 1983.
20. Banker, B. Q., and Victor, M. Dermatomyositis (systemic angiopathy) of childhood. Medicine *45:* 261, 1966.
21. Paulson, O. F., Engel, A. G., and Gomez, M. R. Muscle blood flow in Duchenne type muscular dystrophy, limb girdle dystrophy, polymyositis and in normal controls. J. Neurol. Neurosurg. Psychiatry *37:* 685–690, 1974.
22. Jerusalem, F., Rakusa, M., Engel, A. G., and MacDonald, R. D. Morphometric analysis of skeletal muscle capillary ultrastructure in inflammatory myopathies. J. Neurol. Sci. *23:* 391–402, 1974.
23. Morgan, G., Peter, J. C., and Newbould, B. B. Experimental allergic myositis in rats. Arthritis Rheum. *14:* 599–609, 1971.
24. Manghani, D., Partridge, T. A., and Sloper, J. C. The role of the myofibrillar fraction of skeletal muscle in the production of experimental polymyositis. J. Neurol. Sci. *23:* 489–503, 1974.
25. Partridge, T. A., Manghani, D., and Sloper, J. C. Antimuscle antibodies in polymyositis. Lancet *1:* 676, 1973.
26. Whitaker, J. N. Inflammatory myopathy: a review of etiologic and pathogenetic factors. Muscle Nerve *5:* 573–592, 1982.
27. McDevatt, H. O. Regulation of the immune response by the major histocompatibility system. N. Engl. J. Med. *303:* 1514–1517, 1980.
28. Marsh, D. G., Meyers, D. A., and Bias, W. B. The epidemiology and genetics of atopic allergy. N. Engl. J. Med. *305:* 1551–1559, 1983.
29. Hirsch Enlow, R. W., Bias, W. B., and Arnett, F. C. HLA-D related (DR) antigens in various kinds of myositis. Hum. Immunol. *3:* 181–186, 1981.
30. Behan, W. M. H., Behan, P. O., and Dick, H. A. HLA-B8 in polymyositis. N. Engl. J. Med. *298:* 1260–1261, 1978.
31. Johnson, R. L., Fink, C. W., and Ziff, M. Lymphotoxin formation by lymphocytes and muscle in polymyositis. J. Clin. Invest. *51:* 2435–2449, 1972.

32. Lisak, R. P., and Zweiman, B. Mitogen and muscle extract induced in vitro proliferative responses in myasthenia gravis dermatomyositis and polymyositis. J. Neurol. Neurosurg. Psychiatry *38:* 521–524, 1976.
33. Dawkins, R. L., and Mastaglia, F. L. Cell mediated cytotoxicity to muscle in polymyositis. N. Engl. J. Med. *288:* 434–438, 1973.
34. Haas, D. C. Absence of cell mediated cytotoxicity to muscle cultures in polymyositis. J. Rheumatol. *7:* 671–676, 1980.
35. Behan, W. M., Behan, P. O., Micklem, H. S., and Durward, W. F. Abnormalities of lymphocyte subsets in polymyositis. Br. Med. J. *287:* 181–182, 1983.
36. Rowe, D. J., Isenberg, D. A., McDougall, J., and Beverly, P. C. Characterization of polymyositis infiltrates using monoclonal antibodies to human leucocyte antigens. Clin. Exp. Immunol. *45:* 290–298, 1981.
37. Arahata, K., and Engel, A. G. Monoclonal antibody analysis of mononuclear cells in myopathies; I. Quantitation of subsets according to diagnosis and sites of accumulation and demonstration and counts of muscles fibers invaded by T cells. Ann. Neurol. *16:* 193–208, 1984.
38. Engel, A. G., and Arahata, K. Monoclonal antibody analysis of mononuclear cells in myopathies; II. Phenotypes of autoinvasive cells in polymyositis and inclusion body myositis. Ann. Neurol. *16:* 209–215, 1984.
39. Whitaker, J. N., and Engel, W. K. Mechanisms of muscle injury in idiopathic inflammatory myopathy. N. Engl. J. Med. *289:* 107–108, 1973.
40. Whitaker, J. N., and Engel, W. K. Vascular deposits of immunoglobulin and complement in idiopathic inflammatory myopathy. N. Engl. J. Med. *286:* 333–338, 1972.
41. Behan, W. M., Barkas, T., and Behan, P. O. Detection of immune complexes in polymyositis. Acta Neurol. Scand. *65:* 320–334, 1982.
42. Nishikai, M., and Homma, M. Circulating autoantibody against human myoglobin in polymyositis. J.A.M.A. *237:* 1842–1844, 1977.
43. Mathews, M. B., and Bernstein, R. M. Myositis autoantibody inhibits histidyl-tRNA synthetase: a model for autoimmunity. Nature *304:* 177–179, 1983.
44. Travers, R. L., Hughes, G. R. V., Cambridge, G., and Sewell, J. R. Coxsackie-B neutralization titers in polymyositis-dermatomyositis. Lancet *1:* 1268, 1977.
45. Hendrickx, G. F. M., Verhage, J., Jennekens, F. G. I., and Van Knapen, F. Dermatomyositis and toxoplasmosis. Ann. Neurol. *5:* 393–395, 1979.
46. Nagid, S. K., and Kagen, L. G. Serologic evidence for acute toxoplasmosis in polymyositis/dermatomyositis. Increased frequency of specific antitoxoplasma IgM antibodies. Am. J. Med. *75:* 313–320, 1983.
47. Rowland, L. P., Clark, C., and Olarte, M. Therapy for dermatomyositis and polymyositis. Advan. Neurol. *17:* 63–97, 1977.
48. Riddoch, D., and Morgan-Hughes, J. A. Prognosis in adult polymyositis. J. Neurol. Sci. *26:* 71–80, 1975.
49. De Vere, R., and Bradley, W. G. Polymyositis: its presentation morbidity and mortality. Brain *98:* 637–666, 1975.
50. Henriksson, K. G., and Sandstedt, P. Polymyositis: treatment and prognosis. A study of 107 patients. Acta Neurol. Scand. *65:* 280–300, 1982.
51. Bunch, P. W. Prednisone and azathioprine for polymyositis; long term follow up. Arthritis Rheum. *24:* 44–48, 1984.
52. Bunch, P. W., Worthington, J. W., Kombs, J. J., Ilstrup, D. M., and Engel, A. G. Azathioprine with prednisone for polymyositis. A controlled clinical trial. Ann. Intern. Med. *92:* 365–369, 1980.
53. Levy, R. J., Kissel, J. T., Mendell, J. R., and Griggs, R. C. Incidents of azathioprine toxicity in neuromuscular disease. Neurology *74* (Suppl. 1): 91, 1984.
54. Engel, W. K., Lichter, A. S., and Galdi, A. T. Polymyositis: remarkable response to total body irradiation. Lancet *1:* 658, 1981.
55. Hubbard, W. N., Walport, M. J., Halman, K. E., Beaney, R. P., and Hughes, G. F. Remission from polymyositis after total body irradiation. Br. Med. J. *284:* 1915–1916, 1982.
56. Schon, F., Thomas, P. K., and Senanayake, L. F. Remission from polymyositis after total body irradiation. Br. Med. J. *285:* 290, 1982.
57. Dau, P. C. The role of plasma exchange in the treatment of idiopathic polymyositis. Prog. Clin. Biol. Res. *106:* 223–232, 1982.
58. Dau, P. C. Plasmapheresis in idiopathic inflammatory myopathy; experience with 35 patients. Arch. Neurol. *35:* 544–552, 1981.
59. Rose, A. L. Childhood polymyositis. Am. J. Dis. Child. *127:* 518–522, 1974.
60. Dubowitz, V. Treatment of dermatomyositis in childhood. Arch. Dis. Child. *51:* 494–500, 1976.

61. Miller, G., Heckmatt, J. Z., and Dubowitz, V. Drug treatment of juvenile dermatomyositis. Arch. Dis. Child. *58:* 445–450, 1983.
62. Arnett, F. C., Whelton, J. C., Zizic, T. M., and Stevens, M. B. Methotrexate therapy in polymyositis. Ann. Rheum. Dis. *32:* 536–546, 1973.
63. Benson, M. D., and Aldo, M. A. Azathioprine therapy in polymyositis. Arch. Intern. Med. *132:* 544–551, 1973.
64. Currie, S., and Walton, J. N. Immunosuppressive therapy in polymyositis. J. Neurol. Neurosurg. Psychiatry *34:* 447–452, 1971.
65. Haas, D. C. Treatment of polymyositis with immunosuppressive drugs. Neurology *23:* 55–62, 1973.
66. Metzger, A. L., Bohan, A., Goldberg, L. S., Bluestone, R., and Pearson, C. M. Polymyositis and dermatomyositis: Combined methotrexate and corticoid steroid therapy. Ann. Intern. Med. *81:* 182–189, 1974.
67. Sokoloff, M. C., Goldberg, L. S., and Pearson, C. M. Treatment of corticosteroid-resistant polymyositis with methotrexate. Lancet *1:* 14–16, 1971.
68. Malaviya, A. N., Many, A., and Schwarz, R. S. Treatment of dermatomyositis with methotrexate. Lancet *2:* 485–488, 1968.

POLYMYALGIA RHEUMATICA

There are many illnesses in which muscle pain is a prominent symptom. Sometimes these illnesses are nebulous and the diagnosis difficult to establish. Often the pain seems to be frankly psychosomatic in origin. At other times the physician may take refuge behind a diagnosis such as fibrositis, which often implies no more than a feeling that the disease is organic but an inability to discover any abnormality, although on occasions abnormalities are noted on fascial biopsy (1). One disease, polymyalgia rheumatica, is a major cause of muscle pain and is now widely recognized (2, 3).

The symptoms of muscle pain and stiffness are so characteristic that different patients will use identical phrases in describing their symptoms. After a period of rest, particularly a prolonged period, the muscles "freeze" or "sets like jelly" and any movement of the muscle produces pain or a tearing feeling within the muscle. With continued use and exercise the muscle stiffness and pain may abate. Thus, the discomfort is greatest early in the morning upon arising and, indeed, may be severe enough to prevent the patient from getting out of bed. Usually the shoulder muscles are more involved than any other muscles and in a surprising number, even among younger patients, there is evidence of cervical arthritis. Women suffer from the illness twice as frequently as men and the disease appears in late life, cases under the age of 55 being quite rare in the literature.

There are often other complaints that go along with muscle stiffness and tenderness. The patient may feel chronically unwell and may run a low grade fever with frequent night sweats. Weight loss is often noted. Temporal arteritis with tender, enlarged, and nodular arteries is a recognized complication of the illness. It is difficult to determine the true incidence of temporal arteritis, but it may be as high as 75%. In a study of 85 patients referred to a regional center, giant cell arteritis was found in 55% of the patients (4). In 28 patients the giant cell arteritis followed the onset of polymyalgia rheumatica after an interval of months to years. Temporal artery biopsies were of no value in predicting those patients who might be expected to develop the complication, although obviously they were important in making a diagnosis during an attack. The authors suggested that the treatment of polymyalgia rheumatica should be undertaken bearing in mind the possible serious consequences in a large proportion of the patients, thus underlining the need for suppressive steroid therapy. Polymyalgia rheumatica may occur with surprising suddenness over a period of a few days. Left without treatment, patients do seem to improve, but this improvement may take place over several years and few are willing to endure the symptoms for that length of time. An association between polymyalgia and neoplasia has been suggested, but this association was not confirmed (5).

Examination of the patient when the symptoms are severe may show the stiffened, cautious walk of a patient in pain. The arms are held close to the side and flexed, protected against any untoward swinging movement, and the legs are moved stiffly and slowly. The muscle is often tender to the touch, although the pain produced with palpation is not as severe as that caused when the patient moves. If the patient is seen late in the day when his symptoms have abated, he may appear relatively normal. When asked, the patient usually describes his pain as a feeling of stiffness and to illustrate this will often move his arms in a manner reminiscent of a boxer loosening his shoulder muscles. If the patient can relax, passive movement of the limbs is normal, although often the patient splints the limb against such movement. For the most part, the large joints in the limbs are not clinically abnormal and periarticular tenderness is not generally a part of the disease. Several studies have pointed to laboratory evidence of synovitis in the joints with the suggestion by one group that this is in fact a disease of the joints and not the muscles (6).

Laboratory Studies

With few exceptions the laboratory studies are normal. The sedimentation rate is elevated, often over 70 mm per hour. For the diagnosis of polymyalgia rheumatica to be made with certainty, the elevated sedimentation rate is an essential parameter. Patients often show a mild hypochromic or normochromic anemia. There is occasional elevation of the α_2-globulin, and sometimes antinuclear antibodies are found. The muscle biopsy may also show mild but nonspecific abnormalities (7). There is an increased incidence of HLA-8 antigen in patients with polymyalgia (8). A study of the HLA-D antigens showed a minor increase in the frequency of DR4 and DRw6 (9).

Treatment

Little is known of the etiology of this disease, and the only evidence that it belongs in the rheumatoid group of diseases is that it shares some of their clinical characteristics. The description of the disease may be mundane, but response to treatment often approaches the spectacular. The illness not only responds to prednisone but does so with alacrity. The patient is free of symptoms within a week and often within 24 hours of the administration of prednisone. We have usually started patients on between 30 and 50 mg of prednisone daily and maintain this dosage for 2 months before decreasing it gradually. These levels of prednisone administration are higher than recommended in the literature, but we have felt that the disease is more effectively suppressed this way and relapses are less common. Maintenance with low doses of steroids, from 10 to 20 mg daily, may be necessary for a year or more. Withdrawal of the medication below this level may exacerbate the symptoms.

REFERENCES

1. Simon, D. B., Ringel, S. P., and Sufit, R. L. Clinical spectrum of fascial inflammation. Muscle Nerve *5:* 525–537, 1982.
2. Hunder, G. G., Disney, T. F., and Ward, L. E. Polymyalgia rheumatica. Mayo Clin. Proc. *44:* 849–875, 1969.
3. Andrews, F. M. Polymyalgia rheumatica. Practitioner *205:* 635–640, 1970.
4. Jones, J. G., and Hazleman, B. L. Prognosis and management of polymyalgia rheumatica. Ann. Rheum. Dis. *40:* 1–5, 1980.
5. von Knorring, J. and Somer, T. Malignancy in association with polymyalgia rheumatica and temporal arteritis. Scand. J. Rheumatol. *3:* 129–135, 1974.
6. O'Duffy, J. D., Hunder, G. C., and Wahner, H. W. A follow up study of polymyalgia rheumatica: evidence of chronic axial synovitis. J. Rheumatol. *7:* 685–693, 1980.
7. Brooke, M. H. and Kaplan, H. Muscle pathology in rheumatoid arthritis, polymyalgia rheumatica, and polymyositis. Arch. Pathol. *94:* 101–118, 1972.
8. Rosenthal, M., Müller, W., Albert, E. D., and Schattenkirchner, M. HL-A Antibodies in polymyalgia rheumatica. N. Engl. J. Med. *292:* 595, 1975.
9. Calamia, R. T., Moor, S. B., Elveback, L., and Hunder, G. HLA-DR locus antigens in polymyalgia rheumatica and giant cell arteritis. J. Rheumatol. *8:* 993–996, 1981.

INCLUSION BODY MYOSITIS

Inclusion body myositis is essentially a diagnosis made by muscle biopsy which most resembles one of the genetic dystrophies with marked variability in the size of fibers, increased fibrosis, some fiber splitting and internal nuclei. There are cellular reactions in many but not all of the biopsies which are more associated with necrotic fibers than they are with blood vessels. The term inclusion body myositis is derived from the presence of many degenerative bodies within the muscle cells (1–4). On occasions these resemble autophagic vacuoles with cellular debris and cytomembranous whorls. In addition, in both the cytoplasm and, to a lesser extent, the nuclei there are masses of filaments ranging between 150 and 180 Å in diameter. They have been thought to represent evidence of a viral infection, but they bear no close resemblance to any of the known filaments associated with such infections.

Out of the 20 or so case reports in literature, the great majority are in males. The onset of the disease has been recognized at all ages, but the majority of patients are 40 years or older. Most often there is a slowly progressive weakness of the limb-girdle musculature which is associated in a significant number with distal weakness. In some cases the distal weakness is the early finding and the disease mimics a peripheral neuropathy or hereditary distal myopathy. Confusion with the latter may be compounded since in addition to the slowly progressive weakness there are also abnormal inclusions in the hereditary distal myopathy. In most of the cases there is no other evidence of a related collagen vascular disease nor any skin rash such as might suggest dermatomyositis. Muscle pains are usually absent. The EMG may show irritable phenomena as well as an underlying myopathic pattern. The CK is often mildly elevated but may be normal. The origin of the disease is obscure. Some have claimed to detect evidence of viral infection in the patients, but most of these reports have been dismissed as coincidental. In 6 selected cases of the illness, mumps virus antigen was demonstrated in the inclusions, including intranuclear inclusions. Of the four cases in whom inquiry was made, all gave a history of a clinical attack of mumps (5). Steroids have been used to treat the illness but without any notable success.

I seem to be alone in the muscle fraternity in my skepticism about this entity, but I am reluctant to accept it with the more usual inflammatory myopathies. I think I would be less reluctant to embrace this diagnosis were it termed inclusion body myopathy rather than myositis. Muscle has such a limited number of possible reactions that different etiological entities may well share common pathological responses. Biopsy evidence of a cellular response is not limited to inflammatory myopathies but is often seen in dystrophies of various kinds. Similar, although not identical, types of bodies are seen in other illnesses which do not have an inflammatory or autoimmune basis. The clinical characteristics are not those of a relapsing remitting disease. The behavior of the serum CK is certainly not typical of the other inflammatory myopathies. On the other hand, studies of the type of cell involved in the destructive process have shown similar changes to those seen in polymyositis (6). Thus, the destructive process seems to be instigated by cytotoxic T cells responding to some, as yet, unidentified antigen on the surface of the muscle fiber.

REFERENCES

1. Carpenter, S., Karpati, G. Heller, I., and Eisen, A. Inclusion body myositis. A distinct variety of idiopathic inflammatory myopathy. Neurology *28:* 8–17, 1979.
2. Hunis, E. J., and Samaha, F. J. Inclusion body myositis. Lab. Invest. *25:* 240–248, 1971.
3. Mikol, J., Felten-Papaiconomou, A., Ferchal, R., Perol, Y., Gautier, B., Haguenau, M., and Pepin, B. Inclusion body myositis; clinicopathological studies and isolation of an adenovirus type II from muscle biopsy specimen. Ann. Neurol. *11:* 576–581, 1982.
4. Julien, J., Vital, C., Vallat, J. M., Lagueny, A., and Sapania, D. Inclusion body myositis. J. Neurol. Sci. *55:* 15–24, 1982.
5. Chou, S. M., and Mizuno, Y. Mumps virus antigen in inclusion body myositis. Neurology *35:* 204, 1985.
6. Engel, A. G., and Arahata, K. Monoclonal antibody analysis of mononuclear cells in myopathies; II. Phenotypes of autoinvasive cells in polymyositis and inclusion body myositis. Ann. Neurol. *16:* 209–215, 1984.

EOSINOPHILIC FASCIITIS

In the mid 1970s Shulman (1) proposed a new syndrome, the hallmark of which was firm, taut skin bound down to the underlying structures. Full thickness biopsy extending from the skin to the fascia revealed a cellular response characterized by eosinophils and this was accompanied by eosinophilia in the peripheral blood. The patients were disabled by pain and stiffness in the affected areas. There have been reports of over 100 patients with this entity since Shulman's original description (2–4). Many of the cases date their onset to a time following unaccustomed physical exertion. It is generally a disease of adult life, although it has also been reported in children. On examination the skin is puckered and dimpled with the appearance of orange peel. In some areas the linear depressions cross the skin like "rivulets." The extremities are the commonest site with the forearm and arm leading the list, but the thighs and legs may also be involved. It is usually, but not always, symmetrical. This disease may start with a focus of firm, undurated fascia and skin in the arms which then gradually spreads to involve the trunk.

There is a constant discussion in the literature as to the similarity between this illness and scleroderma. Some suggest that it may be a variety of scleroderma, others that it may belong to an overlap syndrome, while still others believe it to be of different etiology. Those who believe it to be a unique syndrome point to the rarity of Raynaud's phenomenon in eosinophilic fasciitis and to the fact that the internal organs are spared. The peripheral eosinophilia is also rare in scleroderma. In a handful of patients other hematologic abnormalities have been described. These range from aplastic anemia to myelomonocytic leukemia and idiopathic thrombocytopenic purpura. A carpal tunnel syndrome has been noted on occasion, but this may be coincidental. The muscle is usually spared, although an eosinophilic infiltrate may be noted, and unless an effort is made to obtain fascia at the same time as muscle, the diagnosis may be missed. An elevated sedimentation rate and hypergammaglobulinemia has been noted in a high proportion of patients. Eosinophils may be missing from the inflammatory response in the fascia, although they are noted in over 90% of the patients when the peripheral blood smear is evaluated. This disorder responds quite well to suppressive doses of steroids, although maintenance steroid therapy may be necessary for a long time to prevent a recurrence of the induration.

REFERENCES

1. Shulman, L. E. Diffuse fasciitis and eosinophilia: a new syndrome. Arthritis Rheum. Suppl. *19:* 205–217, 1976.
2. Moore, T. L., and Zucker, J. Eosinophilic fasciitis. Semin. Arthritis Rheum. *9:* 228–235, 1980.
3. Michet, C. J., Doyle, J. A., and Ginsburg, W. W. Eosinophilic fasciitis. Mayo Clin. Proc. *56:* 27–34, 1981.
4. Sills, E. M. Diffuse fasciitis with eosinophilia in childhood. Johns Hopkins Med. J. *151:* 203–207, 1982.

SARCOID MYOPATHY

In sarcoidosis, the disease may be found in the muscle as in other tissues. The diagnosis of sarcoid myopathy rests upon the clinical demonstration of involvement of other organs as well as the pathological demonstration of noncaseating granulomas in the muscle. It has been suggested that sarcoidosis may affect muscle exclusively. This is not well substantiated and a critical review of the literature reveals that, on most occasions, sarcoid myopathy is part of more diffuse disease (1). The myopathy takes one of several forms, of which the commonest is asymptomatic (2, 3). As many as half of all patients with sarcoidosis have some involvement of the muscle even in the absence of muscular symptoms. In those patients with overt muscle disease, the majority have a chronic proximal myopathy. Palpable nodules may be found in the muscle, and occasionally a diffuse hypertrophy of the muscle may occur. Women are more commonly affected than men (4:1). Additionally, the age of onset seems to be later in women than in men so that the illness appears predominantly in the postmenopausal woman. A very acute and fulminating myopathy may be seen with marked elevation of CK, but this is unusual.

Laboratory tests which may substantiate the diagnosis of sarcoidosis include the changes seen in the chest x-ray and the positive skin reaction to the Kveim-Siltzbach antigen. It is also important to differentiate the granulomatous changes produced by sarcoidosis from those produced by an impressive array of chemical and other agents. These vary from beryllium to cork dust and from fungi to spirochetes (4). The treatment of sarcoidosis is no more clear than the treatment of polymyositis, probably less so. There is evidence from the literature that the majority of patients are helped by the administration of steroids or ACTH, but controlled studies are lacking. Gardner-Thorpe (1) suggested that, although steroid therapy had been useful in 20 of 26 cases reported in the literature, the hazards of steroid therapy were too great to allow the routine use of the drug. Nevertheless, in a patient whose weakness is secondary to sarcoidosis, the use of prednisone is probably justified at least as a therapeutic trial.

REFERENCES

1. Gardner-Thorpe, C. Muscle weakness due to sarcoid myopathy. Neurology *22:* 917–928, 1972.
2. Silverstein, A. and Siltzbach, L. E. Muscle involvement in sarcoidosis. Arch. Neurol. *21:* 235–241, 1969.
3. Douglas, A. C., Macleod, J. G., and Matthews, J. D. Symptomatic sarcoidosis of skeletal muscle. J. Neurol. Neurosurg. Psychiatry *36:* 1034–1040, 1973.
4. James, D. G. Modern concepts of sarcoidosis (editorial). Chest *64:* 675–677, 1973.

OTHER INFLAMMATORY CONDITIONS

There are other conditions associated with inflammation of the muscle. In some, the etiology is obscure. For example, some patients with an intestinal malabsorption syndrome and IgA deficiency have developed striking muscle weakness with facial and axial muscle involvement (1). In other patients the inflammatory response is due to direct infection of the muscle by various organisms. Bacterial infections include those seen as part of miliary tuberculosis and with other organisms such as staphylococcus and streptococcus.

In tropical countries pyomyositis is not an uncommon disease. The affecting organism is often *Staphylococcus aureus* and usually the large muscle groups are involved, commonly those of the thigh. The muscle is hot, painful, and swollen, and activity is limited because any movement exacerbates the pain. Systemic signs of bacterial infection with fever and malaise are common. Treatment involves the use of the appropriate antibiotics and surgical drainage of the abscess (2).

Parasitic infestations of muscle are also well known. The larvae of trichinella may find their way into human muscle after ingestion of infected pork. General symptoms of malaise and fever are associated with muscle pains and stiffness. There may be periorbital edema. Involvement of the masseter muscles is common, with pain on attempting to open the jaw or on chewing. Skin rashes, petechial hemorrhages, and retinal hemorrhages have been noted. Subclinical infection is probably commoner than is realized, and estimates of the prevalence of trichinosis in the population are in the neighborhood of 4% (3). Laboratory studies, in addition to showing the presence of the parasite in the muscle biopsies, may show accompanying evidence of hypersensitivity such as eosinophilia and hypergammaglobulinemia. Heavy infestation with the trichinella may be fatal. Suggested treatment involves the administration of prednisone in doses of 60 mg daily together with thiobendazole in doses of 50 mg per kilogram per day for 2 weeks (4).

Cysticercosis may also manifest itself as a disease of muscle. The encysted larvae of the tapeworms may present as a space-occupying lesion with central nervous system complaints. Epilepsy is a common symptom. Muscle symptoms, which may be seen in association with neurological deficit or in isolation, include diffuse aches and pains and palpable nodules in the muscle. An unusual form is the pseudohypertrophic variety in which the muscle becomes massively enlarged (5).

The association between toxoplasma infection and polymyositis has been postulated by some authors (6, 7) (see under "Polymyositis and Dermatomyositis"). Serological evidence of a recent toxoplasma infection was more common in patients with a polymyositis-like illness than in control groups of patients. Some reduction in the titers of antibodies to the organism followed treatment with pyrimethamine and sulfonamides. The clinical response to such treatment was not very striking.

Viral infections of muscle may be much commoner than is realized. It is probable that the diffuse aches and pains which so often accompany an attack of influenza actually represent viral inflammatory disease of the muscle. There are numerous reports of more severe complications associated with viral infections. Acute muscle pains in the legs, especially the calf muscles, have been associated with influenza B virus, recovery taking place over a period of a week or so (8). Severe muscle pains and myoglobinuria have been reported with several viruses, although the causality is not always well established and it is possible that the viral infection was simply incidental. Thus echovirus, influenza A, herpes virus and adenovirus 21 have all been incriminated (9–16). The typical picture is of a viral prodrome followed by the development of muscle pains, swelling and the passage of dark urine. Muscle biopsies, when done during the acute phase have predictably shown the changes of muscle necrosis which accompany myoglobinuria. In those whose symptoms have been less, minor changes with vacuolar degeneration have been noted (10). Infection with coxsackievirus is a well known cause of severe muscle pain.

Involvement of the fascia surrounding the muscle may also produce marked muscle symptoms. One of the commonest complaints of patients arriving in a muscle clinic is the "aches, cramps and pains" syndrome. Simon et al. (17) reviewed some of the associated causes and pointed out that full thickness biopsies from skin to muscle often reveal inflammatory changes in the connective tissue. The diagnosis of "fibrositis" which has become unfashionable might thus be resurrected in the future when confirmed by proper studies.

REFERENCES

1. Carroll, J. E., Silvermann, A., Isobe, Y., Brown, W. R., Kelts, K. A., and Brooke, M. H. Inflammatory myopathy. IgA deficiency and intestinal malabsorption. Pediatrics *89:* 216–219, 1976.
2. Fett, J. D. Staphylococcal pyomyositis. Minn. Med. *56:* 724–725, 1973.
3. Zimmerman, W. J., Steele, J. H., and Kagan, I. G. Trichinosis in the U.S. population, 1966 to 1970. Pub. Health Rep. *88:* 607–623, 1973.
4. Davis, M. J., Cilo, M., Plaitakis, A., and Yahr, M. D. Trichinosis: severe myopathic involvement with recovery. Neurology *26:* 37–40, 1976.
5. Sawhney, B. B., Chopra, J. S., Banerji, A, K., and Wahi, P. L. Pseudohypertrophic myopathy in cysticercosis. Neurology *26:* 270–272, 1976.
6. Kagen, L. J., Kimball, A. C., and Christian, C. L. Serological evidence of toxoplasmosis among patients with polymyositis. Am. J. Med. *56:* 186–191, 1974.

7. Samuels, B. C., and Rietschel, R. L. Polymyositis and toxoplasmosis. J.A.M.A. *235:* 60–61, 1976.
8. Dietzman, D. E., Schaller, J. G., Ray, C. G., and Reed, M. E. Acute myositis associated with influenza B infection. Pediatrics *57:* 255–258, 1976.
9. Marcus, J. C., and Bill, P. L. A. Acute myopathy in three brothers. Neuropaediatrie *7:* 101–110, 1976.
10. McKinlay, I. A., and Mitchell, I. Transient acute myositis in childhood. Arch. Dis. Child. *51:* 135–137, 1976.
11. Josselson, J., Pula, T., and Sadler, J. H. Acute rhabdomyolysis associated with an echovirus 9 infection. Arch. Intern. Med. *140:* 1671, 1980.
12. Kessler, H. A., Trenholme, G. M., Harris, A. A., and Levin, S. Acute myopathy associated with influenza A/Texas/1/77 infection. J.A.M.A. *243:* 461–462, 1980.
13. Minow, R. A., Gorbach, S., Johnson, B. L., and Dornfeld, L. Myoglobinuria associated with influenza A infection. Ann. Intern. Med. *80:* 359–361, 1974.
14. Schlesinger, J. J., Gandara, D., and Bensch, K. G. Myoglobinuria associated with herpes group viral infections. Arch. Intern. Med. *138:* 422–424, 1978.
15. Berlin, B. S., Simon, N. M., and Bovner, R. N. Myoglobinuria precipitated by viral infection. J.A.M.A. *227:* 1414–1415, 1974.
16. Wright, J., Couchonnai, G., and Hodges, G. R. Adenovirus type 21 infection. J.A.M.A. *241:* 2420–2421, 1979.
17. Simon, D. B., Ringel, S. P., and Sufit, R. L. Clinical spectrum of fascial inflammation. Muscle Nerve *5:* 525–537, 1982.

MYOSITIS OSSIFICANS PROGRESSIVA

Ectopic calcification is seen in a variety of conditions. Abnormalities of parathyroid function, the late stages of polymyositis, an excessive intake of vitamin D, and repeated trauma may all cause abnormal calcification. The disease myositis ossificans progressiva is set apart from these by a clinical picture which is so different as to be almost instantly recognizable. Although traditionally termed myositis, the illness is not truly one of muscle, but an ossification of the fascial planes, tendons, and aponeuroses. It is an extremely rare condition afflicting both sexes and probably inherited as an autosomal dominant with varying penetrance.

The lesions begin with an area of the muscle which becomes acutely hot, swollen, and tender. As this subsides, progressive ossification occurs over the subsequent weeks and the final result is a bony plaque which impedes the action of the muscle and results in a contracture (Figs. 6.10–6.14). It is not clear why such bone formation occurs, but some events are clearly provocative. Thus, trauma to the muscle or a strain of the muscle is often followed by an area of ossification. One patient developed an extensive plaque of calcification in the area underlying a tuberculin skin test. The disease always commences in the first decade, usually within the first 2 years of life.

In a survey of a large number of cases (1, 2), the muscles of the neck were the first affected in a quarter of the patients. The muscles of the paraspinal region, of the face, and of the shoulders and arms were the initial site of involvement in order of decreasing frequency. The hips and legs were not usually the location of early lesions. The muscles of the eyes, larynx, perineum, diaphragm, and tongue are said to be normal, and the heart is also fortunately spared (3). As the disease progresses, deformities become increasingly severe and bony ankyloses extend across joints locking the limb into immobility. About the best that may be hoped for is that the limb freezes in a position in which it can still be used, but all too often this is not the case and useful function of the arms and legs is lost. Death, which is frequently due to respiratory embarrassment, is postponed until adult life. In the terminal stage

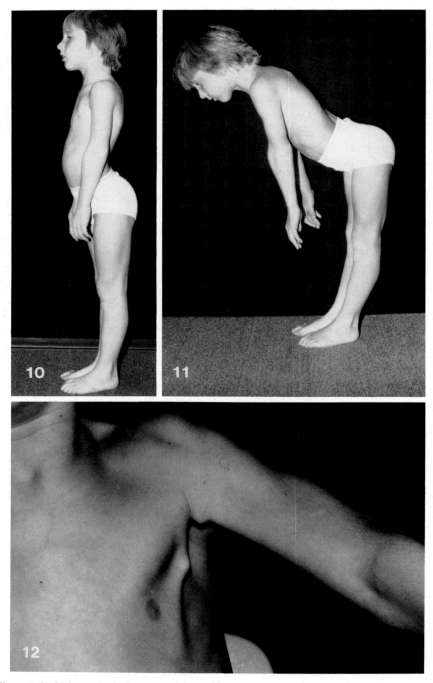

Figures 6.10 through 6.12. Myositis ossificans. Calcification may occur throughout the body and, in this young boy, prevents any flexion of the spine. He still retains movement at the hip but even this is limited. Bony nodules are noticed throughout the body as illustrated in the axilla in Figure 6.12.

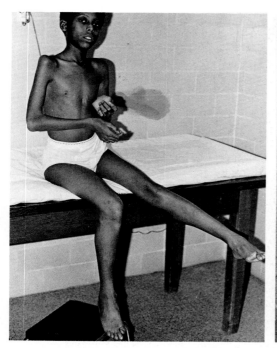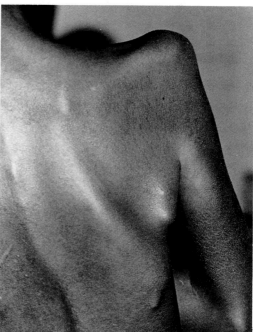

Figures 6.13 (*left*) and 6.14 (*right*).   Myositis ossificans. This patient is fixed in the position shown (Fig. 6.13) by bony bridges extending across the joints. These deposits of bone are easily palpable and often visible (Fig. 6.14). Notice the shortened great toes.

the patient is completely immobile. Although this is an extraordinary and dramatic disease, it has not received more than passing attention in the medical literature. Perhaps this is due to its rarity. The first report is usually attributed to Patin, who mentioned in 1692 the case of a woman who became "hard as wood." No one has had the temerity to cite Lot's wife as another early case.

The associated bony abnormalities are common enough to aid the diagnosis. Most of the patients have microdactyly or adactyly, especially of the big toe and thumb. The proximal phalanges may also be shortened. Other abnormalities which have been described are hallux valgus, exostoses, absent ear lobes, and spina bifida. Associated deafness has been reported, perhaps associated with ossification of the muscles of the inner ear.

The pathological changes are best described as centers of ossification occurring between fascicles or in association with tendons and aponeuroses. There are changes in the muscle itself, but these are nonspecific and may be secondary. A muscle biopsy is probably not a wise procedure in patients with myositis ossificans because such trauma to the muscle is almost always followed by ossification. Various medications have been used including steroids, EDTA, sodium citrate, and injections of parathyroid extract. None of these seems to have been of any value. Recently there has been some interest in the use of diphosphonate. This substance is related to pyrophosphate but is resistant to chemical and enzymatic hydrolysis. In experimental situations in animals it has been thought to prevent soft tissue calcification and reduce bone absorption. In higher doses it prevents the mineralization of the bone matrix. Sodium ethane 1-hydroxydiphosphonic acid (EHDP) or sodium etidronate has been used in myositis ossificans in doses of 20 mg per kilogram of body weight per day. Some reports have suggested that the development of calcification was impeded (4) and have even suggested that some improvement has occurred while on the medication (5). Others have failed to confirm this (6), but it may be worthwhile trying this medication in a severe or rapidly progressive case.

There may also be a benign entity associated with ossification of a muscle. Four patients were reported in each of whom one area of ossification occurred which did not follow any provocative episodes (7).

REFERENCES

1. Lutwak, L. Myositis ossificans progressiva. Am. J. Med. *37:* 269–293, 1964.
2. Illingworth, S. Myositis ossificans progressiva (Münchmeyers disease). Arch. Dis. Child. *46:* 264–268, 1971.
3. Simpson, A. J., and Friedman, S. Myositis ossificans progressiva. Mt. Sinai J. Med. N.Y. *38:* 416–422, 1971.
4. Russell, G. G., Smith, R., Bishop, M. C., Price, D. A., and Squire, C. M. Treatment of myositis ossificans progressiva with a diphosphonate. Lancet *1:* 10–12, 1972.
5. Weiss, I. W., Fisher, L., and Phang, J. M. Diphosphonate therapy in a patient with myositis ossificans progressiva. Ann. Intern. Med. *4:* 933–936, 1971.
6. Bland, J. H., Kirshbaum, B., O'Connor, G. T., and Horton, E. Myositis ossificans progressiva. Arch. Intern. Med. *132:* 209–212, 1973.
7. Samuelson, K. M., and Coleman, S. S. Nontraumatic myositis ossificans in healthy individuals. J.A.M.A. *235:* 1132–1133, 1976.

7

metabolic muscle diseases

EXERCISE*

Most of the muscle diseases described before the 1950s were characterized by pathological changes noted under the microscope. The muscle was thus severely damaged and the nature of the changes so fundamental that it would be irrational to expect the muscle to function in any normal way. On the other hand, the changes allowed the pathologist to work hand-in-hand with the clinician and develop a classification of muscle disease in an orderly fashion. Morphologic studies have told us very little about the origins of the disease and almost nothing at all about how to treat them.

In more recent times the characterization of new muscle diseases has followed the detection of aberrations in chemistry or function. Muscle is a splendidly intricate piece of machinery designed to translate the energy contained in chemical molecules into mechanical work. This complexity carries with it the probability that something will go wrong, a probability confirmed by the large numbers of patients who experience their symptoms during or following exercise, whose muscle biopsies appear normal, and whose diagnosis remains obscure. Prior to the last decade attempts to probe their illness were hampered by a lack of knowledge of the biochemistry and physiology of exercise. As exercise techniques are transferred from the laboratory to the clinic and as the application of biochemical techniques in muscle biopsy becomes more widespread a new phase in muscle disease is being broached. Although only a handful of biochemical defects have so far been identified, there is now an increasing interest in the patient who presents with fatigue, muscle cramps, and other evidence of reversible muscle abnormalities during exercise. To be able to understand these illnesses in any sensible way requires a knowledge of normal exercise. The first section of this chapter will, therefore, deal with the normal individual, not the person with muscle disease.

The central theme in understanding exercise is to understand the necessity for maintaining adenosine triphosphate (ATP) above a critical level. Since ATP levels are important for the very integrity of the tissue itself and not simply for the performance of muscular exercise, they actually cannot be allowed to fall without resulting in tissue damage. This is self-evident in any tissue, but only in muscle does the demand for ATP fluctuate so widely. Complicated mathematical problems may tax the brain cells, but need nowhere as much ATP as picking up a 5-lb weight. Because extraordinary

---

* This is a superficial review of the subject. For a better understanding, references 1–3 should be consulted.

demands may be placed on the ATP supply, the muscle has developed equally extraordinary ways of fulfilling them. There are really three pools from which ATP may be replenished. The first is the immediately available energy rich creatine phosphate within the muscle. The second comes from other intrinsic stores by the metabolism of glycogen and intracellular lipids. The third is brought to the muscle from without and would include sugar and triglycerides. In addition, adenosine diphosphate (ADP), the product of ATP degradation, may be converted back to ATP by the adenylokinase reaction, although this reaction is wasteful and may be thought of as a "desperation" measure.

Exactly which is used and when is a matter of crucial importance since it holds the key to the symptoms of patients with aberrations in their biochemistry. If you are, at present, sitting down reading this book, it is likely that your muscles will be using predominantly fatty acids which is the normal mode of the resting muscle. Should you glance through the window just in time to see your car being side-swiped and, in response, sprint down to the end of the street in a futile attempt to catch the license plate of the offender, you would be using your intramuscular stores of glycogen. Should you be unsuccessful and decide to work off your frustrations by jogging for 10 miles of mindless exercise in the nearby park, your muscles will gradually switch over from using glucose and you will return home burning predominantly fatty acids. This is the gist of the problem and little more is needed to interpret patients' symptoms. There are various mechanisms for preventing the depletion of ATP which inevitably occurs if muscular activity is forced beyond a certain point. Some of these involve the central regulation of exercise, simply that an individual cannot "push" himself beyond a certain point. There are safety mechanisms that are built in which are under neurogenic control and which lead to "fatigue" at a point before the muscle becomes damaged. In other instances, there may be regulation of the enzyme systems by metabolic products that shut down the process.

Instant Supply

Creatine Phosphate

There are about 17 μmol/g of phosphocreatine in normal muscle. Phosphocreatine interacts with ADP to reform ATP. The reaction is reversible and is catalyzed by the enzyme creatine kinase, which is present in large amounts in the sarcoplasm, and is biased in favor of the production of ATP. Even if all the available store of phosphocreatine were used, it would sustain exercise for no longer than a few seconds. Its function is to provide a buffer to support ATP during periods of brief intense exercise far beyond the capability of the other mechanisms. One might imagine this mechanism playing a part in weight lifting or the dash for the goal line in football.

Short-term Support System

Adenylate Kinase and Adenylate Deaminase (Fig. 7.1)

With the breakdown of ATP during contraction, ADP accumulates. The ATP to ADP ratio is an indication of the anaerobic stress to which the muscle

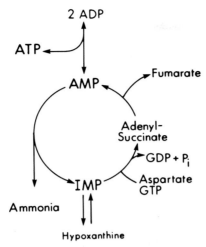

Figure 7.1.   The adenylate kinase, adenylate deaminase and purine nucleotide cycle. Two molecules of ADP are converted into ATP and AMP by the action of adenylate kinase. The AMP forms IMP and ammonia under the influence of adenylate deaminase. The ascending limb of the cycle resynthesises AMP.

is being subjected. ATP can be salvaged from ADP by the reaction catalyzed by adenylate kinase. One molecule of ADP is converted to AMP and the other to ATP. The disposal of adenosine monophosphate (AMP) is accomplished by adenylate deaminase with the resultant formation of inosine monophosphate (IMP) and ammonia. IMP is then degraded to hypoxanthine which appears in the blood. Relatively large amounts of ammonia and hypoxanthine appear in the blood following strenuous exercise. The total absence of this in patients with adenylate deaminase deficiency suggests that this is the major route of formation of the compounds. The subsequent fate of hypoxanthine is to be degraded to uric acid.

Although this reaction replenishes the ATP supply, it is, in essence, wasteful and there is a net loss of purines from the muscle. The IMP formed can be reconverted to ATP via adenylosuccinate by the purine nucleotide cycle (4). The two limbs of the cycle may not be active synchronously. In situ stimulation of rat muscle showed that conversion of AMP to IMP is active during intense exercise in fast muscle and formation of AMP from IMP takes place during the recovery phase (5). Stimulation of slow muscle (soleus) did not result in IMP formation which may indicate that this cycle is only active in fast muscle. Hypoxanthine is not formed in muscle itself in vitro, as judged from stimulation studies (6), but does appear in the blood following exercise in humans. Since high levels of ATP inhibit one of the 5'-nucleotidases that control the initial step of the degradation of IMP to hypoxanthine, and since a high level of IMP itself will inhibit the adenylosuccinate synthetase during periods of intense work, the reaction should favor the production of hypoxanthine. This is clinically substantiated by the marked increase in hypoxanthine noted in the venous blood after intensive forearm exercise. The puzzling aspect is that this elevation is maximal 10–15 minutes after the exercise. There is no proven explanation for this, although it is possible that, since phosphorylated compounds are not transported across membranes, the rise of IMP in the muscle occurs a good deal earlier than the rise of hypoxanthine in the blood.

Intermediate Support System

Glycogen

Glycogen stores within the muscle fiber provide one of the most important sources of readily available energy. The actual amount of glycogen in the muscle varies depending upon diet and other factors, but is around 1–2 g per 100 g of muscle. Glycogen is a large molecule made up of glucose units arranged in a daisy chain fashion by means of α_{1-4}-linkages. At about every 10th glucose molecule, a different bond, the α_{1-6}-linkage, occurs to form branch points at which new chains start. The breakdown of muscle glycogen is accomplished by phosphorylase, an enzyme associated with a complicated activating system. It cleaves the α_{1-4}-links to start the process leading to the formation of pyruvate as indicated in Figure 7.2. The controlling enzyme in the pathway to pyruvate is phosphofructokinase (PFK); its action might be likened to a valve which, being opened or closed, controls the flow through this metabolic sequence. High concentrations of ATP, which is a negative modulator of PFK, shut the system down, but ADP, which is a positive modulator, has the reverse effect.

Three molecules of ATP are generated during this reaction. A problem occurs in the oxidation of glyceraldehyde 3 phosphate since this generates the reduced form of its coenzyme, reduced nicotinamide-adenine dinucleotide (NADH). If the glycolytic process is to provide a continuing source of ATP, the coenzyme will be increasingly converted to its reduced form. Tying up the coenzyme in this fashion is not acceptable to the cell, which has to recycle it to its oxidized form. There are two ways of doing this. The most efficient, from the cell's point of view, is to couple the surplus electrons to oxygen by means of the mitochondrial respiratory chain. If oxygen is unavailable, as it might be in some forms of intense exercise in which the workload outstrips the blood supply's capacity to provide the necessary oxygen, another way of recycling NADH comes into play through the formation of lactate. The NADH reduces pyruvate to lactate leaving NAD^+, its oxidized form. The problem of accumulation of NADH has been solved, but is now replaced by the accumulation of lactate. On the other hand, the cells can cope with an excess of lactate much more easily than an undersupply of NAD^+.

What is valid in terms of glycogen is also true in terms of glucose. The only difference is that glucose must enter the process in its phosphorylated form and 1 ATP molecule is used to accomplish this. Therefore, the net ATP production from glucose is only two-thirds that from glycogen.

Long-term Energy Supply

In muscle that has an adequate supply of oxygen for its energy needs, the mechanisms are different. This is true of resting muscle and in endurance exercise, such as bicycling, when the workload is not excessive. In endurance exercise, the blood supply to the muscle is markedly increased (up to 20-fold) to cope with the increased energy demand. In this situation, both carbohydrates and fats are utilized, although as time goes on, the carbohydrate oxidation is diminished and the oxidation of fat is increased.

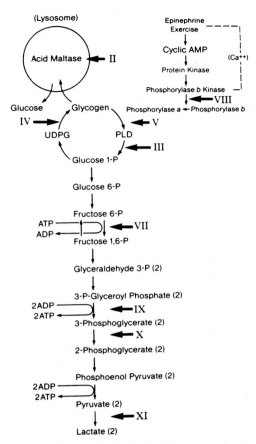

Figure 7.2. Glycogen metabolism and glycolysis. The *arrows* indicate enzyme defects producing disease in the human; *II*, acid maltase; *III*, debranching enzyme; *IV*, branching enzyme; *V*, phosphorylase; *VI*, phosphofructokinase; *VII*, phosphorylase *b* kinase; *VIII*, phosphoglycerate kinase; *IX*, phosphoglycerate mutase; and *X*, lactate dehydrogenase (*UDPG* = uridine diphosphate glucose, *PLD* = phosphorylase limit dextrin). (Courtesy Dr. S. DiMauro.)

Carbohydrates

Aerobic glycolysis proceeds in an exactly similar fashion to anaerobic glycolysis down to the level of pyruvate. Pyruvate is oxidatively decarboxylated by means of a very complex enzyme system, pyruvate dehydrogenase, to form acetyl coenzyme A. With this irreversible reaction begins the entry into the tricarboxylic acid cycle, by which is accomplished the complete breakdown of pyruvate to carbon dioxide and water. The cycle is a one-way cycle since another irreversible oxidative decarboxylation occurs when α-ketoglutarate is converted to succinic acid. During each turn of the cycle, there are three steps that produce NADH and one step that produces reduced flavin adenine dinucleotide (FADH). These reduced coenzymes enter the respiratory chain on the mitochondrial cristae, and the electrons are transferred in a cascading series of reactions involving different cytochromes, the final accepter being oxygen. The net result of this is to regenerate NAD^+ and

FAD^+ and form water. In the course of the reaction, the energy released is stored in the form of new ATP, 3 molecules of ATP being associated with the reoxidation of NADH and 2 molecules with FADH. The net formation of ATP resulting from the complete breakdown of 1 glucose molecule is 38 molecules. ADP and ATP concentrations influence the pyruvate dehydrogenase complex. When ATP concentrations are high, the enzyme complex is inhibited, whereas it is activated by high concentrations of ADP.

Fat (Fig. 7.3)

The potential energy stored in the body as fat far exceeds that available from carbohydrate stores. A triglyceride molecule is a combination of glycerol with three fatty acids and this represents the basic building block of the fat stores. Under the action of various lipases, fatty acids are split off and enter the circulation together with glycerol. This release of fatty acids from the fat stores is promoted by catecholamines such as epinephrine and norepinephrine, as well as by glucagon and growth hormone. During exercise, these hormones are sharply increased resulting in a surging tide of fatty acids. The increase in blood levels, together with the increase in the blood supply to the muscle tissue, all combine to make fatty acids increasingly available for energy metabolism. In man, palmitic and oleic acids are the principal ones involved and, like other fatty acids, they do not travel across the mitochondrial

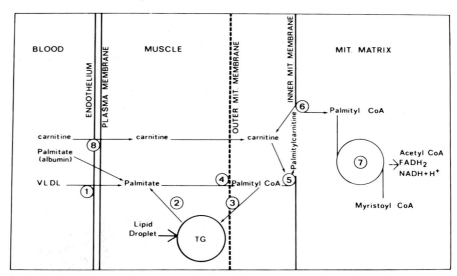

Figure 7.3. Scheme of lipid metabolism. Fatty acid (exemplified by palmitate) arrives in the blood either bound to albumin or as triglycerides in the very low density lipoproteins (*VLDL*). *TG* represents the endogenous lipid stores which are triglycerides. The fatty acids pass through the mitochondrial membrane to the mitochondrial matrix where they undergo β-oxidation. The numbers in the figure indicate the enzymes or enzyme complexes involved in the process: *1*, lipoprotein lipase; *2*, tri-, di-, and monoglyceride lipase; *3*, synthesis of triglycerides from long chain acyl CoA involves glycerol-1-phosphate and the three enzymes glycerol phosphate acyltransferase, phosphatidate phosphatase, and diglyceride acyltransferase; *4*, palmityl-CoA synthetase; *5*, carnitine palmityltransferase I; *6*, carnitine palmityltransferase II; *7*, β oxidation; and *8*, active transport system of carnitine in to muscle. (Courtesy Dr. D. C. DeVivo.)

membrane by themselves, but need a carrier system in order to undergo further metabolism. This carrier is carnitine. Carnitine is hooked on to palmitic acid by means of the enzyme carnitine palmityl transferase (CPT I). The conjugated form of palmityl carnitine is shuttled across the membrane, and the carnitine is unhooked on the other side by CPT II. Medium chain triglycerides probably have a different system of transportation.

Once the fatty acid is in the mitochondrion, it is subject to β oxidation. Basically this process clips successive pairs of carbon atoms from the end of the chain and forms acetyl CoA. The first step in the procedure is an energy-dependent one in which the fatty acid is activated by the formation of acyl CoA. This undergoes dehydrogenation by acyl CoA dehydrogenase and a double bond is formed between the two carbon atoms. Fatty acids of various chain lengths have their own acyl CoA dehydrogenase, four in all, and all work in conjunction with FAD. The reduced FADH is recycled to FAD via the intramitochondrial respiratory chain as noted previously. The unsaturated derivative produced by this reaction is now hydrated by enoyl CoA hydratase forming the β-hydroxyacyl CoA derivative, which is again dehydrogenated by β-hydroxyacyl CoA dehydrogenase, this time using NAD as the coenzyme, and the β-ketoacyl derivative is finally cleaved by the enzyme thiolase producing acetyl CoA and an acyl CoA which is now two carbon fragments shorter than the original. Each turn of beta oxidation produces FADH and NADH which will form ATP during their reoxidation by the respiratory chain and a molecule of acetyl CoA which will enter the Krebs' cycle precisely as before. It should be noted that fatty acid oxidation can in no way result in carbohydrate formation or lactate formation since the essential step would be the conversion of acetyl CoA to pyruvate and this is not possible. Parenthetically, the reverse (fat formation from carbohydrates) is quite possible since fats can be built up from acetyl CoA. The complete oxidation of palmitic acid in this fashion will produce 129 moles of ATP from each mole of palmitate metabolized.

The Final Common Pathway

The cytochrome chain or the electron transport chain is the final common pathway for the oxidation of fuel. This system is a series of iron containing compounds embedded in the cristae of the inner mitochondrial membrane. The iron undergoes a cyclical change in valence as electrons are handed from one to the other. Only the terminal cytochrome a_3 (cytochrome c oxidase) is capable of reducing molecular oxygen directly. There are three points in this chain at which ATP is formed during the sequential transfer of electrons. The system thus acts to control the flow of electrons toward oxygen in an orderly fashion. It harnesses what might otherwise be wasted energy in the same way that a series of locks can be used to control the flow of a river and allow the orderly progression of river traffic. There are four functional constituents of the respiratory chain. The first (complex I) couples the oxidation of NADH to the reduction of coenzyme Q and is NADH-CoQ reductase. The prosthetic group is flavin mononucleotide which acts in concert with several nonheme iron containing sulfur centers. These iron sulfur centers are redox systems necessary for the efficient transfer of electrons. Complex II acts in parallel to complex I and couples succinate to coenzyme Q (succinate CoQ reductase). This complex contains flavin adenine dinucleotide as well as nonheme iron centers. Complex III is the reduced coenzyme Q-cytochrome c reductase and contains cytochrome b and c_1. Cytochrome b consists of at least two types, one of which is rapidly oxidized (b_k), the other more slowly (b_t). The ultimate link in this chain is complex IV which effects the final transfer to oxygen. This is cytochrome c oxidase which is also composed of different units including cytochrome a and a_3, copper atoms, and various other subunits. Coenzyme Q moves back and forth between the first two complexes and complex III as it is alternately reduced and oxidized. Cytochrome c likewise ferries between complex III and IV.

The synthesis of ATP is coupled to the reoxidation of the electron carriers in the respiratory chain. The exact mechanism is not clear but an ATP synthesizing enzyme (ATP synthase) is embedded in the inner mitochondrial membrane and in some fashion harnesses the energy released by the movement of electrons from one carrier to another to form ATP. The sequence is shown in Figure 7.4. ATP is formed at 3 sites, one of which is associated with complex I activity. Thus the oxidation of succinate will liberate 2 molecules of ATP whereas an NADH linked reaction will involve complex I and liberate a "bonus" ATP. Substances which interfere with the activity of this chain, such as amytal, antimycin A or cyanide, have a potent effect on the organism, as do many of the illnesses associated with electron transport defects.

Exercise and the Individual

The effects of exercise on the cellular chemistry are accompanied by changes such as an increase in breathing and heart rate which are noticed by the individual. These changes are easy to measure and since the clinical changes are indirectly produced by the biochemical changes, measuring the one may be a simple way of obtaining information about the other. Most patients given the choice between having their pulse taken, or having their mitochondria collected would opt for the former, on economic if not any other grounds. The problem, as usual, is to determine how accurate the relationship is and

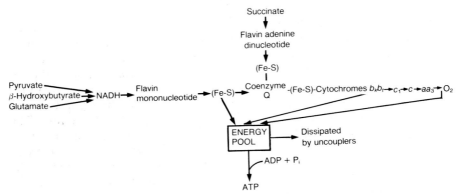

Figure 7.4. Diagram of the cytochrome chain. NAD and FAD linked substrates enter the chain at different places. "*Fe-S*" indicates the nonhaem iron sulfur proteins. (Adapted from J. A. Morgan-Hughes et al.: *Journal of the Neurological Sciences, 43:* 27, 1979.)

in what detail extrapolation may be made to predict biochemical anomalies. It is obvious that detailed information on the activity of the iron sulfur containing centers of the cytochrome chain is not going to be obtained by analysis of the breathing rate, but nevertheless, such measurements might be useful to predict which patients could be usefully subjected to further analysis. This concept of the development of simple procedures, which will allow us to screen patients for further and more complicated tests, is basic to the whole problem of the clinical evaluation of neuromuscular disease and introduces the subject of the normal response of the individual to exercise.

The availability of oxygen in muscle tissue is the major limiting factor in any exercise other than that of very brief duration. Since oxygen supply is synonymous with blood supply, it is obvious that a major factor in any evaluation of exercise is an evaluation of the cardiovascular status. It is equally apparent that the blood which arrives in the muscle must be normally oxygenated, which presupposes normal respiratory function. It requires no particular clairvoyance to predict that, during any steady bout of exercise, the pulse will rise, there will be a redistribution of blood supply in the body so that it favors the muscles, cardiac output will be increased, and an increase in the frequency of respiration will be needed to keep pace with the additional blood flow through the lungs.

If one sets off jogging, the additional demand for energy in the muscle is immediate. The increase in pulse, cardiac output, and respiratory rate is not instantaneous and lags behind. Within a few minutes at a steady jogging pace, these parameters will reach a steady state. The oxygen uptake, pulse, cardiac output and respiratory rate will be appropriate to the level of exercise being demanded. In the interval between the start of exercise and the physiological responses reaching steady state, the energy will have to be supplied by other sources, presumably from intramuscular stores. During this time, the individual develops an oxygen "deficit." The reverse occurs upon the cessation of exercise. The energy requirements drop immediately, but only sometime later do the cardiovascular and respiratory responses return to their resting levels. During this time, which is the time of repayment of the oxygen "debt," the muscles are presumably restoring the level of the supplies which were used to sustain exercise during the period of oxygen deficit.

The higher the work load, the longer the period of oxygen deficit and, at extreme levels, the physiological responses may never catch up to the muscle's need for oxygen, in which case the muscle will fail. It should be emphasized that this is not an abnormal response. Indeed, championship long distance runners probably push themselves very close to this point which, hopefully, will occur just after they finish the race and not just before. The period of time when the oxygen debt is being repaid, i.e., the patient is recovering from the effects of exercise, is roughly proportional to the amount of the deficit generated during the time of exercise. The physiological changes are quite remarkable. The cardiac output at rest, is very variable but is around 5 liters/minute, of which about 15% is sent in the direction of the muscles. With exercise, the output may rise to 20–30 liters/minute or more in the trained athlete. Of this amount, 80% may be consigned to the muscle. Direct measurement of blood flow in the muscles confirms this very large increase during exercise. Forearm exercise of 10–15 minutes may be associated with an increase in blood flow of 20 times the resting level. Much of this change in blood flow arises from local dilatation of the muscle capillaries. The mechanisms involved are not entirely clear, but the accumulation of local metabolites, particularly potassium, and the change of the pH within the muscle may act as powerful vasodilators. Skin vessels also dilate during exercise, which aids in the necessary dissipation of heat from the working muscles.

There is obviously a practical limit to the amount of exercise any individual can do. This will depend upon the individual's sex, state of health, and state of training. The maximum amount of work possible will also depend upon the period of time during which the effort must be sustained. The practical aspects of this are discussed below under the exercise testing.

From all of the preceding, it is obvious that an individual's work capacity will depend on many factors other than his muscle strength. Cardiac or respiratory disease, anemia, or peripheral vascular problems will all deprive the muscle of the necessary oxygen and will limit the patient's exercise ability as surely as if he had an abnormality of the muscle itself.

There are other effects of exercise, which are not apparent to the individual, but which can easily be measured. During the time of oxygen deficit, there is a brisk elevation of lactate in the serum. For obvious reasons, this is usually most marked in the earliest phases of endurance exercise or following short-term intense exercise. It also depends, to some extent, upon the subject's motivation. There are those who are able to "push" themselves further than others and they may be expected to generate more lactate. Conversely, the subject who abandons exercise at the first signs of discomfort is unlikely to have very high lactate levels. Another metabolite which is noted in the blood stream early in exercise is ammonia. Like lactate, this probably reflects the inability of blood-borne oxygen to keep up with the energy demands and is an indicator of the body's attempt to maintain ATP levels through the adenylokinase/adenylate deaminase reactions. Hypoxanthine in the serum shows a marked elevation following short-term exercise, but it is not so noticeable at the end of endurance exercise. This is probably generated through the same pathways responsible for ammonia but, in practical terms, it is probably more reliable since ammonia is not only volatile, but becomes incorporated in the body's buffering systems. There is an odd delay in the appearance of hypoxanthine in the blood. It reaches peak levels several minutes after the period of exercise, rather than during exercise. This may be, in part, due to the fact that it is derived from IMP, a substance that is not transported easily across the muscle membrane.

During the course of endurance exercise, catecholamines are released into the blood stream. The amount of insulin is decreased and fat is mobilized. This results in an increasing level of fatty acids, which seems to be less dependent upon the intensity of the exercise than on the duration of the exercise. Even in patients who are poorly motivated, exercising at low work levels, but who are able to exercise for a long period of time, the fatty acid levels are equivalent to those exercising at much higher workloads.

Myoglobin and creatine kinase (CK) are released into the blood stream following exercise, but the mechanics of their release are obscure. Because of the association of high levels of myoglobin and CK with severe muscle diseases, we are used to thinking of their presence in the serum in ominous terms. Actually, the release of these two compounds in the serum after exercise is a normal phenomenon and they may reach very high levels indeed. The peak levels of CK following exercise is delayed for 12–18 hours after the exercise. This often corresponds to a time when the muscles are sore and aching from unaccustomed exertion. Myoglobin levels peak earlier, within 2–3 hours. There is an association between the intensity of exercise in any given subject and the levels of CK and myoglobin which are attained. The most extreme elevations of CK follow a type of exercise which has been termed "eccentric" exercise (7, 8). In this type of exercise the muscle is actually doing work while lengthening, a paradoxical situation which is best illustrated by thinking of the action of the quadriceps muscle while stepping down off a high step, or walking downhill. It probably accounts for the often voiced complaint of mountain hikers that the worst part of the climb is when they come back down again and the ground slopes sharply away under them. The other unusual aspect of the CK elevation in this situation is that it is extremely delayed up to 4–5 days.

The state of training of the individual makes a tremendous difference to the physiological and biochemical responses. Regular endurance training increases the aerobic capacity of the muscle, the maximum oxygen consumption, the workload, and even the maximum heart rate (although it slows the heart rate for any given level of exercise). It also reduces the amount of lactate appearing in the serum and may obliterate the CK and myoglobin rise in the serum. Thus, the trained individual has to be evaluated in a different fashion from the sedentary person.

The previous paragraphs have been intentionally vague in order to give the reader an outline of the principles involved in exercise physiology. These comments would be useless were it not for our ability to make specific measurements. There are several types of tests which allow us to look at the different aspects of exercise.

The incremental exercise test allows us to determine the maximum workload, maximum oxygen consumption, the respiratory exchange ratio or respiratory quotient, the "anaerobic" or ventilatory threshold, and the maximum heart rate. Cardiac output can be measured noninvasively in this test, although it requires more sophisticated equipment.

The forearm exercise test measures the acute performance of the forearm muscles under relatively anaerobic conditions and the prolonged exercise test measures the performance under endurance conditions and is useful in assessing fatty acid metabolism and changes in serum muscle enzymes in response to exercise. The details of these tests are as follows.

Incremental Exercise Test

The first point to emphasize is that no incremental exercise test is done until the subject's fitness to perform such a test has been evaluated. This should include a stress test with the proper EKG monitoring. It should also be borne in mind that a patient who is suspected of having a biochemical defect of muscle may be vulnerable to exercise-provoked myoglobinuria.

An incremental exercise test is easiest to perform on a bicycle ergometer, although it can be done using other exercise devices. There must be some means of measuring the volume, oxygen content and carbon dioxide content of the inspired and expired air. This can be done by either collecting the air in Douglas bags or on a breath by breath basis using more elaborate equipment. Heart rate and EKG are monitored throughout the test. The initial level of work is set low enough to be fairly comfortable and the patient exercises for 4 or 5 minutes to reach steady state. The exercise is then increased by steps every minute until the subject is no longer capable of sustaining the level of exercise demanded. The size of the increments as well as the starting level requires some judgment on the part of the tester. As the work load increases, the oxygen consumption and the heart rate increase. The "$\dot{V}O_{2max}$" or maximum oxygen consumption is the point at which an increase in the workload no longer causes an increase in oxygen consumption. It is obvious at this stage that the patient is entering an "anaerobic" phase of exercise. In practice, not everyone can attain this level, in which case the $\dot{V}O_{2max}$ is the highest level attained by the end of the test. Since the patient himself decides when the test shall be stopped, motivation plays a major part in its proper performance. The $\dot{V}O_{2max}$ and maximum heart rate attained with this type of testing may be slightly different from that seen with other methods such as running uphill. The normal values are influenced by age as well as by the state of training and vary from 35 to 50 ml oxygen/kg body weight/minute. These values are based on studies carried out by volunteers who were motivated in the direction of exercise and one should expect levels at the lower end of this range in an unselected population. Maximal heart rate also declines with age. It is approximately 200 in a 20-year-old and declines roughly 1 point for every year thereafter. There is a proportionally larger fall between the ages of 40 and 50. It is around 165 at 50 years of age.

There are other interesting aspects to the incremental exercise test. At submaximal levels of exercise, there is a relationship between the amount of oxygen consumed and the amount of work done (Fig. 7.5). This is to be expected since the increase in work has to be paid for by increasing oxygen consumption. The relationship is a linear one and the slope of this line is a measure of the efficiency of the muscle in converting oxygen to work. This is approximately 1.6 ml additional oxygen for every additional kilopond meters (kpm) (9).

The respiratory exchange ratio (RER, respiratory quotient) can also be calculated from measurements of oxygen and CO_2. When carbohydrates are burned, the oxidation of the 6 carbon molecules consumes 6 molecules of O_2 and produces 6 molecules of CO_2. The respiratory exchange ratio is the quotient of the amount of CO_2 produced to the amount of O_2 consumed. Thus when the body is burning predominantly carbohydrate, the respiratory exchange ratio will be close to 1. When fat is oxidized, the 16 or 18 chain length fatty acids require greater amounts of oxygen (for example, a 16 carbon fatty acid requires 23 molecules of oxygen and will produce 16 molecules of CO_2). The respiratory exchange ratio for fat is usually considered to be 0.70. With intense exercise, the RER may be appear to be greater than 1 because the output of CO_2 may not precisely reflect the cellular production of CO_2. The body's buffering mechanisms and the use of internal carbohydrate stores may result in a tide of CO_2 being released into the expired air which does not directly reflect what is going on in the cell. Similarly, voluntary overbreathing

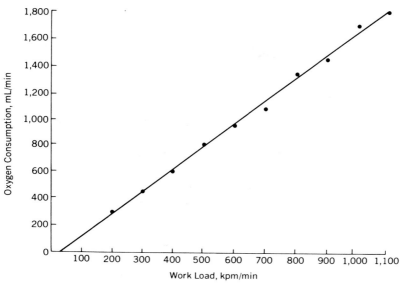

Figure 7.5. Oxygen consumption during an incremental exercise test. Increasing amounts of oxygen are needed for increasing levels of work. There is a linear relationship as indicated by this graph.

toward the end of exercise may "wash out" CO_2 from the body, producing a falsely high result.

The hyperventilation threshold or "anaerobic" threshold is a phenomenon which is related to this (10). During submaximal exercise, the gradual increase in the workload is associated with an increase in oxygen consumption and also with an increase in the respiratory rate, which can be measured as the volume of air expired in 1 minute (minute ventilation). There is a linear relationship between the oxygen consumption and the minute ventilation during the early part of exercise. At a level somewhere around 60% of the $\dot{V}O_{2max}$, untrained subjects begin to use anaerobic glycolytic mechnisms and lactic acid will reach the bloodstream from the muscle. This excess of lactic acid is dealt with by the bicarbonate buffering system and carbon dioxide is released. Both the slight change in pH and the release of carbon dioxide are potent stimuli of ventilation and the previous linear relationship between ventilation and oxygen consumption is disturbed as respiratory rate and excursions now increase out of proportion to the increase in oxygen consumption. The point at which this break in the relationship occurs has been called the hyperventilation threshold or anaerobic threshold. In most people, the hyperventilation threshold coincides with the appearance of lactate in the circulation. That it does not depend solely on the presence of lactate in the blood has been determined by a patient with McArdle's disease who had neither an increase in lactate nor any acidosis, but who had a perfectly normal hyperventilation threshold (11). This probably means that lactate is only one of several different stimuli associated with exercise which increase ventilation. The anaerobic threshold can also be determined by the measurement of end tidal oxygen pressure (Fig. 7.6). The hyperventilation previously mentioned is over and above that necessary to provide oxygen. Therefore the oxygen in

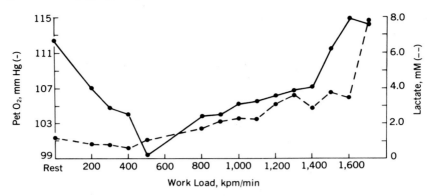

Figure 7.6. A demonstration of the hyperventilation threshold or "anaerobic" threshold. Increasing levels of work (indicated on the horizontal axis) are initially associated with a fall in the end tidal O_2 concentrations. This is easy to understand on the basis of increasing oxygen needs. After a certain work load, respiration increases at a rate greater than necessary for oxygen consumption. This results in an *increase* in the end tidal oxygen pressure. The point in which this change occurs is known as the "hyperventilation" or "anaerobic" threshold. This also coincides with the appearance of lactate in the venous blood as indicated by the *dashed line.*

the inspired air is not reduced as much as it might be and the concentration in the end tidal sample rises.

The incremental exercise test can thus be used to give indirect information in regard to an individual's muscle metabolism and function. The maximum work load (W_{max}) is a measure of the mechanical strength of the muscle. Oxygen consumption at rest as well as the slope of the increase in oxygen consumption with varying work loads, indicates the muscle's efficiency in converting oxygen to work. The respiratory exchange ratio gives some information as to the type of fuel being used and the anaerobic threshold is a useful measure which indicates the point at which the muscle has to change from oxidative metabolism to draw upon its intramuscular supplies in an anaerobic fashion. As will be mentioned later, it varies quite considerably with regard to the state of training of the individual.

Forearm Exercise

The ischemic forearm exercise test was one of the first tests to be designed with the specific aim of screening for a neuromuscular disease (phosphorylase deficiency), when, in the 1950s, it was realized that the absence of muscle phosphorylase led to a predictable absence of lactate in the venous circulation from exercising muscle. The forearm is used because it is convenient to obtain a sample of blood from the antecubital vein and the exercise of repetitive gripping is one which uses all of the muscles in the forearm. Because anaerobic glycolysis is tested in this system, the test is often done with a cuff inflated around the upper arm to cut off the circulation to the forearm.

One-Minute Maximum Forearm Exercise Test

Munsat (12) has suggested a standardized forearm ischemic exercise test which has proved useful. A catheter is placed in a superficial vein and a cuff around the upper arm is inflated to a level above systolic pressure. The patient is then asked to grip an ergometer or dynamometer repetitively at about 60 strokes per minute sufficient to produce a work load of 4–7 kpm. The test was found to be reliable as long as work exceeded 4 kpm. After 1 minute the exercise is stopped and the cuff is deflated. In addition to a resting sample obtained before the test, the venous blood is collected at intervals of 1, 3, 5, 10, and 20 minutes after the cessation of work. The peak lactate level occurs in normal subjects at about 3 minutes and should be 3–5 times normal. In patients with McArdle's disease, as with some of the other enzyme deficiencies mentioned below, there is no rise in the lactate level.

The inflation of the cuff around the arm may not actually be necessary. The work required from forearm muscles in exerting the maximum grip is far beyond the capability of the blood supply to sustain. After several minutes of exercise, of course, the blood supply increases up to 15–20-fold. But in the first minute the test is, to all intents and purposes, "ischemic" without placing a cuff around the upper arm. If the test is carried out with the circulation unobstructed, the patient should be instructed to grip with their maximum force. Obviously, if the patient does not feel like exerting his maximum strength, the resting blood flow may well support the activity and the test will be a failure, but all tests of exercise depend upon the patient's cooperation for their proper interpretation.

In the forearm exercise test as we perform it, the patient sits with his forearm resting on the table, gripping a device in which two upright metal bars are attached to a rigid frame and the leading bar is also attached to strain gauge. Substituting such items as a rolled up towel, piece of foam rubber or a pair of old socks for the proper measurement of grip strength will result in a failure of the test. It is imperative to be able to measure the output. Resting blood is obtained from an indwelling catheter in the antecubital vein and the patient then grips repetitively sustaining his maximum strength for 1.5 seconds, then relaxing the hand completely for 0.5 seconds. This continues for 1 minute and blood is sampled as at intervals of 2, 5, 10, 15, 30, and 60 minutes following the cessation of exercise.

We found no real difference in lactate generation between the two methods. In some patients whose cooperation is elusive there may be slightly higher lactate levels with the cuff inflated, but the test is still not satisfactory. The normal response to this test is a rise of lactate from a typical value of 1 μM/ml to around 4 μM/ml within 3 minutes after the end of exercise. The minimum acceptable rise is a doubling in lactate levels. Ammonia production from muscle is also usually noted and is proportional to the rise in lactate. Ammonia will often reach levels of 1 to 1.5 μg/ml from a resting level of less than 0.5 μM/ml. Peak levels of ammonia usually occur slightly later than those of lactate, but still within 4 or 5 minutes following exercise.

Incremental and Exhaustive Forearm Tests (13)

Although the elevation of lactate following the 1-minute maximum forearm test is predictable, elevation of ammonia is often irregular. Since an absence of adenylate deaminase may cause a lack of ammonia production by muscle, it is important to have a test which may reliably detect this. We have therefore replaced the standard forearm test with an incremental forearm exercise test, which employs a graded series of work loads, and gives more information. The maximum grip strength is first determined, preferably more than 15 minutes before the test begins. The setup is otherwise identical to the routine forearm exercise test. A technique has to be available to program the work load so that the subject may anticipate the level. The easiest way to accomplish this is to present the output from the strain gauge as a trace on an oscilloscope. The desired work load for each time period is then represented on the oscilloscope by a second trace, and the subject has to match the two traces. Using this technique, the initial work load is set at 10% of the maximum. This level is increased by 10% every minute using the same repetitive grip technique as described above. The subject will gradually tire and the test is discontinued when he can no longer attain more than 50% of the demanded load. This usually occurs after 6 or 7 minutes (about 60% of the maximum work load) (Fig. 7.7).

An alternate method of this type of forearm testing, which is roughly equivalent, is to exercise the forearm at 50% of the maximum load until the subject can no longer squeeze the grip device, which occurs at 8–11 minutes. This is an exhaustive forearm test.

Both these tests result in the appearance of lactate, ammonia and hypoxanthine in the venous blood (Fig. 7.8). The lactate appears first, followed by ammonia which is first noted at 3–4 minutes in the incremental exercise test, and finally hypoxanthine. Since hypoxanthine and ammonia are produced by the same pathway, one would expect them to be proportional to each other and to the amount of exercise. Although this is so, there is an interesting difference in the time at which the peak levels occur. For hypoxanthine this

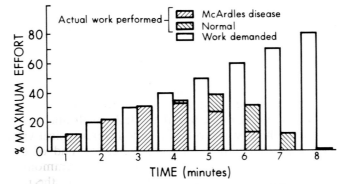

Figure 7.7. Mechanical performance during the incremental forearm test. The test is conducted by having the patient squeeze a device which programs the amount of effort required. The subject is asked to match the work demanded. At the beginning of the test, during the first minute, the work demanded is 10% of maximum and is increased 10% in each successive minute. The work demanded is represented on the graph by the *white bars*. The *shaded bars* represent the actual work performed by 15 normal subjects as well as by a patient with McArdle's disease. During the first 3 min at a low work level there is no difference. (The shaded block representing the normal is "hidden" behind the shaded block representing the McArdle patient.) Fatigue occurs in both McArdle disease individual and the normal individuals. Both groups fatigue slightly at 4 min but the phosphorylase-deficient patient fatigues much more rapidly as the work load increases.

is 10–20 minutes after the exercise is over. The reason for this is unclear. Perhaps since hypoxanthine is produced from IMP, a phosphorylated compound which passes across the membrane only with difficulty, the delay has to do more with membrane transport than it does with an actual delay in hypoxanthine production. Levels of CK are not affected in the normal individual. Myoglobin is slightly elevated over resting levels 60 min after the conclusion of exercise, but is not in the "abnormal" range (Fig. 7.9).

The forearm test gives information with regard to the glycolytic pathways and the adenylokinase-adenylate deaminase reactions during acute intensive exercise. It can also be used to screen for illnesses in which exercise-induced muscle damage occurs. Any defect in the glycolytic chain will be expressed as an absence of lactate production. Excessive lactate production at low levels

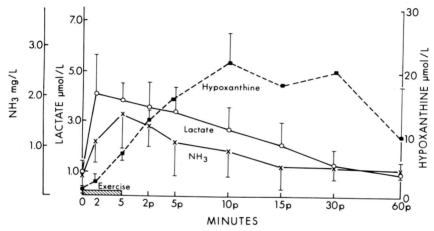

Figure 7.8. The appearance of metabolites in the venous blood in the working forearm. The subject exercises at increasing work loads as indicated by the *shaded area*. Venous blood is sampled during and after the exercise as indicated on the horizontal axis. The *bars* represent the standard deviation ($N = 12$).

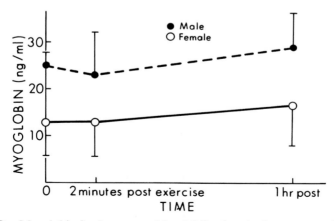

Figure 7.9. Myoglobin in the venous blood following the incremental forearm test. There is a minor increase in levels of myoglobin. The *bars* represent the standard deviation ($N = 12$).

of work may be associated with abnormalities of oxidative phosphorylation as seen in mitochondrial disorders. An absence of ammonia and hypoxanthine production is seen in adenylate deaminase deficiencies (14).

Since the production of hypoxanthine probably reflects activity of the adenylate kinase reaction, a reaction which is called into play to bolster failing supplies of ATP, one woud expect any metabolic disorder in which energy metabolism was defective to be mirrored in high levels of hypoxanthine. This was found to be true in a patient with McArdle's disease (15), but confirmation is needed in other illnesses. An abnormal elevation in myoglobin will indicate a muscle which is susceptible to exercise-induced "damage."

Prolonged Exercise

Endurance exercise can be evaluated using a bicycle ergometer. To be useful, the exercise probably has to continue for more than an hour. Thus it is a test which should be used with caution in people who are at risk for myoglobinuria, although for the normal patient it presents no particular risk. Venous blood is drawn after 30 minutes, 1 hour, 90 minutes, and again 30 minutes after the completion of exercise (16). Serum CK can be monitored every 6 hours or alternatively a single sample may be obtained 12–18 hours after the exercise. The exercise load is set at a level high enough to be taxing, but not so high as to cause exhaustion. For most individuals this level is about 50–60% of the patient's maximum ability as measured with the incremental exercise test. The subject rides at this load for 90 minutes. The load can be reduced if the subject finds it intolerable. During the first half-hour there is a marked increase in the lactate level in the blood. This is followed by an increasing change to fatty acid oxidation and the lactate level may fall. In a subject with the ability to push himself beyond the barriers set by the discomfort of exercise, anaerobic glycolysis still provides an important part of the energy supply and the lactate remains elevated. During the 90-minute period there is a progressive elevation of fatty acid levels in the normal subject. This elevation seems to depend not upon the intensity of the exercise, but only on the duration. There are also changes in hormone levels with a decrease in insulin and an increase in catecholamines. In the untrained individual, both CK and myoglobin may be markedly elevated. Levels of serum CK in men may exceed 1,000 IU/ml, but the effect is less pronounced in women. The peak values are delayed from 12 to 18 hours after the end of the exercise. Myoglobin is similarly elevated although this elevation occurs much earlier, within 2–3 hours of the exercise (Fig. 7.10). The prolonged exercise test is not as useful as the preceding two tests because of the variability of individual responses in the normal subject, but it is helpful in screening for some exercise-induced myopathies in which the CK and myoglobin elevation is often higher than normal. In addition, the peak levels of CK occur at an earlier time point in patients with myopathies, within 2–3 hours in some cases. The prolonged exercise test should also be useful in detecting abnormalities in fatty acid mobilization but so far none are known.

Effects of Training

Repetitive muscle work results in a training effect improving the performance of both muscle and the cardiovascular system. There are many different

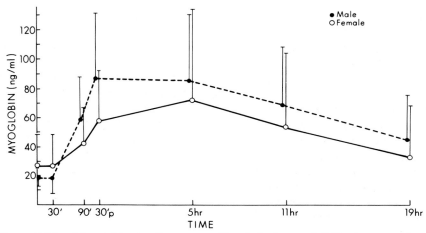

Figure 7.10. Myoglobin in the venous blood during and following a prolonged exercise test. The exercise consist of 90 min of bicycle riding at half the maximum load. The *bars* represent the standard deviation ($N = 10$). There is obviously considerable variability in the level but all subjects showed some rise of myoglobin.

types of training, but most is known about endurance training. In this type of training, exercise is performed at a submaximal work load, usually around 60% of the maximum. The training period is at least 30 minutes and this is repeated at least 4 times a week. The literature on the effect of this is voluminous and what follows is a very simple summary.

The oxidative capacity of the muscles is greatly increased due to an increase in the blood supply and an increase in the mitochondrial oxidative enzyme systems. This results in higher values for the W_{max} and in the $\dot{V}O_{2max}$. The oxygen consumption per unit of work is unchanged. Lactate production is blunted, particularly in the prolonged exercise test, because the muscle does not depend so much on anaerobic glycolysis (Fig. 7.11). Fatty acid utilization is increased.

The heart rate at any given absolute level of exercise is decreased, although it remains the same when considering the work load relative to the new W_{max}. Thus exercise at 60% of the maximum work load will still produce about the same degree of tachycardia. However, the work load which represents 60% of the maximum is higher than in the untrained state.

One of the most constant findings is that the CK elevation seen following prolonged exercise in the untrained state is markedly reduced following training (Fig. 7.12). Whether this signifies a beneficial effect on the muscle in terms to its resistance to exercise stress is uncertain.

REFERENCES

1. Astrand, P. O., and Rodahl, K. *Textbook of Work Physiology.* McGraw Hill, New York, 1977.
2. McArdle, W. D., Katch, F. I., and Katch, V. L. *Exercise Physiology.* Lea & Febiger, Philadelphia, 1981.
3. Edwards, R. H. T. (editor). *Human Muscle Fatigue: Physiological Mechanisms* (Ciba Foundation Symposium 82). Pitman Medical, Belmont, Calif., 1981.
4. Lowenstein, J. M. Ammonia production in muscle and other tissues: the purine nucleotide cycle. Physiol. Rev. *52:* 382–414, 1972.

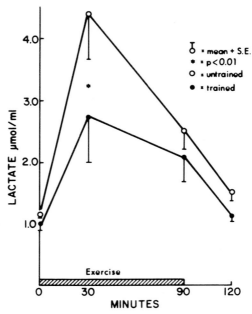

Figure 7.11. The effect of training on the lactate response to exercise. The provocative test was a prolonged exercise test for 90 min on a bicycle at ½ the maximum work load. Venous blood was drawn at rest, 30 min into the exercise, at the end of exercise, and ½ hour following exercise. Training consisted of four 30-min periods each week during which the subjects exercised at 60% of their maximum work load.

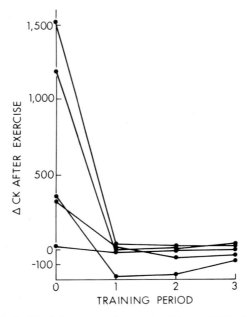

Figure 7.12. The effect of training on peak creatine kinase (CK) elevation following a prolonged exercise test in 5 normal controls. The change in CK is markedly reduced following training. The training periods are indicated in months. Training consisted of bicycle exercise 3 times a week at 60% of the maximum work load.

5. Meyer, R. A., and Terjung, R. L. Differences in ammonia and adenylate metabolism in contracting fast and slow muscle. Am. J. Physiol. *237:* C111–C118, 1978.
6. Brooke, M. H., Choksi, R., and Kaiser, K. K., IMP production is proportional to muscle force in vitro. Neurology, 1986 (in press).
7. Newham, D. J., Jones, D. A., and Edwards, R. H. T. Large delayed plasma creatine kinase changes after stepping exercise. Muscle Nerve *6:* 380–385, 1983.
8. Schwane, J. A., Johnson, S. R., Vandenakker, C. B., and Armstrong, R. B. Delayed onset muscle soreness and plasms CPK and LDH activities after downhill running. Med. Sci. Sports Exerc. *15:* 51–56, 1983.
9. Carroll, J. E., Hagberg, J. M., and Brooke, M. H. Bicycle ergometry and gas exchange measurements in neuromuscular disease. Arch. Neurol. *36:* 457–461, 1979.
10. Wasserman, K., Whipp, B. J., Koyal, S. N., and Beaver, W. L. Anaerobic threshold and respiratory gas exchange during exercise. J. Appl. Physiol. *35:* 236–243, 1973.
11. Hagberg, J. M., Coyle, E. F., Carroll, J. E., Miller, J. M., Martin, W. H., and Brooke, M. H. Exercise hyperventilation in patients with McArdle's disease. J. Appl. Physiol. *52:* 991–994, 1982.
12. Munsat, T. L. A standardised forearm ischemic exercise test. Neurology *20:* 1171–1178, 1970.
13. Patterson, V. H., Kaiser, K. K., and Brooke, M. H. Forearm exercise increases plasma hypoxanthine. J. Neurol. Neurosurg. Psychiatry *45:* 552–553, 1982.
14. Patterson, V. H., Kaiser, K. K., and Brooke, M. H. Exercising muscle does not produce hypoxanthine in adenylate deaminase deficiency. Neurology *33:* 784–786, 1983.
15. Brooke, M. H., Patterson, V. H., and Kaiser, K. K. Hypoxanthine and McArdle disease: a clue to metabolic stress in the working forearm. Muscle Nerve *6:* 204–206, 1983.
16. Brooke, M. H., Carroll, J. E., Davis, J. E., and Hagberg, J. M. The prolonged exercise test. Neurology *29:* 636–643, 1979.

BIOCHEMICAL DEFECTS CAUSING EXERCISE INTOLERANCE

There are a group of disorders in which a known biochemical defect is associated with symptoms of exercise intolerance. There may be other associated problems, but the cardinal feature is that normal exercise is impossible for the patient because of the development of disabling symptoms. These are usually of two kinds; fatigue and muscle pains. The fatigue is easily understandable in an illness in which the energy supply is unable to sustain the exercise in a normal fashion. There is, as yet, no clear explanation for the muscle pains. These pains are of varying severity and often associated with a tight muscle which is firm to palpation. In some of the illnesses a frank muscle contracture, which is an electrically silent shortening of the muscle, is noted. Such muscle pains are often associated with necrosis of muscle fibers and with the appearance of large amounts of myoglobin and CK in the blood. In extreme cases myoglobinuria and renal damage subsequent to this may be noted.

It is possible for a normal subject to exercise to such an extent that the energy stores of muscle are markedly depleted. Fatigue is then prominent, but muscle pains are usually not noted until some hours following such exercise. The immediate development of muscle pain and contracture, which characterizes so many of the biochemical defects, is absent. One might speculate that there is built into normal muscular activity a series of safety mechanisms which allow the muscle to deplete its energy supplies in a predictable and orderly fashion. The ensuing fatigue protects the muscle against further exercise which might be harmful. Perhaps specific enzyme defects disturb this normal sequence and allow part of the machinery to run at full throttle, while other parts are totally shut down. I always have a weakness for simplistic analogies which turn out to be meaningless when analyzed in any detail, but one might think of depressing the accelerator pedal to the floor while in an automobile. If this is done with the car traveling down the highway in a normal fashion, it will result in a satisfying surge of speed. If it is done with the transmission disengaged, it will result in frighteningly high rpms and bits of the pistons appearing over the landscape. One might think of the transmission in this case as being the biochemical step which controls the orderly flow of energy. Its absence results in a disintegration of the motor, which might be equivalent to the muscle contracture. It is also obvious that this disintegration does not occur with the motor idling, but only in response to the floored accelerator pedal or the demands of excessive exercise. We shall now move back from the garage to the clinic and outline these disorders in sequence.

Abnormalities of Glycogen Metabolism

Myophosphorylase Deficiency (McArdle's Disease, Type 5 Glycogenosis)

Phosphorylase is a complicated enzyme. Myophosphorylase cleaves the bonds between the glucose molecules of the glycogen chain making the hexose sugar available for further metabolism in glycolysis. A defect in this enzyme leads to a patient who is unable to utilize glycogen as a source of energy and gives predictable difficulties during heavy or intensive short-term exercise, such as carrying a piano upstairs, when glycogen is normally the chief substrate utilized. The illness occupies a special place in the constellation of biochemical disorders, since it was the first of the enzyme defects to be suspected on clinical grounds and the unraveling of the basic defect established principles which hold true of all disorders of energy metabolism (1–3).

The illness is inherited as a autosomal recessive or rarely as an autosomal dominant (4). It is commoner in the male than female. Usually before the child is 10 years old, he starts to complain of fatigue and an inability to keep up with others of his age. There may be mild aching in the legs, but this symptom is often noted for the first time in early adolescence. It then becomes increasingly severe and may be provoked by anything more than the mildest exertion. Often, at some stage in teenage life, a particularly heavy bout of exercise will be accompanied by painful cramps in the muscles which have been used. These pains will last for several hours, even overnight, and the patient may notice that his urine becomes the color of a Burgundy because of the attendant myoglobinuria. At the stage in his life when muscle pain becomes severe, the patient's activity may be severely curtailed and even walking the length of a city block is arduous. A muscle that is exercised hard enough to produce a cramp becomes shortened and cannot be stretched passively without producing severe pain. As the years progress, with repeated bouts of muscle pain, a permanent weakness of the proximal muscle may be found.

Quite early in the disease, patients notice that their exercise tolerance may be increased enormously if they slow down immediately upon the initial sensation of muscle fatigue. When they then resume exercise at a slow rate, they experience a "second wind" as does the long distance runner. Many patients with McArdle's disease are able to tell exactly when this occurs and can exercise for long periods of time at a rate which would have totally disabled them if attempted initially. One patient referred to this as a "barrier" and said that the initial exercise was accompanied by a sense of laboring and tightness in the muscles, but once the barrier was broken, he had a sense of ease and relaxation and could exercise for as long as he wished.

Patients may also notice a rapid acceleration of heart rate and of breathing with the beginning of exercise. In spite of the tachycardia, there is only rarely evidence of any abnormality of the heart itself (5). Since the absence of the enzyme is limited to muscle, no other organs suffer from the primary effects of the disease. Secondary involvement of the kidney and even acute renal failure may be seen after myoglobinuria (6, 7). Most patients are aware of the amount of exercise which can produce this degree of damage and assiduously avoid situations which might demand it.

Initial examination of the patient reveals little untoward. There is no apparent wasting; indeed, some patients are unusually muscular. Weakness is detected only in the older patients and the reflexes are all normal. It is only when exercise testing is carried out that the abnormalities become apparent. The forearm exercise test is markedly abnormal. It should be emphasized that exercise tests in patients with McArdle's disease, as in the other abnormalities of glycolysis, are not benign tests. The contracture and the pain that are produced are indicative of muscle damage, and occasionally frank myoglobinuria may be produced. Although it is vital to employ this test in the diagnosis, it should not be used in frivolous demonstrations. When the forearm muscles are subjected to high intensity exercise, as described previously (see p. 256), they fatigue rapidly within 1 or 2 minutes. The pattern of this fatigue is quite abnormal. In the average person, the grip tires after 5 or 6 minutes, and if exercise is continued until the hand is paralyzed, the muscles of the forearm are completely limp. The wrist and fingers can be moved passively without any resistance. In the patient with McArdle's disease, as the paralysis occurs, the muscles become increasingly tight and the wrist becomes fixed in flexion with the fingers gripped firmly around the dynamometer or whatever object is being used in the exercise. The wrist and fingers cannot then be passively straightened, but remain locked in an iron grip. This is a true contracture since placement of an EMG needle in the tightened muscles reveals no electrical activity whatsoever. The chemical accompaniment of this is the absence of rise in lactate levels in the venous blood from the exercised forearm. Ordinarily, the breakdown of glycogen, which is provoked under conditions of heavy intensive exercise or under ischemic conditions, results in the production of lactate. Since it is impossible for the patient to break down glycogen, no lactate is produced. One would expect that forearm exercise would cause a decline in levels of ATP with the development of fatigue. Actual measurements have not confirmed this (8), although one might suspect that this was due either to technical difficulties, or to the fact that a detectable reduction in ATP levels would result not in symptoms of fatigue and pain, but in actual death of the muscle. Be that as it may, there is evidence that the biochemical support systems, which are used to bolster ATP levels, are depleted. Thus, a decrease in creatine phosphate levels was detected by means of nuclear magnetic resonance studies (9). Similarly, there is an abnormally high production of hypoxanthine during the forearm test, suggesting that the adenylate kinase/adenylate deaminase reactions, which promote the formation of ATP from ADP, are working overtime (10). With a little planning, it is possible to carry out a single exercise test and combine the clinical, electrical, and biochemical studies (and perhaps even Grand Rounds!). This avoids the necessity of repeated ischemic tests.

Since an absence of lactate production following forearm exercise is noted in several of the enzyme defects in glycolysis, the exact diagnosis of phosphorylase deficiency depends upon the biochemical and histochemical demonstration of the enzyme's absence in the muscle itself. A biopsy may also show anatomical changes within the muscle fibers (Figs. 7.13–7.17). Subsarcolemmal deposits of glycogen and scattered necrotic fibers are common. Biochemical measurement of glycogen shows an increase from the normal 1% to around 3% or, in occasional patients, as much as 5% of the muscle weight.

Bicycle exercise presents a more severe challenge to the patient. The cardiac output is excessively high for the amount of work being done. The simplest evidence of this is a pulse rate, which is higher than seen in the normal patient for the equivalent given level of exercise. A more detailed measurement shows that the cardiac output, which should increase approximately 5–6 liters for every additional liter of oxygen used in performing the work, actually increases at over double that rate (11, 12). This abnormal response is not an indication

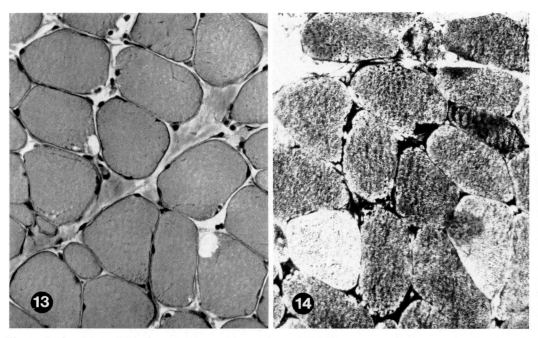

Figure 7.13. McArdle's disease. The routine stains of the biopsy may show nonspecific changes consequent upon myoglobinuria. In addition, there are often subsarcolemmmal blebs. These blebs lie immediately under the sarcolemma and have eaten away part of the underlying muscle fiber (Verhoef-Van Giesen stain).

Figure 7.14. With the PAS stain for glycogen these subsarcolemmal blebs often stain intensely. Unfortunately, one has to be cautious in the interpretation because the PAS stain normally has a tendency to accumulate in the spaces between the fibers unless the technique is faultless. In this photograph, for example, one subsarcolemmal bleb is clearly seen in the fiber toward the top of the photograph as it erodes into the substances of the muscle fiber. In some other areas of the photograph the stain is less convincing since it seems to be merely filling in the gaps between the fibers.

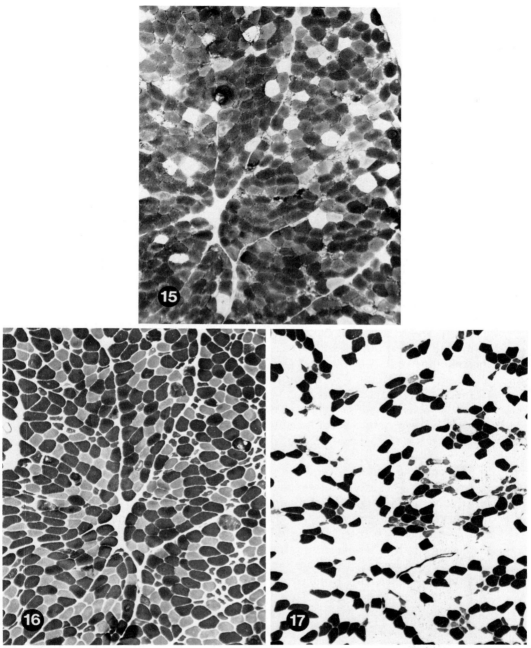

Figure 7.15. In addition, some fibers in the PAS reaction are totally devoid of stain because they are necrotic.

Figures 7.16 and 7.17. ATPase reactions show numerous Type 2C fibers characteristic of regenerating muscle. They can be found by comparing Figure 7.16 with Figure 7.17. Figure 7.16 is a routine ATPase reaction in which the Type 1 fibers are light and the Type 2 fibers are dark. There are many scattered small fibers which are a shade lighter then the normal Type 2 fiber. With the modified ATPase following preincubation at pH 4.3 (Fig. 7.17) the Type 1 fibers are darkly stained and the normal Type 2 fibers are unstained. The Type 2C fibers can again be seen as an intermediate staining fiber scattered throughout the biopsy.

of cardiac damage, but is probably due to unusual changes in the vascular bed or other abnormal vasoregulatory responses. It is possible that the blood circulation to the muscle is affected by the metabolites produced by exercise. In one patient, if exercise were sufficient to increase the oxygen uptake to greater than 60% of the maximal value, the heart rate became maximal after 2 minutes. The administration of glucose which might be expected to bypass the biochemical abnormality tended to lessen this phenomenon (13). The second wind phenomenon occurred only if the initial blood flow on resuming exercise was more than thrice the normal resting level.

In the normal subject, an incremental exercise test produces a "hyperventilation threshold." At this point, the linear increase in respiration associated with the increasing work load accelerates out of proportion to the increasing level of exercise. This has been ascribed to the effects of lactate produced by the working muscle. McArdle's patients, however, have a pronounced threshold, even in the absence of lactate production which suggests that the explanation for this phenomenon should be sought elsewhere (14).

The nature of the "second wind" phenomenon is also obscure. It has been suggested that it is associated with a change in the supply of fatty acid to the muscle (15). This is logical since the only source of energy for the muscle other than carbohydrate is derived from fat. The "second wind" is usually associated with a rise in fatty acid, and exercise tolerance is reduced by nicotinic acid (a drug that blocks the release of free fatty acids and glycerol from fat), and is increased by isoproterenol and norepinephrine (which increase the free fatty acid levels). On the other hand, the second wind occurs after only a few minutes of exercise, which is an unlikely time for fatty acid metabolism to change. It has been suggested that the phenomenon is more closely associated with the change in the blood flow to the muscle. In the forearm exercise test, a local "second wind" occurred only in the muscles being exercised (16). If the "second wind" is truly associated with the arterial level of free fatty acids, it will be a general phenomenon and not one localized at the exercising muscle.

Treatment. The exercise tolerance of patients has been augmented by intravenous glucose and the oral administration of fructose. The sublingual administration of isoproterenol has also been recommended, as has coenzyme Q_{10} in oral doses of 0.15 g (17). The latter was proposed to boost mitochondrial oxidation. None of these measures seems to be of universal therapeutic value. Although occasional patients are helped by sublingual isoproterenol, most find the side effects more troublesome than the disease. Honey, which is rich in fructose, has been given to patients, but again without notable success. One facet of the illness, which is not explained, is the fluctuation in the degree of severity. I have seen patients who have led active lives, going to school and participating in social activities, who only 2 months later have had severe limitation to their exercise capacity and have been confined to a wheelchair. Recovery from this state can be equally abrupt. One possible explanation for this type of change was noted in a patient whose leg symptoms became incapacitating so that she could no longer climb even a few steps without severe pain. Any attempt to walk was accompanied by subsequent myoglobinuria. This turned out to be due to occlusion of the femoral artery (18). The reduction of the blood supply to the leg increased the muscle's dependence upon intracellular glycogen stores and exacerbated a situation which was already bad.

Biochemical Ramifications. Phosphorylase is one of those enzymes whose subtle complexities seem never ending, like an intricately carved series of nested boxes. Phosphorylase itself exists in two forms. The active form, phosphorylase *a*, which is a tetramer and the inactive dimer, phosphorylase *b*. The conversion of the inactive to the active form is catalyzed by phosphorylase kinase. This enzyme is itself activated by a protein kinase and the protein kinase is activated by cyclic AMP, which is produced under the influence of adenyl cyclase. There is, thus, a cascading series of reactions and a defect in any one of these might result in an absence of phosphorylase activity. One, therefore, cannot assume that an absence of phosphorylase activity implies an absence of the enzyme.

Different molecular etiologies for the disease are suggested by the finding of patients with McArdle's disease in whom a protein was detected immunologically or electrophoretically which resembled the phosphorylase protein, but without enzyme activity (6, 19). In other patients, no such protein was detected.

There are different forms of phosphorylase in the heart and liver, as well as a fetal isoenzyme of muscle phosphorylase which disappears after birth. There are three isoenzymes in the heart, one of which is the muscle form, another characteristic of the heart, and a third which is a hybrid of the other two. When muscle from a patient with myophosphorylase deficiency is cultured, the enzyme activity returns. This is due to the presence of the fetal isoenzyme in tissue culture, which is not present in the adult muscle (20). This may also be the explanation for scattered phosphorylase positive fibers in patients with McArdle's disease (21). As the necrotic fibers regenerate, they go through a phase in which the fetal isoenzyme is present and reactive.

Clinical Variety. A case which was difficult to explain was that reported by Kost and Verity (22) of a 60-year-old woman, with phosphorylase deficiency, whose life-long activities had included sports and mountain climbing, who suddenly, at the age of 60, developed disabling cramps and was shown to have deficiency of phosphorylase including an absence of the protein on sodium dodecyl sulfate (SDS) gel electrophoresis. Why such a patient would develop symptoms for the first time at this age is totally unclear. Phosphorylase deficiency is also being added to a growing list of abnormalities of glycogen metabolism associated with severe weakness and hypotonia in infancy. One such girl was normal at birth and for the first 4 weeks of life, but then began to have increasing difficulty with feeding, respiratory function deteriorated, and movements of the arms and legs decreased. Mentally she appeared to be normal. Within 2 months, she was dead from aspiration pneumonia and progressive respiratory failure. The enzyme protein was absent when detection was attempted using immunodiffusion techniques (23). Phosphorylase deficiency has also been reported as the cause of progressive proximal weakness occurring for the first time in middle age and unassociated with myoglobinuria, muscle cramps, or fatigue (24).

Phosphorylase Kinase Deficiency. Phosphorylase kinase was undetectable in a boy who was noted to be quite floppy during the first few months of his life, and then developed exercise induced pains in the legs in early childhood.

Another case was reported from Japan with a similar early history of hypotonia and a delayed motor development. This child was not yet old enough to determine whether she had exercise intolerance or not (25, 26).

REFERENCES

1. McArdle, B. Myopathy due to a defect in muscle glycogen breadown. Clin. Sci. *10:* 13–33, 1951.
2. Schmid, R., and Mahler, R. Chronic progressive myopathy with myoglobinuria; demonstration of a glycogenolytic defect in the muscle. J. Clin. Invest. *38:* 2044–2058, 1959.
3. Mommaerts, W. F. H. M., Illingworth, B., Peason, C. M., Geuillory, P. J., and Seraydarian, K. A functional disorder associated with the absence of phosphorylase. Proc. Natl. Acad. Sci. *45:* 791–797, 1959.
4. Chui, L. A., and Munsat, T. L. Dominant inheritance of McArdle syndrome. Arch. Neurol. *33:* 636–641, 1976.
5. Engel, W. K., Eyerman, E. L., and Williams, H. E. Late onset type of skeletal muscle phosphorylase deficiency. N. Engl. J. Med. *268:* 135–141, 1963.
6. Ratinov, G., Baker, W. P., and Swaimam, K. F. McArdle's syndrome with previously unreported electrocardiographic and serum enzyme abnormalities. Ann. Intern. Med. *62:* 328–334, 1965.
7. Grunfeld, J. P., Ganeval, D., Chanard, J., Fardeau, M., and Dreyfus, J. C. Acute renal failure in McArdle's disease. N. Engl. J. Med. *286:* 1237–1241, 1972.
8. Rowland, L. P., Avaki, S., and Carmel, P. Contracture in McArdle's disease. Arch. Neurol. *13:* 541–544, 1965.
9. Ross, V. D., Radda, G. K., Gadian, D. G., Rocker, G., Esiri, M., and Falconer-Smith, J. Examination of a case of suspected McArdle's syndrome by P nuclear magnetic resonance. N. Engl. J. Med. *304:* 1338–1342, 1981.
10. Brooke, M. H., Patterson, V. H., and Kaiser, K. K., Hypoxanthine and McArdle disease: a clue to metabolic stress in the working forearm. Muscle Nerve *6:* 204–206, 1983.
11. Haller, R. G., Lewis, S. F., Cook, J. D., and Blomqvist, C. G. Hyperkinetic circulation during exercise in neuromuscular disease. Neurology *33:* 1283–1287, 1983.
12. Haller, R. G., Lewis, S. F., Cook, J. D., and Blomqvist, C. G. Myophosphorylase deficiency impairs muscle oxidative metabolism. Ann. Neurol. *17:* 196–199, 1985.
13. Andersen, K. L., Lund-Johansen, B., and Clausen, G. Metabolic and circulatory responses to muscular exercise in a subject with glycogen storage disease (McArdle's disease). Scan. J. Clin. Lab. Invest. *24:* 105–113, 1969.
14. Hagberg, J. M., Coyle E. F., Carroll, J. E., Miller, J. M., Martin, W. H., and Brooke, M. H. Exercise hyperventilation in patients with McArdle's disease. J. Appl. Physiol. *52:* 991–994, 1982.
15. Porte, D., Crawford, D. W., Jennings, D. B., Aber, C., and McIlroy, M. B. Cardiovascular and metabolic responses to exercise in a patient with McArdle's syndrome. N. Engl. J. Med. *275:* 406–412, 1966.
16. Pernow, B. B., Havel, R. J., and Jennings, D. B. The second wind phenomenon in McArdle's syndrome. Acta Med. Scand. Suppl. *472:* 294–307, 1967.
17. Nono, N., Mineo, I., Sumi, S., Shimizu, T., Kang, J., Nonaka, K., and Tarui, S. Metabolic basis of improved exercise tolerance. Neurology *34:* 1471–1476, 1984.
18. Wheeler, S., and Brooke, M. H. Vascular insufficiency in McArdle disease. Neurology *33:* 249–250, 1983.
19. Feit, H., and Brooke, M. H. Myophosphorylase deficiency: two different molecular etiologies. Neurology *26:* 963–967, 1976.
20. DiMauro, S., Arnold, S., Miranda, A. F., and Rowland, L. P. McArdle disease; the mystery of reappearing phosphorylase activity in muscle culture: a fetal isoenzyme. Ann. Neurol. *3:* 60–66, 1979.
21. Roelofs, R. L., Engel, W. K., and Shauvin, P. B. Histochemical phosphorylase activity in regenerating muscle fibers from myophosphorylase deficiency patients. Science *177:* 795–797, 1972.
22. Kost, G. J., and Verity, M. A. A new variant of late onset mild phosphorylase deficiency. Muscle Nerve *3:* 195–201, 1980.
23. DiMauro, S., and Hartlage, P. L. Fatal infantile form of muscle phosphorylase deficiency. Neurology *28:* 1124–1129, 1978.
24. Engel, W. K., Eyerman, E. L., and Williams, H. E. Late onset type of skeletal muscle phosphorylase deficiency. N. Engl. J. Med. *268:* 135–141, 1963.
25. Strugalska-Cynowska, M. Disturbances in the activity of phosphorylase *b* kinase in a case of McArdle myopathy. Folia Histochem. Cytochem. *5:* 151–156, 1967.
26. Ohtani, Y., Matsuda, I., Iwamasa, T., Tamari, H., Origuchi, and Y., Miike, T. Infantile

glycogen storage myopathy in a girl with a phosphorylase kinase deficiency. Neurology *32:* 833–838, 1982.

Phosphofructokinase Deficiency (Type 7 Glycogenosis)

The enzyme PFK is responsible for the conversion of fructose-6-phosphate to fructose-1,6-diphosphate, a reaction which is essential in the glycolytic process. It is the rate limiting step and gycolysis is turned on or off by factors which control the activity of PFK. The absence of this enzyme is associated with an illness which closely resembles phosphorylase deficiency, for the obvious reason that the defect is in the same chain of metabolic reactions. The patients experience the early onset of fatigue and aching pains in the muscles. With more strenuous exertion, severe muscle pains, contractures, and myoglobinuria occur. In most patients, the episodes are more severe than seen in McArdle's disease and the attack may be associated with nausea and vomiting (1–3). The pattern of inheritance, as with many of the glycogenoses, is of an autosomal recessive disorder and decreased levels of enzyme activity in the heterozygote betray the carrier state even though such a person is asymptomatic (4). The laboratory investigations show changes similar to those found in phosphorylase deficiency. There is no rise in venous lactate following forearm exercise and the development of muscle contractures are noted.

The CK is often abnormal and the muscle shows sarcolemmal blebs which contain glycogen. Glycogen is also found lying free within the muscle cell. In addition to biochemical methods for diagnosing PFK deficiency, a histochemical technique is also available (5). A finding which differentiates the biopsy from that of McArdle's disease is the presence of unusual structures in some of the muscle fibers. These consist of an abnormal polysaccharide which is resistant to diastase digestion and is brightly staining with PAS. Histochemical reactions indicate an abnormal polysaccharide without acidic groups, perhaps an insoluble form of glycogen. Under electron microscopy, these structures have a fine filamentous appearance, such as might be associated with long chains of polysaccharides. This may be due to activation of the enzyme glycogen synthase by the elevated concentrations of glucose-6-phosphate which occur subsequent to the enzyme deficiency. Glycogen synthase elongates the polysaccharide chains of glycogen and may form an abnormal polysaccharide with long side chains (6).

The patients also suffer from evidence of a mild hemolytic anemia as evidenced by an increased level of bilirubin and increased reticulocytes in the blood. Gouty arthritis was described in one patient (4) and high levels of uric acid in the blood were noted. The reason is uncertain. Increased purine degradation and uric acid production associated with the mild hemolysis, as well as an overproduction of urate stimulated by increased levels of fructose-6-phosphate acting on the pentose phosphate shunt, might result in elevated uric acid levels. An alternative explanation, one which is unproven in this case, is that the increased levels of hypoxanthine which follow exercise in McArdle's disease, are also seen in PFK deficiency. This is then degraded to uric acid.

The enzyme PFK is analogous to phosphorylase, being comprised of subunits which combine to form an active tetramer. There are two types of subunits, M and R. Muscle PFK is composed of identical M subunits, whereas the enzyme in the erythrocyte is normally made up of both types of subunit. Muscle PFK deficiency results in a disappearance of the activity of the M subunit. The activity of the enzyme in the red blood cell is only partially affected since the R subunit is still preserved. Nevertheless, this abnormality is presumably responsible for the mild hemolysis. Although the enzyme is inactive, its presence in one case of the disease was suggested by a positive immunological cross reaction with PFK antibody at least in one case (4). In another patient, immunological studies failed to show the presence of any detectable enzyme protein (2). Whether this was due to the use of a less sensitive technique, or whether the situation is similar to that seen in phosphorylase deficiency with two different forms of the illness is not, at present, clear. There seems to be no successful treatment for this condition.

Clinical Variety. As in McArdle's disease, PFK deficiency has been described in a totally different clinical setting (6). A woman in her 60s was noted to have increasing difficulty with proximal weakness for the preceding 6 years or so. In retrospect, the patient had never been very athletic and had been noted in childhood to fatigue more readily than her playmates. On the other hand, exercise intolerance and muscle cramps were absent and myoglobinuria had never been noted. She had a life-long diplopia due to a congenital Duane syndrome and was noted to have prominent proximal weakness on examination.

Another patient with congenital weakness of the limbs, mental retardation and a corneal ulceration died of respiratory insufficiency at the age of 4. Although glycogen was not immediately apparent under the light microscope, electron microscopic and biochemical studies demonstrated an increase in the muscle cell content. There was a marked decrease in PFK levels of the muscle. Phosphorylase *b* kinase was reduced to about one-third of the normal value, a level which should be adequate for normal muscle function. The rest of the biopsy appeared to resemble one of the congenital muscular dystrophies, as did the patient's clinical picture, an impression which was reinforced by the presence of joint contractures (7).

Two other reports also stressed a picture of a fixed myopathy without exercise-provoked symptoms (8, 9).

REFERENCES

1. Tarui, S., Okuno, G., and Ikura, Y. Phosphofructokinase deficiency in skeletal muscle; a new type of glycogenosis. Biochem. Biophys. Res. Commun. *19:* 517–523, 1965.
2. Layzer, R. B., Rowland, L. P., and Ranney, H. M. Muscle phosphofructokinase deficiency. Arch. Neurol. *17:* 512–523, 1967.
3. Tobin. W. E., Huijing, F., Porro, R. S., and Salzman, R. T. Muscle phosphofructokinase deficiency. Arch. Neurol. *28:* 128–130, 1973.
4. Agamanolis, D. P., Askari, A. D., DiMauro, S., Hays, A., Kumar, K., Lipton, M., and Raynor, A. Muscle phosphofructokinase deficiency: two cases with unusual polysaccharide accumulation and immunologically active enzyme protein. Muscle Nerve *3:* 456–467, 1980.
5. Bonilla E., and Schotland, D. L. Histochemical diagnosis of muscle phosphofructokinase deficiency. Arch. Neurol. *22:* 8–12, 1970.
6. Hays, A. P., Hallett, M., Delfs, J., Morris, J., Sotrel, A., Shevchuk, M. M., and DiMauro, S. Muscle phosphofructokinase deficiency: abnormal polysaccharide in a case of late onset myopathy. Neurology *31:* 1077–1086, 1981.
7. Danon, M. J., Carpenter, S., Manaligod, J. R., and Schliselfeld, L. H. Fatal infantile glycogen storage disease: Deficiency of phosphofructokinase and phosphorylase-*b*-kinase. Neurology *31:* 1303–1307, 1981.
8. Guibaud, P., Carrier, H., and Mathieu, M. Observation familiale de dystrophie musculaire

congenitale caractarisee par deficit en phosphofructokinase. Arch. Fr. Pediatr. *35:* 1105–1115, 1978.

9. Serratrice, G., Morges, A., and Roux, H. Forme myopathique du deficit en phosphofructokinase. Rev. Neurol. *120:* 271–277, 1967.

Phosphoglycerate Kinase Deficiency (Type 9 Glycogenosis) (1)

The enzyme phosphoglycerate kinase (PGK) transfers the phosphate from 3-phosphoglyceroyl phosphate to ADP forming 3-phosphoglycerate and ATP. This reaction is again part of the glycolytic process and a deficiency gives the predictable picture of exercise intolerance. A 14-year-old boy was described who had repeated complaints of muscle pains and weakness after vigorous exercise, such as running and biking. At the age of 14, he had severe pain and weakness of the leg muscles after running in the snow for 15 minutes. Two hours later, he had vomiting and pigmenturia. His CK level increased to over 400,000 within 24 hours and renal function was compromised. He had noted a "second wind" phenomenon on several occasions. The patient thus presented with a picture indistinguishable from phosphorylase or PFK deficiency. In contradistinction, the muscle biopsy appeared relatively normal with normal glycogen concentrations and some mild increase in lipid droplets. Forearm exercise test produced no rise in venous lactate, as would be expected. PGK activity in the muscle was found to 5% of the normal value. The enzyme was also deficient in the red blood cells and the abnormality was reproduced in tissue culture of muscle and fibroblasts. PGK is a single polypeptide and other abnormal variants have been described, most of which produce abnormalities in the red blood cell. The muscle abnormality was felt to be due to a mutant PGK. Since the enzyme is controlled by a gene on the X chromosome, it is possible that it is an X-linked recessive disorder. A reduction in the PGK activity of the red blood cells in the patient's mother but not in his father supported this possibility.

REFERENCE

1. DiMauro, S., Dalakas, M., and Miranda, A. F. Phosphoglycerate kinase deficiency, another cause of recurrent myoglobinuria. Ann. Neurol. *13:* 11–19, 1983.

Phosphoglycerate Mutase Deficiency (Type 10 Glycogenosis)

The rather monotonous litany of exercise induced symptoms is also used in describing this illness. Three patients have been described; two men aged 52 and 24 and a 17-year-old girl. All had recurrent myoglobinuria after intense exercise. In the case of the 52-year-old man, he also had typical attacks of gouty arthritis for which he was treated with colchicine and allopurinol (1–3).

Forearm exercise testing in two of these patients showed a decreased lactate production in the venous blood, although it was not absent. The serum CK was mildly elevated, except during frank attacks of muscle pain and myoglobinuria when it was, of course, markedly elevated. With forearm exercise testing in the 24-year-old, the development of contractures in the muscle coincided with an elevation of venous lactate to almost double the slightly high baseline values (a blunted response). Incremental exercise testing on a bicycle provoked a normal rise in lactate and showed that all the other physiological measurements such as V_{O_2max} and heart rate were also normal, a finding not easily explained.

Changes noted on the muscle biopsy included increased staining with PAS stain for glycogen. Eighteen days after a bout of myoglobinuria, the biopsy from the 24-year-old showed variation in fiber size, groups of regenerating fibers, and tubular aggregates. Biochemical evaluation of glycogen showed a slight increase in the amount, up to 2 g per 100 g muscle.

Phosphoglycerate mutase is an enzyme which exists as a dimer. There is a subunit which is characteristic of muscle (the M subunit) and one which is characteristic of brain (the B subunit). The predominant form in normal muscle is an MM form in which the two subunits are identical. In the illness, the M subunit is missing. A small amount of residual activity in the patient's muscle is due to the existence of the BB form, which accounts for approximately 3% of the normal activity. When muscle was cultured, the enzyme activity returned, but this is simply because in normal muscle cultures, as well as in the patient's culture, the enzyme is present in the BB form.

Evaluation of the parents' biopsies in the second case showed that both had a decreased activity in the muscle, indicating the heterozygote state and showing that the illness is inherited as an autosomal recessive. The activity in the red blood cells is normal because the predominant form of the enzyme there is the BB form.

Of interest is the appearance of gout and atherosclerosis with cardiac symptoms in the first patient. It is not clear whether these are related to the enzyme defect, but they have been described in other patients with glycolytic disorders.

REFERENCES

1. DiMauro, S., Miranda, A. F., Olarte, M., Friedman, R., and Hays, E. P. Muscle phosphoglycerate mutase deficiency. Neurology *32:* 584–591, 1982.
2. Bresolin, N., Ro, Y. I., Reyes, M., Miranda, A. F., and DiMauro, S. Muscle phosphoglycerate mutase (PGAM) deficiency: a second case. Neurology *33:* 1049–1053, 1983.
3. Kissel, J. T., Beam, W., Bresolin, N., Gibbons, G., DiMauro, S., and Mendell, J. R. Physiologic assessment of phosphoglycerate mutase deficiency: incremental exercise tests. Neurology *35:* 828–833, 1985.

Lactate Dehydrogenase Deficiency

An 18-year-old man presented with a complaint of exercise intolerance, fatigue, and myoglobinuria. His symptoms were found to be due to a complete deficiency of the muscle form of lactate dehydrogenase (LDH) (1). A discrepancy was noted between the elevation of CK and the elevation of LDH in the serum. Ordinarily, these two enzymes fluctuate with some degree of synchrony since both leak from damaged muscle. The marked elevation of CK without an accompanying change in LDH suggested a possible deficiency in this enzyme. Forearm exercise tests produced a slight elevation of lactate in the venous blood, but not anywhere near the normal range. Pyruvate levels, on the other hand, were markedly elevated. This would be expected in a deficiency of LDH since the glycolytic pathway down to pyruvate is intact and only the conversion of pyruvate to lactate is deficient. Therefore, the pyruvate increases in a situation analogous to water being held back behind a dam.

LDH is made up of four subunits. Each subunit may have one of two different forms, either M which is characteristic of muscle, or H. This gives rise to different isoenzymes with composition of M_4, M_3H, M_2H_2, MH_3, and

H_4 (H = heart). As compared with this normal pattern of five isoenzyme bands, the patient demonstrated only one band which had the characteristics of H_4 and was found in both the muscle and the blood cells. This same abnormality, with LDH existing as a single isoenzyme, was found in three of the patient's siblings. Two other siblings and the parents had an increase in the ratio between H and M subunits in the red blood cell LDH, which would suggest a heterozygote state and indicate an autosomal recessive method of inheritance. It also provides a simple test for the detection of the heterozygote state.

REFERENCE

1. Kanno, T., Sudo, K., Takeuchi, I., Kanda, S., Honda, N., Nishimura, and Y., Oyama, K. Hereditary deficiency of lactate dehydrogenase M subunit. Clin. Chem. Acta *108:* 267–276, 1980.

Abnormalities of Lipid Metabolism

The metabolism of fatty acids in muscle is effected by a system equally as complex as that which handles carbohydrates. Long chain fatty acids, such as palmitate and oleate, are the predominant sources of energy, but the muscle also has mechanisms for breaking down medium chain fatty acids. There are some differences in the two systems because of the existence of enzymes which are specific to fatty acids of a particular chain length. Fatty acids are carried to the muscle in the blood, either bound to albumin or in the form of triglycerides, in the very low density lipoprotein fraction. Lipoprotein lipase in the capillary endothelium, working in conjunction with an apolipoprotein in the plasma, frees up the individual fatty acids from the triglycerides. Another lipase associated with the adipose tissue in the body is activated by lipolytic hormones and mobilizes fatty acids from fat stores. It is influenced by cyclic AMP levels. In this fashion, the increased levels of catecholamines seen in exercise are responsible for fatty acid mobilization from the fat stores. In addition, small lipid droplets, which are easily visible under the microscope, form the intracellular fat stores in the muscle and have their own system of enzymes responsible for synthesis and degradation. As might be expected, lipid droplets are more numerous in the highly oxidative or Type 1 fibers.

Once the free fatty acids arrive in the muscle, they have to be "primed" in order to enter the metabolic process. This is accomplished by forming the coenzyme A derivative (palmityl CoA in the case of palmitate), a reaction which is catalyzed by fatty acyl CoA synthetase on the mitochondrial membrane. The cell now encounters another problem since the mitochondrial membrane is impermeable to this form of fatty acid. In order to allow its passage across the membrane, it has to be hooked up to carnitine which carries it into the mitochondrial matrix. The enzyme which accomplishes this reaction is carnitine palmityl transferase. It exists in two forms; I on the outer face of the inner mitochondrial membrane which hooks the compounds together, and II on the inner surface of the inner mitochondrial membrane which uncouples the compound, producing palmityl CoA and free carnitine. The carnitine is again available to shuttle more fatty acids across the membrane. Once in the matrix, an orderly sequence of reactions split off pairs of carbon atoms from the fatty acid chain by β oxidation, so-called because the cleavage occurs at the β position (see p. 249). Acetyl CoA is produced by this process and enters the Krebs' cycle as outlined previously. One would imagine, in view of the complicated network of enzyme reactions involved, that there would be as many biochemical defects producing exercise intolerance on the basis of lipid metabolism as there are affecting carbohydrate metabolism. So far, only one has been recognized, although other disorders of lipid metabolism cause overt muscle weakness. Some consolation may be derived from the fact that the disorder which has been described, carnitine palmityl transferase deficiency, produces symptoms which are satisfyingly close to those which would be predicted from a knowledge of exercise physiology and biochemistry.

Carnitine Palmityl Transferase Deficiency

There have now been several reports of a disorder in which muscle pains and subsequent myoglobinuria have occurred recurrently and in association with relatively prolonged exercise. (See DiMauro et al. (1) for review.) Typically, the patient is a young adult male. Only one female patient has so far been described. Often the patient has experienced bouts of muscle pain in childhood, sometimes associated with pigmenturia. These symptoms are provoked by situations quite different from that seen in disorders of glycogen metabolism. The patient with carnitine palmityl transferase (CPT) deficiency has no problem with strenuous exertion and short-lived bouts of highly intensive exercise are well tolerated. A patient with CPT deficiency is no different from the normal individual, but none of us can sustain high level exercise near our maximum work load for more than 10 or 15 minutes. This may give the patient a false sense of security since the muscle function is so obviously normal for activities which are often regarded as the true test of muscle function by the layman. But serious problems arise when less intense exercise is prolonged for an hour or so. The patients with CPT deficiency develop their symptoms during prolonged cross country running, mountain climbing (it is hard to abandon all further exercise when you are half way up a mountain), or five set tennis matches. In all of these situations, of course, the exercise is prolonged so that the muscle depends upon fatty acid for its fuel supply rather than carbohydrate. It is obviously exactly this situation which is hardest for the patient with CPT deficiency to tolerate.

There is also a difference in the significance of the symptoms as interpreted by the patient. A patient with phosphorylase deficiency sensing the onset of a severe muscle contracture knows instinctively to stop all exercise. The muscle is in an acute situation and makes its discomfort immediately known. In CPT deficiency, the pains are milder and contractures are not noted. By the time severe muscle pain is noted by the patient, it is already too late. the pain persists many hours after exercise and myoglobinuria is inevitable.

There is another situation in which the body becomes dependent on fatty acids, which is unrelated to exercise. During fasting, in order to preserve the glucose supplies for vital tissue such as the brain, the rest of the body's metabolism switches over increasingly to fatty acids. This results in the mobilization of fat stores and, pari passu with the increasing levels of fatty acid in the blood, the muscle spares glucose and metabolizes fat. Fatty acids are also metabolized in the liver, the result of which is the production of ketone bodies in the blood. The situation which would, in theory, put the patient with CPT deficiency in the greatest danger is prolonged exercising in the fasting state. This, indeed, has been substantiated by the patients. Prolonged fasting alone and without exercise may result in symptoms in some. One student at a military academy, who was required to run 6 miles before breakfast had his first bout of fulminant myoglobinuria with renal failure. The patient may tacitly recognize the situation and may carry candy bars with him for use during any exercise.

In some older patients following repeated bouts of myoglobinuria, a mild fixed weakness may develop. This may be similar to weakness seen in other forms of recurrent myoglobinuria and may simply be the result of repeated insults into the muscle over a number of years. It should be stressed, however, that the typical picture of CPT deficiency does not include weakness. The onset of severe myoglobinuria is heralded by symptoms no different from those seen with other causes. The muscles are swollen, extremely tender and there may be profound weakness of the affected muscle during an attack. Respiratory weakness has also been noted during such attacks, and assisted ventilation may be necessary.

The disorder is suspected to be due to an autosomal recessive inheritance, since the abnormalities have been noted in siblings. The male proponderance is difficult to explain on this basis and the possibility of CPT deficiency being an X-linked recessive disorder has not been ruled out.

Laboratory Studies. The muscle biopsy is surprisingly normal, although an increased lipid deposition has been reported as part of the disease. Sophisticated morphometric analysis may be necessary to show such a change, and it is, perhaps, safest to assume that the finding of a normal muscle biopsy does not rule out CPT deficiency. Obviously there may be secondary changes due to the necrosis associated with myoglobinuria and the recovery process which ensues.

There is no abnormality noted in forearm exercise testing. This is expected since the forearm test addresses glycogen metabolism rather than lipid metabolism. During the incremental exercise test, the oxygen cost in terms of the amount of oxygen consumed per unit work performed is higher than normal. Because the patient with CPT deficiency has difficulty metabolizing fatty acids, one would expect the respiratory exchange ration (RER, respiratory quotient) would be higher or more characteristic of carbohydrate metabolism than fatty acid metabolism. The resting RER in one such patient was over 0.9 compared to the normal value at rest of around 0.8. Furthermore, the hyperventilation threshold or anaerobic threshold was higher than the normal value. The fact that it occurred closer to the point of maximum work capability or exhaustion, suggests perhaps a more efficient than normal utilization of carbohydrate (2). With the prolonged exercise test, there is an abnormal increase in serum CK for the level of exercise undertaken. It should be stressed that prolonged exercise testing in the patient with CPT deficiency runs the risk of producing myoglobinuria. Fasting is also a provocative test in this disorder and is probably safer than the prolonged exercise test. It may not be entirely without risk, however. An increase in CK and serum myoglobin may be noted during the fast. There is also a deterioration in the work performance of patients after fasting. One patient, who was able to carry out a normal exercise test before a fast, was unable to exercise at all following a 38-hour fast.

In addition to the abnormality in muscle CPT, the liver may also be involved. Oxidation of fatty acids by the liver results in the production of ketone bodies, which appear in the blood. The normal ketonemia and ketonuria produced by a 38-hour fast is absent in some patients with CPT deficiency (1, 3).

REFERENCES

1. Dimauro, S., Trevisan, C., and Hays, A. Disorders of lipid metabolism in muscle. Muscle Nerve *3:* 369–388, 1980.
2. Carroll, J. E., Brooke, M. H., DeVivo, D. C., Kaiser, K. K., and Hagberg, J. M. Biochemical and physiologic consequences of carnitine palmityl transferase deficiency. Muscle Nerve *1:* 103–110, 1978.
3. Bertorini, T., Yeh, Y. Y., Trevisan, C., Stadlan, E., Sabesin, S., and DiMauro, S. Carnitine palmitate transferase deficiency: myoglobinuria and respiratory failure. Neurology *30:* 263–271, 1980.

Other Abnormalities of Lipid Metabolism

This section should be much larger than it actually is. There are undoubtedly numerous other abnormalities of lipid metabolism, which give rise to exercise-induced symptoms. Unfortunately, they have yet to be characterized. Part of the problem lies in the inherent difficulties in assaying mitochondrial function. Unlike carbohydrate metabolism, which takes place in the cytoplasm as well as in the mitochondria, the interesting parts of fatty acid oxidation take place mostly within the mitochondria. There are many problems in accurate measurement of mitochondrial function, ranging from the large sample needed for adequate preparation of mitochondria to the undoubted fragility of the mitochondria themselves. This results in two sets of problems. On the one hand, abnormalities may be reported which are simply due to damage to the mitochondria during the preparation. On the other hand, biochemical defects may be missed due to the variability seen in the behavior of normal mitochondria.

We must, therefore, rely a great deal on indirect evidence and clinical suspicions to point to the presence of a lipid disorder. Undoubtedly, this situation will improve in the future.

One of the first case reports of exercise-induced symptoms of a lipid disorder involved two sisters (1). Eighteen-year-old identical twin girls had aching of the muscles with cramps since childhood. These were occasionally severe and sometimes associated with myoglobinuria. The pains could come on at any time of the day or night, were often related to some preceding exercise hours before. The discomfort lasted for several hours to several days. Neither weakness nor wasting was noticed, and no other abnormality was found. Ischemic exercise tests showed a normal rise in lactate. The symptoms were made worse by a 60-hour fast, during which time the serum CK and other "muscle" enzymes became abnormal. Additionally, the patients failed to produce ketone bodies in the urine during the fast, in contrast to normal controls in whom the production of ketone bodies occurred within 36 hours. The plasma cholesterol was normal and the triglycerides were at the lower limit of normal. The lipoprotein pattern was also unchanged. When the patients were fed triglycerides containing medium chain fatty acids, there was not only some amelioration of the symptoms, but ketone bodies were readily produced. Some increase in lipid deposition was noted in the muscle. These patients were described before CPT deficiency had been identified. Ironically, it was this case report which lead to speculation about the existence of CPT deficiency, and yet when the enzyme was assayed in these girls, it was found to be normal (cited in DiMauro et al. (2)).

An attempt to approach the problem from the opposite end was made by studying palmitate oxidation in 200 consecutive human muscle biopsies (3). The ability of a biopsy specimen to oxidize palmitate with a radioactive label on the first carbon atom (^{14}C-1-palmitate) was compared with its ability to oxidize palmitate with a radioactive label that might be at any position along the carbon chain (uniform label or U-^{14}C-palmitate). A defect occurring somewhere in β oxidation might allow the removal of the first carbon atom, in which case the radioactive label from ^{14}C-1-palmitate would be fully recovered. Carbon atoms labeled further down the chain might not be removed in the presence of a defect in a subsequent step, and there would be an incomplete recovery of the radioactive label from U-^{14}C-palmitate. This would be expressed by a change in the ratio of the oxidation of labeled ^{14}C-1-palmitate to the oxidation of the U-^{14}C form. Among the nine biopsies identified as having an abnormally high ratio, there were three teenage males, all of whom had been active athletically, who had noticed a deterioration of their performance with exercise intolerance. The serum CK levels were extremely high (up to 22,000) and the biopsies were of the type showing active degeneration and regeneration, although none of the patients had overt myoglobinuria or renal failure. In one of the other patients, a 53-year-old woman, there was a 10-year history of exercise precipitated muscle pain, although the CK was normal and the biopsy was not indicative of an active process. No abnormal storage of lipid was noted in any of these muscle biopsies. CPT estimations in these biopsies were either normal, or if the CPT assay was not available, the ratio of palmitate oxidation to pyruvate oxidation was normal, indicating that there was no selective defect in the initial steps of palmitate oxidation (i.e., including the reaction catalyzed by CPT). Other disorders of lipid metabolism have also been postulated (4–6), but, with lipid storage in the muscle biopsies and with weakness a permanent part of the clinical picture and exercise intolerance a relatively minor one, these patients' symptoms more resembled those of the lipid storage myopathies such as carnitine deficiency.

REFERENCES

1. Engel, W. K., Vick, N. A., Glueck, C. J., and Levy, R. I. A skeletal muscle disorder associated with intermittent symptoms and a possible defect of lipid metabolism. N. Engl. J. Med. *282:* 697–704, 1970.
2. Dimauro, S., Trevisan, C., and Hays, A. Disorders of lipid metabolism in muscle. Muscle Nerve *3:* 369–388, 1980.
3. Shumate, J. B., Brooke, M. H., Carroll, J. E., and Choksi, R. M. Incomplete palmitate oxidation: a possible source of human myopathy. Arch. Neurol. *39:* 561–564, 1982.
4. Jerusalem, F., Spiess, H., and Baumgartner, G. Lipid storage myopathy with normal carnitine levels. J. Neurol. Sci. *24:* 273–282, 1975.
5. Bradley, W. G., Jenkison, M., Park, D., Hudgson, P., Gardner-Medwin, D., Pennington, R. J. T., and Walton, J. N. A myopathy associated with lipid storage. J. Neurol. Sci. *16:* 137–154, 1972.
6. Johnson, M. A., Fulthorpe, J. J., and Hudgson, P. Lipid storage myopathy, a recognizable clinical, pathological entity. Acta Neuropathol. *24:* 97–106, 1973.

Mitochondrial Abnormalities

Some years ago, it appeared that we were to be inundated with diseases in which structural abnormalities of the mitochondria were associated with particular clinical entities. "Pleoconial" and "megaconial" myopathies vied with other muscle diseases with atypical mitochondria and the result was a series of remarkable pictures of ultrastructural changes that would have graced the walls of the Museum of Modern Art. The belief that each would characterize a particular clinical entity has turned out to be no more than a pious hope, but surviving from this early work are a series of pathological changes seen with the muscle biopsy which characterize mitochondrial disorders in general. Under the light microscope, scattered muscle fibers are seen with a heavy granular deposit which stains red or purple with the modified Gomori trichrome stain. Descriptively these are called "ragged red" fibers. With the more conventional hematoxylin and eosin stain, the network is colored blue. Under the electron microscope these granular clumps are seen to be collections of abnormal mitochondria. The mitochondria may be hypertrophied with a decreased number of cristae or cristae which are tightly packed. There may be a relatively lucent matrix. There are often inclusions ranging from round osmiophilic bodies to bizarre paracrystalline bodies with well marked periodicity or striations. Since no particular change has been associated with a particular biochemical or clinical finding, in the subsequent section the term "ragged red" fiber will be used to refer to these changes collectively.

As biochemical techniques are being developed to unlock the reactions occurring down the respiratory chain, it is becoming apparent that there are disorders of mitochondrial function in muscle, which share common clinical symptoms and in which the mitochondria are morphologically abnormal, although such abnormalities are not characteristic for any one of them.

The majority of case reports showing biochemical abnormalities of the electron transport chain, are of patients with severe fixed deficits and these will be referred to later. There are also, however, well documented reports of defects in mitochondrial function which produce exercise related symptoms as their predominant feature. Paradoxically, we shall start this section with a discussion of an illness which is really in neither category, but its clinical presentation can be correlated to a disturbance in mitochondrial function in very obvious ways. The same correlation can then be applied to the other disorders of mitochondrial function, although the relationship becomes increasing subtle.

Luft's Disease

Luft's disease is regularly mentioned in the neuromuscular literature, even though there are few cases and the muscular symptoms are minor. Two women have been described, both suffering from a similar clinical disorder (1, 2). They experienced fever, profuse sweating, and heat intolerance. One preferred to spend her time in a cold room at 4°C. Thirst and appetite were excessive; polyuria was also noted. The general physical examination showed a tachycardia with rapid respirations, profuse sweating, and warm, flushed skin. Blotchy erythematous changes of the skin over the legs were seen. Some degree of muscle weakness was noted in both patients, although this was mild and generalized.

This is obviously a hypermetabolic state. Somehow or other, the patient's thermostat had been turned up and laboratory studies provided the confirmation. The basal metabolic rate was elevated, although thyroid studies were entirely normal.

In contrast to the rather mild clinical involvement of muscle, morphological studies showed striking changes. Ragged red fibers were numerous. Ultrastructural studies revealed the mitochondria to be more numerous than usual and many were enlarged. They contained tightly packed cristae with paracrystalline and round osmiophilic inclusions.

Biochemically, the disease was characterized by defective respiratory control, indicating a relative uncoupling of oxidative phosphorylation from the energy needs of the body. Ordinarily, the reduction of substrates and the passage of electrons down the electron transport chain is tightly coupled to a need for ATP. Adding the appropriate substrates and ADP to a mitochondrial preparation will increase its uptake of oxygen, which will then decrease again as ADP is converted to ATP. It is apparent in Luft's disease, that this oxidative phosphorylation has become uncoupled and is now no longer under the control of the usual influences. A study of one patient (3) suggested that mitochondria were incapable of retaining calcium once it had been taken up and that all of the respiratory activity, instead of being usefully coupled to the provision of energy rich phosphates, was used in a futile attempt to retain calcium within the mitochondria. The constant and uncontrolled mitochondrial respiratory activity resulted in heat production and was probably the basis of the rest of the patients symptoms and signs.

There was no family history of any similar illness in these cases and laboratory studies were not very helpful. Serum muscle enzymes were within normal limits. The EMG showed a pattern which was "consistent with a myopathy" (4). There was also a progressive decline in the mechanical force of contraction of the muscle with continued activity. This may mirror a feature seen in some of the other mitochondrial myopathies.

There are important principles to be gained from this disease. The function of the electron transport chain in the mitochondria is not controlled by the usual mechanisms. It is, therefore, free running, expending large amounts of energy in seemingly "useless" work. Nevertheless, the mitochondrial mechanisms seem capable of handling this work and the only deleterious by product is heat, which the patient has to dissipate. The excessive demand for energy is compensated for by increasing the food and water intake. In the subsequent two illnesses, another step is added; namely, that the respiratory chain is not adequate to keep up with the demands placed on it.

REFERENCES

1. Luft, R., Ikkos, D., Palmieri, G., Urnster, L., and Afselius, B. A case of severe hypermetabolism of nonthyroid origin with a defect in the maintenance of mitochondrial respiratory control; a correlated clinical, biochemical and morphological study. J. Clin. Invest. *21:* 1776–1804, 1962.
2. Haydar, N. A., Conn, H. L., Afifi, A., Wakid, N., Ballas, S., and Fawaz, K. Severe hypermetabolism with primary abnormality of skeletal mitochondria: Functional and therapeutic effects of chloramphenicol treatment. Ann. Intern. Med. *74:* 548–558, 1971.
3. DiMauro, S., Bonilla, E., Lee, C. P., Schotland, D., Scarpa, A., Conn, H., and Chance, B. Luft's disease; further biochemical and ultrastructural studies of skeletal muscle in the second case. J. Neurol. Sci. *27:* 217–232, 1976.

4. deJesus, P. V. Neuromuscular physiology in Luft's syndrome. Electromyogr. Clin. Neurophysiol. *14:* 17–27, 1974.

NADH-CoQ Reductase Deficiency (Complex I)

An illness manifesting Complex I defects associated with pain, weakness, and fatigue has been described in two sisters, a mother and daughter, and a few unrelated patients (1–4). In the sisters, the symptoms developed in childhood and both weakness and excessive fatigue were noted. Exercise was often associated with a heavy feeling in the limbs and muscle aches were frequent. After exercise, the patients became tired, nauseated, and breathless. Recurrent bouts of weakness were also noted, often accompanied by headache, nausea and vomiting. Over the years, there was progression of the illness and the patients were only capable of a limited amount of exercise as young adults. The acute attacks were a feature of this illness and could be brought on by unaccustomed activity, fasting, or small quantities of alcohol. In one such episode, a patient was admitted to the hospital so weak that she was unable to lift her legs off the bed or to stand. She had bilateral ptosis, extraocular weakness, and nystagmus in all directions of gaze with a profound generalized weakness of all muscle groups. A blood lactate level taken 5 days after the admission was still almost 18 mM. The patient recovered after treatment of the lactic acidemia with intravenous sodium bicarbonate and potassium supplements. Muscle biopsy showed subsarcolemmal deposits of abnormal mitochondria and some increase in stippling of the more central parts of the fibers when stained with the oxidative enzymes. The mitochondria were increased in number with obvious structural abnormalities and crystalline inclusions.

Studies on the exercise bicycle showed a pronounced increase in heart rate for the level of exercise with an abnormal increase of lactate and pyruvate. Both sisters had to be helped from the bicycle at the end of the exercise, because their weakness was so severe. These responses are not abnormal in themselves. An untrained individual working to exhaustion may also produce large amounts of lactate and have a high pulse rate. What makes it abnormal is the association of these changes with the very low level of work. It requires only a small and logical step to suggest that the root of the abnormal response lies in the electron transport chain which is inadequate to the task demanded. Whereas a similar low level of work could be sustained in the normal individual without even increasing the blood supply, the patient's physiological responses suggest a marked exercise stress. Such a discrepancy between the work load and the capacity of the electron chain to handle it, would have to be due an abnormality in the latter.

Biochemical studies of mitochondrial function showed some marked abnormalities. Oxygen consumption by a normal mitochondrial preparation is tightly coupled to the production of ATP. In the resting situation, the system idles along consuming small amounts of oxygen. If substrate and ADP is added to the medium, there is an immediate increase in the uptake of oxygen as the ADP is converted to ATP. The system then slows back down again. Thus, the state of respiration can be followed by monitoring oxygen consumption. It is also possible to introduce substances such as 2,4-dinitrophenol (DNP) which uncouple this whole process and cause a sharp increase in oxygen uptake regardless of the presence of ADP or other metabolites. The system may be further manipulated by using different substrates which enter different points along the electron chain. Thus, NAD-coupled substrates are linked through the flavin mononucleotide to coenzyme Q and on down the chain. Succinic dehydrogenase is more directly coupled to coenzyme Q and bypasses the flavin mononucleotide. When succinate was used as a substrate, respiratory control was normal, although the use of NAD-coupled substrates showed the respiratory control to be defective. Secondly, it was possible to couple substrates such as hydroxybutyrate and malate using tetramethylphenylene diamine (TMPD) and ascorbate. This is an artificial way of coupling the substrates directly to cytochrome *c*. Normal amounts of cytochrome *b* were present in the mitochondrial preparation. This suggested that the electron chain was intact beyond cytochrome *b* and that the defect lies somewhere between the NADH dehydrogenase and cytochrome *b*.

A response to oral carnitine was noted in another patient with complex I deficiency (3). This 24-year-old woman noticed progressive weakness during her second pregnancy and was found to have an abnormal amount of lipid in the muscle biopsy. Carnitine in the muscle was 12% and 27% of normal, and when she was treated with oral DL-carnitine, 6 g daily, she had "considerable improvement in muscle strength" after 14 months. Her mother, who had a long history of muscle pain, weakness, and fatigue, had similar changes in the muscle biopsy and also demonstrated a defect in complex I.

One patient, a 13-year-old girl with exercise intolerance and lactic acidosis was successfully treated with 100 mg daily of oral riboflavin (4).

REFERENCES

1. Morgan-Hughes, J. A., Darveniza, P., Landon, D. N., Land, J. M., and Clark, J. B. A mitochondrial myopathy with a deficiency of respiratory chain NADH-Co-Q reductase activity. J. Neurol. Sci. *43:* 27–46, 1979.
2. Land, J. M., Morgan-Hughes, J. A., and Clark, J. B. Mitochondrial myopathy. Biochemical studies revealing a deficiency of NADH-cytochrome *b* reductase activity. J. Neurol. Sci. *50:* 1–13, 1980.
3. Clark, J. B., and Hayes, D. J. Mitochondrial myopathies: disorders of the respiratory chain and oxidative phosphorylation. J. Inherited Metab. Dis. *7* (Suppl. 1): 62–68, 1984.
4. Arts, W. F. M., Scholte, H. R., Bogaard, J. M., Kerrebign, K. F., and Luyt-Houwen, I. E. M. NADH-CoQ reductase deficient myopathy: successful treatment with riboflavin. Lancet *2:* 581–582, 1983.

Cytochrome b Deficiency (Complex III)

A 38-year-old man presented with a complaint of excessive fatiguability since childhood. He was relatively normal until 7 years of age when he had difficulty keeping up with other children and complained of aching pains in the legs after exercise, which were relieved by rest (1). The disorder was progressive and exhaustion came on at shorter intervals so that he was finally able only to walk slowly for a distance of 100 yards before having to rest. He had a mild diffuse weakness, but the striking abnormality was a progressive increase in the muscle weakness during sustained activity which occurred within 30 seconds of contraction against maximal resistance. This additional weakness would recover following rest. Serum CK and most other serum values were normal. The muscle biopsy showed an increased granularity or "stippling" of the muscle fibers with the oxidative enzyme reactions and similar red stippling on the Gomori trichrome stain. The suspicion that these were due to abnormal mitochondria was confirmed by the electron microscopic picture of marked abnormalities in mitochondrial structure, with unusual branching cristae, a relatively electron lucent matrix, and some dense crystalline inclusions.

Exercise studies were carried out on a bicycle ergometer with results similar to those in the previous illness. The patient rode the bicycle for 15 minutes with no load. This is the absolute minimum condition for exercise and should be accomplished with no difficulty by even the least athletic subject. Faced with this task, the patient's heart rate rose to 150 during the first 3 minutes, an enormous rise for this level of effort. Lactate and pyruvate levels in the blood also rose markedly with levels of 12 mM/liter being noted for lactate.

The authors studied the mitochondrial biochemistry in detail. There was no increase in oxygen uptake with either succinate or NAD-coupled substrates and ADP. Nor was oxygen uptake increased by the uncoupling agent flurocarbonyl-cyanide phenylhydrazone (FCCP). Spectrographic analysis of the mitochondria revealed a relative deficiency of cytochrome b, which appeared to be responsible for the illness in this patient.

A similar defect in complex III was found in a 20-year-old Chilean girl who had a life long story of ptosis and fatiguing weakness (2). She tired easily, could not hurry, and became breathless with a mild amount of exertion. She felt weak and stiff in the legs. On examination she had a ptosis but no other external ocular palsies, and mild diffuse weakness. Although she resembled a patient with congenital myasthenia gravis there was no laboratory evidence of this. The muscle biopsy showed ragged red fibers and Type 2B fiber deficiency. The carnitine levels were normal. Increased amounts of lactate were noted in the serum, both at rest and following exercise. Substrate utilization by the mitochondria was low for all substrates unless TMPD was added to the mixture. TMPD bypasses complex III, coupling directly to cytochrome c. Further analysis showed a decrease in the amount of reducible cytochrome b and an apparent total absence of cytochrome c.

One of the most interesting reports of a patient with complex III deficiency was that of a 17-year-old girl who was well until the age of 9 (3). At this time she developed decreased exercise tolerance and experienced cramps and vomiting after exertion. Her height and weight which had been at the 50th percentile at the age of 7 dropped to the 10th percentile. She had no weakness when the illness commenced. By the time she was 15 she was severely restricted and could walk only 100–200 meters without severe dyspnea. Her muscles were wasted and diffusely weak. She demonstrated high lactic acid levels and, following 3 minutes on a treadmill, her blood lactate was over 13 meq/liter. She had one episode of severe metabolic acidosis associated with prolonged vomiting and a seizure. The biochemical defect was found to be a lack of cytochrome b and other peptide components of complex III. ^{31}P-NMR demonstrated a fall in phosphocreatine levels with exercise and an abnormally prolonged recovery time. The patient was treated with vitamins K_3 (menadione) and C in an attempt to bypass the defect (4). The doses used were 1 g of vitamin C and 10 mg of menadione every 6 hours. Menadione is reduced by coenzyme Q and both menadione and vitamin C may serve as cytochrome c reductants. Thus, in theory the defect in complex III might be bypassed.

Administration of the vitamins to the patient resulted in an almost immediate clinical improvement with increased endurance. There was a more rapid
recovery of phosphocreatine following exercise. The blood lactate, however,
remained elevated. This is the first treatment of mitochondrial myopathy
which seems to have documented improvement. It may well establish the
model for the treatment for other defects in the respiratory chain.

Another ^{31}P-NMR study of patients with mitochondrial myopathies, most
with complex I defects, confirmed the delayed recovery of phosphocreatine
levels depleted by exercise. There was an associated ineffective rephospho-
rylation of ADP (5).

REFERENCES

1. Morgan-Hughes, J. A., Darvenica, P., Kahn, S. M., Landon, D. N., Sherratt, R. M., Land,
   J. M., and Clark, J. B. A mitochondrial myopathy characterized by a deficiency in reducible
   cytochrome *b*. Brain *11:* 617–640, 1977.
2. Hayes, D. J., Lecky, B. R. F., Landon, D. N., Morgan-Hughes, J. A., and Clark, J. B. A new
   mitochondrial myopathy. Brain *107:* 1165–1177, 1984.
3. Kennaway, N. G., Buist, N. R. M., Darley-Usmar, V. M., Papadimitriou, A., DiMauro, S.,
   Kelley, R. I., Capaldi, R. A., Blank, N. K., and D'Agostino, A. Lactic acidosis and
   mitochondrial myopathy associated with deficiency of several components of complex 3 of
   the respiratory chain. Pediatr. Res. *18:* 991–999, 1984.
4. Eleff, S., Kennaway, N. G., Buist, N. R. M., Darley-Usmar, V. M., Capaldi, R. A., Bank,
   W. J., and Chance, B. ^{31}P-NMR studies of improvement of oxidative phosphorylation by
   vitamins K_3 and C in a patient with a defect in electron transport and complex 3 in skeletal
   muscle. Proc. Natl. Acad. Sci. U.S.A. *81:* 3529–3533, 1984.
5. Arnold, D. L., Taylor, D. J., and Radda, G. K. Investigation of human mitochondrial
   myopathies by phosphorus magnetic resonance spectroscopy. Ann. Neurol. *18:* 189–196,
   1985.

Myoglobinuria

Myoglobin is a respiratory pigment with a molecular weight of about
17,000. Related to hemoglobin, it functions as a storehouse of oxygen. Its
dissociation curve is different from hemoglobin and it releases oxygen only
when the PO_2 in the tissue is very low. Therefore during light exercise, oxygen
is retained by myoglobin and is released during heavy exercise. The amount
of myoglobin in the muscle is often related to physical activity. The largest
amount of myoglobin is found in the muscles of diving mammals, such as
the whale.

When there is acute damage to muscle fibers, myoglobin may be released
into the serum and thence into the urine. The renal threshold is low, in the
neighborhood of 0.5 mg/100 ml. Under extreme circumstances, the release
of myoglobin is sufficient to cause the urine to become dark, reddish brown,
and the accumulation of pigment casts in the renal tubules may be associated
with tubular necrosis and renal failure.

Clinical Aspects. Myoglobin is released from normal muscle under the
stress of exercise. Forty percent of naval recruits demonstrated increased
quantities of myoglobin in the serum during the first 6 days of training camp
(1), and an unusually strenuous exercise program was associated with six
cases of overt myoglobinuria in a Marine camp (2).

Muscle is susceptible to damage in situations other than excessive exercise.
Sometimes the stress is an external one, such as a crush injury. At other
times, a metabolic anomaly is responsible. Various classifications have been

proposed; one of the most useful differentiates the hereditary myoglobinurias from the sporadic (3). The hereditary causes of myoglobinuria are probably all associated with a metabolic defect in energy metabolism such as those which have already been discussed.

Other illnesses in which the precise metabolic defect has not yet been identified are characterized by symptoms similar to those seen in the known disorders of metabolism. One entity was characterized by fatigue, pain, and myoglobinuria with exercise (4, 5). It was inherited as an autosomal recessive. In childhood the affected members had a limited ability to exercise. There were periods of exacerbation when only a few steps would provoke muscle pain and fatigue and further exercise was not tolerated. Exercise also gave rise to an abnormal tachycardia and dyspnea. If exercise were forced on the patient during such times, myoglobinuria resulted. Some of these patients had fixed weakness, while others were normally strong when the muscle was tested with brief contractions. Occasionally, hypertrophy of the calf muscles was noted, but the examination was not otherwise abnormal. Although the illness is reminiscent of McArdle's disease, elevation of lactate levels and more especially of pyruvate levels was noted following exercise. The authors suggested that the predominant feature was a hyperkinetic circulatory state, perhaps due to a reflex effect following the accumulation of abnormal metabolites in the muscle.

In another report (6), a patient suffering from exertional myoglobinuria was described in whom an abnormally high lactate production was noted following exercise. The patient's tolerance for exercise was also reduced because of aching and fatigue of the muscles which developed after a few minutes on a treadmill. The picture was complicated by a history of high alcoholic intake, at least at the beginning of the studies. The authors suggested that oxidative phosphorylation may have been uncoupled and the dependence upon anaerobic metabolism resulted in the excessive lactate production.

The sporadic occurrence of myoglobinuria is often seen with unusual or forced exercise. Various picturesque names, such as "squat jump" myoglobinuria, have been coined to indicate the provocative exercise. Myoglobinuria may also be seen in the muscle damage sustained during severe electric shock or after convulsions. Crush injuries such as those caused by falling masonry may also be associated with myoglobinuria, hardly a surprising finding in view of the enormous damage which may occur. Others have suffered from crush injuries from the weight of a body lying on an arm. In this case, a combination of factors is probably responsible. Ordinarily a person will turn over even during deep sleep, otherwise the discomfort will lead to awakening. This type of crush injury is therefore more readily seen in comatose patients, particularly when the coma is due to heroin or alcohol, drugs which may themselves be toxic to muscle.

Interruption of the blood supply to a muscle causes infarction and widespread muscle destruction. For this reason embolism of a major artery is sometimes associated with myoglobinuria. Many drugs are associated with disturbances of oxidative metabolism and may place an additional strain on the necessary energy supplies to muscle. Carbon monoxide, various narcotics, and barbiturates have all been responsible for myoglobinuric episodes, as have other metabolic derangements such as diabetic acidosis and non-ketotic hyperglycemic hyperosmolar coma. Toxins, such as plasmocid, damage the muscle directly and may cause widespread necrosis. ε-Aminocaproic acid has been used in patients with subarachnoid bleeding to reduce the incidence of further bleeding. It is an antifibrinolytic agent and its use has now been associated with several cases of severe myopathy (7). Other toxic causes of myoglobinuria vary from the mundane, such as alcohol, to the exotic, such as a bite from the Malaysian sea snake. Licorice, succinylcholine, and amphotericin B are also agents which have been associated with muscle breakdown. Contamination of fish with industrial toxins was thought to cause myoglobinuria in the outbreak of the illness known as Haff disease. Other precipitating events include hypokalemia, heat stroke, and high fever. Rarely an acute muscle illness such as polymyositis may be accompanied by myoglobinuria.

The symptoms of exercise-provoked myoglobinuria are rather stereotyped. The patient has a sense of aching and fatigue in the muscles while exercising. Often this exercise is forced, either because the patient is in a situation, such as the military, where the exercise is compulsory or because the activity has to be continued for the patient's safety, as in mountain climbing. With the continuation of exercise, the muscles become weaker and the patient feels generally unwell with headache, nausea, and, not infrequently, vomiting. Exercise while fasting is particularly liable to provoke attacks in susceptible individuals. The patient may collapse and be admitted to the hospital in a coma. The combination of coma and anuria due to the attendant renal damage may mask the underlying muscle destruction unless an accurate history can be obtained. In less severe cases, the muscle pain and weakness are followed by pigmenturia, which may occur up to 24 hours afterwards. The relationship of the symptoms to exercise is illustrated by a case of a 22-year-old girl who attempted a difficult hike up a mountain. Half way to the summit, her legs became fatigued and painful, but she had no symptoms in her arms. Her companion carried her on his back much of the rest of the way, and she had to use her arms for support. Thereupon fatigue and pain developed in her arms, so that by the time she arrived at the top of the mountain she was totally incapacitated. The muscles most often affected are the large muscles of the limbs. The cranial muscles are seldom involved, perhaps because they are never subject to the forceful contractions that are demanded of the limb muscles under conditions of unusual exertion.

Patients who have myoglobinuria which is unrelated to exercise may not notice the onset of the muscular symptoms, perhaps because many of the provocative causes are associated with a disturbance of consciousness.

Upon examination of a patient during an acute bout of myoglobinuria the muscles are painful, swollen, and indurated. Weakness is always present in such muscles and may amount to a total paralysis. In general, the degree of weakness parallels the pain and swelling.

Laboratory Studies. The identification of myoglobin in the urine is necessary in order to make the diagnosis. The urine should be freshly voided and neutralized to prevent the breakdown of myoglobin. Myoglobinuria can be confused both with hemoglobinuria and with the urine seen in porphyria. Myoglobin and hemoglobin react with the benzidine test for heme pigment, a reaction which is not seen in porphyria. In hemoglobinuria, red cells may be detected in the urine. If they are not seen, it would imply that the destruction of red blood cells must have taken place in the circulation, in which case the serum should be pink. In myoglobinuria, the serum is not tinted. The most reliable identification of myoglobin depends upon electrophoresis and immunoprecipitation by an antibody prepared against purified myoglobin or by the more sensitive radioimmunoassay.

Supporting evidence for myoglobinuria is an extreme elevation of the levels of serum "muscle" enzymes. These are high initially, with CK levels often over 50,000, and then they decline over a period of days. Renal failure is the most serious complication of myoglobinuria. The patient's survival depends upon the early recognition of this and the appropriate treatment with dialysis. Even in those patients without overt clinical evidence of renal failure there is often a decrease of renal function. Creatinine clearance may be abnormal and increased levels of blood urea nitrogen may be found.

After an acute attack, the patient's muscle function returns to normal within 1–3 weeks. Renal function may be impaired much longer, and it may take up to 6 or 7 weeks before creatinine clearance returns to normal values. Some degree of hyperkalemia is also seen in myoglobinuria and may be severe. The muscle biopsy may show signs of fiber necrosis (Figs. 7.18–7.22).

The treatment of the acute attack of myoglobinuria is largely supportive.

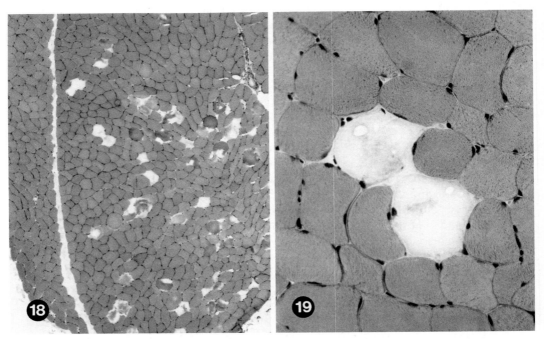

Figure 7.18.   In myoglobinuria of various causes, whether associated with toxic drugs or metabolic disorders, there are certain common changes. This is a hematoxylin and eosin stain of a biopsy from a patient with recurrent myoglobinuria. Overall, the biopsy appears relatively normal but scattered throughout the biopsy are isolated fibers which have undergone necrosis. In the extreme form these simply appear as spaces where the fibers used to be.

Figure 7.19.   Is a higher power view to show that the "spaces" are not entirely empty but are filled with a pale homogeneous staining material.

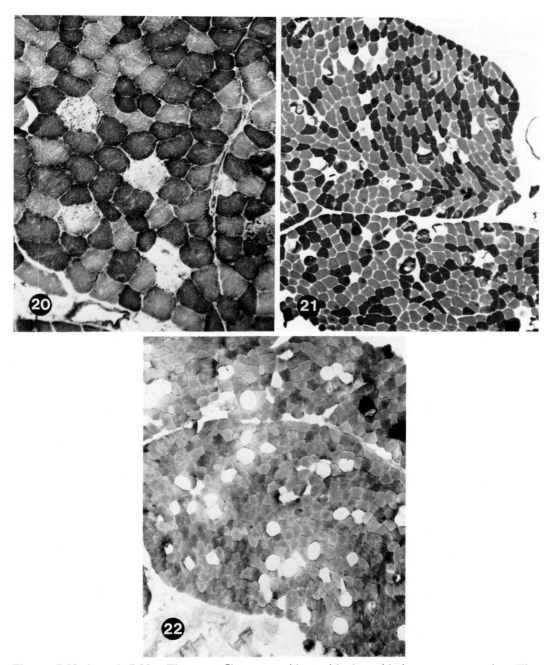

Figures 7.20 through 7.22. The same fibers are evident with the oxidative enzyme reaction (Fig. 7.20), with the ATPase reaction (Fig. 7.21), and with the PAS stain for glycogen (Fig. 7.22). This last stain is of particular interest since glycogen depletion is one of the earliest signs of a fiber in metabolic difficulties.

It is important to keep the patient at rest to prevent further stress on the muscles. Renal function should be closely monitored and dialysis carried out where appropriate. The administration of mannitol to promote diuresis has been recommended in those patients whose renal function is relatively well preserved.

REFERENCES

1. Olerud, J. E., Homer, L. D., and Carroll, H. W. Serum myoglobin levels predicted from serum enzyme values. N. Engl. J. Med. *293*: 483–485, 1975.
2. Demos, M. A. and Gitin, E. L. Acute exertional rhabdomyolysis. Arch. Intern. Med. *133*: 233–239, 1974.
3. Rowland, L. P. and Penn, A. S. Myoglobinuria. Med. Clin. North. Am. *56*: 1233–1256, 1972.
4. Larsson, L. E., Linderholm, H., Muller, R., Ringqvist, T., and Sornas, R. Hereditary metabolic myopathy with paroxysmal myoglobinuria due to abnormal glycolysis. J. Neurol. Neurosurg. Psychiatry *27*: 361–380, 1964.
5. Linderholm, H., Muller, R., Ringqvist, T., and Sornas, R. Hereditary abnormal muscle metabolism with hyperkinetic circulation during exercise. Acta Med. Scand. *185*: 153–166, 1969.
6. Kontos, H. A., Harley, E. L., Wasserman, A. J., Kelly, J. J., and Magee, J. H. Exertional idiopathic paroxysmal myoglobinuria; evidence for a defect in skeletal muscle metabolism. Am. J. Med. *35*: 283–292, 1963.
7. Kennard, C., Swash, M., and Henson, R. A. Myopathy due to epsilon-aminocaproic acid. Muscle Nerve *3*: 202–206, 1980.

Malignant Hyperpyrexia (Malignant Hyperthermia)

Clinical Aspects. Man shares with the pig an unusual illness in which an explosive rise in temperature is associated with muscular rigidity and necrosis. The disorder is also well known in veterinary circles and zoos where an animal may collapse and die abruptly after being chased and captured—the so-called "capture myopathy" (1). The onset in humans is provoked by anesthesia, especially by the administration of halothane and succinylcholine, and it usually occurs in a patient whose prior history gives no clue to the existence of the illness. Following the infusion of succinylcholine the muscles may fasciculate, and tone in the muscles may be increased. This is particularly true of the masseter muscles, and a clenched jaw during the induction of anesthesia is an ominous sign. A short time thereafter there commences an extraordinary rise in body temperature, which may climb at a rate of 2°C per hour. An intense rigidity appears in all muscle groups, and a progressive metabolic acidosis develops. Untreated patients usually die. Convulsions are common shortly before death. Sometimes the same event may occur following exposure to heat and exercise culminating in what appears to be "heat stroke."

Although the development of malignant hyperpyrexia is unusual (between 1 in 15,000 and 1 in 50,000 anesthetics) (2), its severity has prompted attempts to define the susceptible population. In many cases the disease is inherited as an autosomal dominant. At times overt signs and symptoms of muscle disease have been found. Hypertrophy of thigh muscles, atropy of the distal part of the thighs, lumbar lordosis, mild hip weakness, and diminished deep tendon reflexes have all been observed. Myotonia has been noted on several occasions. The lack of specificity of the signs reduces their diagnostic value unless the family history indicates that the patient is at risk. Malignant hyperthermia has complicated central core disease, myotonia congenita and Duchenne dystrophy. The King-Denborough syndrome is a particular constellation of findings including malignant hyperthermia and is described below.

Laboratory Studies. Persistently high values of serum CK have been recorded in some patients and if a patient about to undergo surgery has a family history of malignant hyperthermia, CK testing is mandatory. Unfortunately, there may be susceptible patients who have normal levels of CK. Ellis et al. (3) suggested that patients prone to malignant hyperthermia could be detected by the action of halothane with or without the addition of succinyl choline on an excised strip of muscle. Ordinarily this does not cause any contraction of the muscle, but the authors found that, in patients with malignant hyperthermia, the muscle underwent contracture. Since then, reports on this aspect have been contradictory (4, 5). Perhaps some of the differences found by various investigators may be due to differences in the proportion of different muscle fiber types in the tested muscle, since the Type 1 muscle fiber is more sensitive than the Type 2 muscle fiber to the caffeine-induced contracture (6).

Early work in the pharmacology of the illness centered around caffeine to which the muscle seemed to demonstrate an abnormal sensitivity. The caffeine contracture was potentiated by halothane, a phenomenon occurring in both normal individuals and in patients with malignant hyperthermia. It was not unnatural in an illness in which the excitation contraction coupling seemed to be abnormal that attention turned towards to the sarcoplasmic reticulum and calcium release. By loading the sarcoplasmic reticulum with calcium, even normal fibers may be made abnormally sensitive to the development of a caffeine contracture (7). Calcium transport in the sarcoplasmic reticulum is under a very complicated control system. To a large extent, this is regulated by adenylate cyclase, an enzyme localized almost completely to the sarcolemmal membranes. Adenylate cyclase controls the formation of cyclic AMP which in turn governs the action of protein kinase. Phosphorylation of a 22,000 dalton protein, phospholamban seems to control the influx of calcium. It is a long chain of events, but it is possible that the adenylate cyclase ultimately controls the transport of calcium. In the muscle from patients with malignant hyperthermia, the adenylate cyclase activity was found to be increased. It is difficult to understand how an illness, which is genetically determined, might be caused by an overactivity of an enzyme, rather than its absence. Neither is it clear why halothane and succinyl choline ignite the catastrophic events in malignant hyperthermia since one would have thought that the increased enzyme activity would be a constant phenomenon. As Willner and co-authors (7) pointed out, though, in vivo the majority of adenyl cyclase is dormant most of the time.

The remarkable production of heat in the illness is due to a metabolic aberration, the nature of which is not clear. In pigs, a progressive loss of ATP and an accumulation of phosphate in the blood have been described (8). There is also an increase in "cycling" of fructose-6-phosphate to fructose-1,6-diphosphate and back. With each turn of this cycle ATP is hydrolyzed and heat is generated. Halothane increases the rate of cycling. There are, however, differences between the human disease and that of a pig and the etiology may be quite different.

Treatment. The treatment of the illness depends upon its early recognition. The development of hyperpyrexia and muscle stiffness during anesthesia is an indication to discontinue the surgical procedure. Untreated, the illness is usually fatal. As soon as the diagnosis is suspected, all anesthetic agents are discontinued, and 100% oxygen is given by endotracheal tube. The patient is cooled by all possible means and the metabolic acidosis is controlled with bicarbonate (9). The specific agent used in treatment is an intravenous preparation of dantrolene sodium, which may be given in doses up to 7 mg/kg without major side effects. In a recent multicenter study, the average dose given to patients with definite malignant hyperthermia was 2.5 mg/kg. Using this regimen, all 11 patients so treated recovered without sequelae. When the drug was given more than 24 hours after the diagnosis, there was some reversal of the clinical signs, but there was still a 75% mortality (10). The same drug is effective in the treatment of the porcine malignant hyperthermia. Malignant hyperthermia may be complicated by myoglobinuria with renal failure and by hyperkalemia, as potassium and myoglobin are released from the damaged muscle.

King-Denborough Syndrome

An unusual syndrome occurs in which malignant hyperthermia is associated with several other abnormalities. Originally described in 1973 in four boys, the disorder is a mild nonprogressive myopathy with multiple congenital abnormalities (11, 12). The children are all short statured and their motor development is delayed. Their IQ seems to be normal, but they have a moderate degree of muscle weakness both of the hips and of the shoulders. Some scapular winging may be noted. The body habitus is unusual. In addition to short stature, there is webbing of the neck and pectus carinatum. The face is abnormal with underdevelopment of the cheek bones and mandible causing micrognathia. Their palpebral fissures slant downwards. There is often ptosis and the ears appear to be low set (Fig. 7.23). A speech defect occurs. The teeth are crowded together. Cryptorchidism is frequently noted. As the child grows older, a kyphoscoliosis is seen. Muscle biopsy shows mild nonspecific abnormalities which suggest a congenital myopathy. Only one of the cases reported has been a girl (13). Since this patient was studied mostly postmortem, few details are available.

REFERENCES

1. Chalmers, G. A., and Barrett, M. W. Capture myopathy. In: *Noninfectious Disease of Wildlife*, edited by G. Hoff and J. Davis. Iowa State University Press, Ames, Iowa, 1982, pp. 84–93.
2. Britt, B. A., and Kalow, W. Malignant hyperthermia: a statistical review. Can. Anaesth. Soc. J. *17*: 293–315, 1970.
3. Ellis, F. R., Keane, N. P., Harriman, D. G. F., Summer, D. W., Kyei-Mensah, K., Tyrrell, J. H., Hargreaves, J. B., Parikh, R. K., and Mulrooney, P. L. Screening for malignant hyperpyrexia. Br. Med. J. *3*: 559–561, 1972.
4. Britt, B. A., Kalow, W., Gordon, A., Humphrey, J. G., and Rewcastle, N. B. Malignant hyperthermia; an investigation of five patients. Can. Anaesth. Soc. J. *20*: 431–467, 1973.
5. Isaacs, H., and Heffron, J. A. A. Morphological and biochemical defects in muscles of human carriers of the malignant hyperthermia syndrome. Br. J. Anaesth. *47*: 475–481, 1975.
6. Brownell, A. K. W., and Szabo, M. The in vitro caffeine contracture test: influence of muscle histochemical profile on test results. Can. Anesth. Soc. J. *29*: 218–226, 1982.
7. Willner, J. H., Cerri, C. G., and Wood, D. S. High skeletal muscle adenylate cyclase in malignant hyperthermia. J. Clin. Inv. *68*: 1119–1124, 1981.
8. Clark, M. G., Williams, C. H., Pfeifer, W. F., Bloxham, D. P., Holland, P. C., Taylor, C. A., and Lardy, H. A. Accelerated substrate cycling of fructose-6-phosphate in the muscle of malignant hyperthermic pigs. Nature *245*: 99–101, 1973.
9. Maisel, R. H., Sessions, D. G., and Miller, R. N. Malignant hyperpyrexia during general anesthesia. Successful management of a case. Ann. Otol. Rhinol. Laryngol. *85*: 729–733.

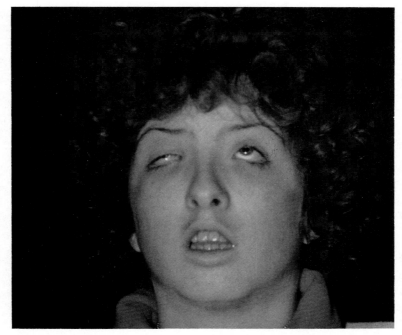

Figure 7.23. A patient with the King-Denbrough syndrome showing a reverse slant of the eyes and ptosis.

10. Kolb, M. E., Horne, M. L., and Martz, R. Dantrolene in human malignant hyperthermia: a multicenter study. Anesthesiology *56*: 254–262, 1982.
11. King, J. O., and Denborough, M. A. Anesthetic induced malignant hyperpyrexia in children. J. Pediatr. **83**: 37–40, 1973.
12. Kaplin, A. M., Bergeson, E. S., Gregg, S. A., and Curless, R. G. Malignant hyperthermia associated with myopathy and normal muscle enzymes. J. Pediatr. *91*: 431–433, 1977.
13. Mcpherson, E. W., and Taylor, C. A. The King syndrome: malignant hyperthermia myopathy and multiple anomalies. Am. J. Med. Genet. *8*: 159–165, 1981.

BIOCHEMICAL DEFECTS CAUSING FIXED ABNORMALITIES

This section deals with the known biochemical disorders in which exercise-induced symptoms are a relatively minor part of the clinical picture if they occur at all. It is not entirely reasonable that some illnesses should simply cause muscle fatigue and cramps while other defects cause widespread lesions of the central nervous system and permanent damage to the muscle with the production of wasting and weakness. Presumably, the perturbation of function caused by diseases in the latter category crosses some hypothetical threshold and cause irreparable muscle damage, whereas the perturbation in the first type of illness is either self-limiting or easily repaired.

Abnormalities of Carbohydrate Metabolism

Acid Maltase Deficiency (Type 2 Glycogenosis)

Maltase (α-1,4-glucosidase) is an enzyme with widespread distribution in various tissues. Its activity varies with the pH, and this variation is compatible with the existence of two or possibly more forms. One, with a pH optimum

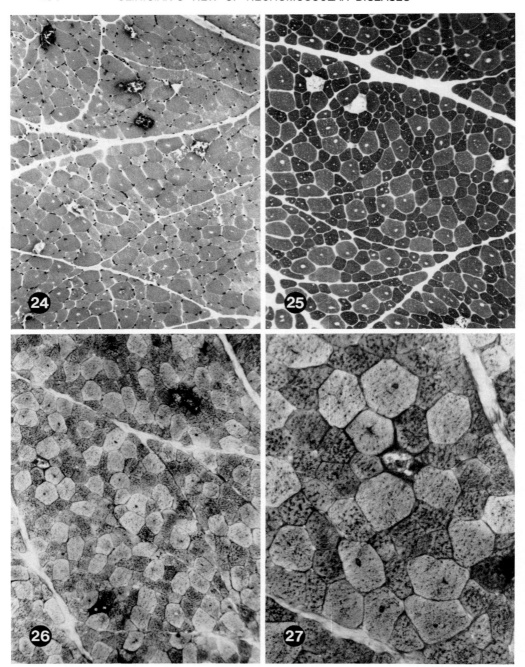

Figure 7.24. Acid maltase deficiency. With the hematoxylin and eosin stain the most striking finding is the presence of vacuoles in many of the fibers. In addition, fibers which are entirely replaced by glycogen can be seen, indicated by the intensely staining granular material towards the top of the photograph. There is also an abnormal variability in the size of the fibers.

Figure 7.25. An ATPase stain of a biopsy in acid maltase deficiency clearly demonstrates the vacuoles. The necrotic fibers also are demonstrated as empty spaces formerly occupied by muscle fibers. In this patient there is a mild degree of Type 2 fiber atrophy, the dark fibers tend to be smaller than the light ones.

of 4.5–5, is known as acid maltase. Although the biochemical activity of the enzyme is known, the specific function of maltase in the scheme of carbohydrate metabolism is not clearly understood. It is a lysosomal enzyme and its absence in the disease acid maltase deficiency is associated with the accumulation of glycogen in lysosomes as well as free in the tissue (1).

The infantile variety of acid maltase deficiency (Pompe's disease) was the first to be described. The children may be normal for a few weeks after birth but then develop severe hypotonia and enlargement of the heart, tongue, and liver owing to the accumulation of glycogen in these organs. The disease is inherited as an autosomal recessive. There is a reduction in acid maltase levels in the muscle and skin fibroblasts of the heterozygote carrier (2). The disease is progressive; the children become intermittently cyanotic and usually die from either cardiac or respiratory failure before 1 year of age.

A milder form of the illness is seen in children whose symptoms begin in infancy or early childhood but whose decline is much slower. Many of these patients survive for several years, although not beyond the second decade (3). A proximal weakness develops, and the muscles may feel firm or rubbery. This makes it difficult to distinguish the disease clinically from Duchenne muscular dystrophy, a problem which is compounded by a tendency to develop ankle contractures. There is no involvement of the heart in this form. Death usually occurs due to respiratory failure.

The adult variety of acid maltase deficiency begins later and the hereditary basis of the illness appears to be autosomal recessive (2–5), with the gene located on chromosome 17. Decreased levels of acid maltase have been found in the carrier state (2, 6, 7). A proximal weakness is noted, greater in the hips than in the shoulders. The heart and liver are not abnormal, and only one patient has been described with enlargement of the tongue. A clue to the diagnosis may be found in the involvement of the respiratory muscles. In general the illness resembles limb girdle dystrophy or polymyositis, but severe respiratory involvement is unusual in the early phase of these two conditions. Patients may have frankly anoxic symptoms from their respiratory weakness, such as nightmares disturbing their sleep, before the hip weakness presents a major problem.

The diagnosis rests with laboratory studies. There is often mild elevation of the serum "muscle" enzymes. The EMG shows irritable muscles with high frequency repetitive potentials and myotonia. This is more pronounced in the infantile variety. In the adult form, EMG changes may be restricted to the paraspinal muscles or other truncal muscles. Clinical myotonia is usually absent. The muscle biopsy shows a striking myopathy in which the muscle fibers are peppered with vacuoles (Figs. 7.24–7.27).

EKG studies are abnormal in the infantile variety; there is a depression of the ST segment with inversion of the T waves. There may be giant QRS complexes, and the PR interval is usually shortened.

Figure 7.26. The PAS stain for glycogen often shows a central spot in the muscle fibers. In addition, there is an abnormal stippling of the muscle fibers indicating the deposition of glycogen in small packets. The necrotic fibers are filled with glycogen indicated by the areas of intense stain in this low power view.

Figure 7.27. High power view of the biopsy shown in Figure 7.26 illustrating the changes in more detail.

Acid maltase activity in muscle is lacking in all the varieties of this disease. Interestingly, there is no difference in the enzyme activity of muscles which are severely affected and those which are relatively spared. Even in those with a normal histologic appearance, the enzyme is deficient. An increase in glycogen content accompanies the vacuolar changes. The glycogen appears to be of normal structure except in occasional cases where reduction in the length of the outer chain is noted. The defect has been reproduced in tissue culture of muscle suggesting that it is a true primary myopathy (8).

In view of the difference in severity, one might expect some differences in the biochemistry of the three types of illness. Acid maltase is absent in the infantile and childhood varieties. In the adult disease, very small amounts of lysosomal enzyme are present (6). The presence of neutral maltase may be responsible for some of the differences. The latter enzyme is decreased in both liver and muscle of patients with the infantile variety but not the adult form of the illness. Perhaps its activity compensates, in part, for that of the absent acid maltase (9). In the childhood form, neutral maltase is normal in the muscle in the heart but decreased in the liver. It has been suggested that a decrease in the ratio of acid maltase to neutral maltase may be helpful in the diagnosis of adult acid maltase deficiency. Acid maltase activity has also been studied in the urine and found to be reduced.

In an illness marked by accumulation of glycogen and in which the usual degradative pathways are preserved, attempts to mobilize tissue glycogen with epinephrine injections and to limit the intake of dietary carbohydrates are worthwhile. Unfortunately, the results obtained with this treatment over a period of years were something less than dramatic, although possible benefit was obtained in two adults (3).

Heterozygote carriers show a reduction in urinary enzyme activity and in the activity in skin fibroblasts which is important in genetic counseling (10). Some reduction of acid maltase activity was also noticed in leukocytes.

Prenatal diagnosis is possible since fetal cells cultured from fluid obtained by amniocentesis lack enzyme activity.

This section should be closed with a cautionary paragraph. Although superficially, the accumulation of glycogen in the muscle is easy to attribute to an enzyme which is responsible for its breakdown, it is not a tidy explanation. It is as if the piece of the jigsaw puzzle fits exactly, but when in place, the pattern is wrong. In the first place, acid maltase is a lysosomal enzyme and it is less easy to explain the occurrence of pools of glycogen outside the lysosomes. One might, perhaps, disregard this by as simply due to the rupture of lysosomes allowing the glycogen to escape. There is no explanation for the varying severity of the illness in its different forms, and even worse, there is no satisfactory explanation for why these two forms occur in the same family, in which case both forms are presumably related to the same gene (7). Further confusion has arisen with the description of four boys from three different families with a lysosomal glycogen storage disease very similar to acid maltase deficiency of the childhood type whose acid maltase levels were normal. The only major difference was the involvement of the cardiac muscle and severe mental retardation (11, 12).

REFERENCES

1. DiMauro, S. Metabolic myopathies. In: *Handbook of Clinical Neurology,* edited by P. J. Vinken and G. W. Bruyn. North-Holland, Amsterdam, 1979, Vol. 41, p. 175.

2. Engel, A. G., and Gomez, M. R. Acid maltase levels in heterozygous acid maltase deficiency and in non-weak and neuromuscular disease controls. J. Neurol. Neurosurg. Psychiatry *33*: 801–804, 1970.

3. Engel, A. G., Gomez, M. R. Seybold, M. E., and Lambert, E. H. The spectrum and diagnosis of acid maltase deficiency. Neurology *23*: 95–106, 1073.

4. Hudgson, P., and Fulthorpe, J. J. The pathology of type II skeletal muscle glycogenosis. J. Pathol. *116*: 139–147, 1975.

5. Martin, J. J., deBarsy, T., and den Tandt, W. R. Acid maltase deficiency in non-identical twins; a morphological and biochemical study. J. Neurol. *213*: 105–118, 1976.

6. Mehler, M., and DiMauro, S. Residual acid maltase activity in late onset acid maltase deficiency. Neurology *27*: 178–184, 1977.

7. Looner, M. C. B., Busch, H. F. M., Koster, J. F., Martin, J. J., Niermeijer, M. F., Schram, A. W., Brouwer-Kelder, B., Mekes, W., Slee, R. G., and Tager, J. M. A family with different clinical forms of acid maltase deficiency: biochemical and genetic studies. Neurology *31*: 1209–1216, 1983.

8. Askanas, V., Engel, W. K., DiMauro, S., Brooks, B. R., and Mehler, M. Adult-onset acid maltase deficiency. N. Engl. J. Med. *294*: 573–578, 1976.

9. Angelini, C., and Engel, A. G. Comparative study of acid maltase deficiency: Biochemical difference between childhood and adult types. Arch. Neurol. *26*: 573–578, 1976.

10. Mehler, J., and DiMauro, S. Late onset acid maltase deficiency. Arch. Neurol. *33*: 692–695, 1976.

11. Danon, M. J., Oh, S. J., DiMauro, S., Manaligod, J. R., Eastwood, A., Naidu, S., and Schliselfeld, L. H. Lysosomal glycogen storage disease with normal acid maltase. Neurology *31*: 51–57, 1981.

12. Riggs, J. E., Schochet, S. S., Gutmann, L., Shanske, S., Neal, W. A., and DiMauro, S. Lysosomal glycogen storage disease without acid maltase deficiency. Neurology *33*: 873–877, 1983.

Amylo-1,6-Glucosidase Deficiency (Debrancher Deficiency, Type 3 Glycogenosis)

An autosomal recessively inherited deficiency of this enzyme is associated with hepatomegaly and a failure to thrive in the first year of life. Frequently, the children are floppy and have poor head control (1). They are mentally unimpaired. The enzyme deficit is associated with the deposition of glycogen in liver, striated muscle, and, to a lesser extent, cardiac muscle. Although, in the majority, the enzyme is lacking in all tissues, it is occasionally detected in muscle or in both liver and muscle of a few patients. There is a slow improvement and the liver may return to normal size by adolescence. The patients then live a normal adult life, but the enzymatic abnormality persists.

Other patients with debrancher deficiency develop muscular weakness with a much later onset. One man presented with an eight month history of distal weakness and wasting beginning at the age of 43 (2). There was a preceding story of muscle fatigue and weakness associated with pain, but this was insubstantial. On clinical examination the disorder resembled a motor neuron disease. A slightly different clinical picture was seen in an 18-year-old patient whose muscle symptoms were those of fatigue, stiffness, and weakness of the leg muscles, a picture compounded by a history of gouty arthritis (3). Five adults with the illness were reported in which slowly progressive weakness was associated with heart and liver abnormalities (4). Four men and one woman complained of weakness, often extending back into childhood, but usually not presenting any noticeable difficulty until adult life. In most, the weakness was proximal, but distal wasting and weakness were noted in two patients and, because there were associated fasciculations, this was felt to represent amyotropic lateral sclerosis (ALS) in one patient. One man only became aware of the weakness at the age of 52. The EKG in all patients showed left ventricular hypertrophy and was associated with congestive heart failure in two. Hepatomegaly was noted in three. The EMG showed a mixed pattern with irritable phenomena including positive sharp waves and fibrillations. Repetitive high frequency discharges and myotonia was noted occasionally. The muscle biopsy is markedly abnormal with glycogen filled vacuoles disrupting the fibers. In addition to an increase in internal nuclei and some necrotic fibers, there were also scattered ring fibers. The CPK was markedly increased, often being over 1,000.

Biochemical estimation of debrancher activity demonstrated its absence in the muscle and liver. The glycogen content of the muscle was elevated to 3–5 times normal and the glycogen itself was abnormal with the characteristic appearance of limit dextrin, having been stripped by phosphorylase until the branch points were reached. The glycogen in the red blood cells is even more increased than that in the muscle. Predictably, since the enzyme is involved in the breakdown of glycogen, the forearm exercise test demonstrated a failure of lactate production. Even though the forearm exercise is markedly abnormal, only a minority of the patients experience exercise intolerance. One man suffered from muscle cramps and another from light-headedness and intense perspiration while exercising. No myoglobinuria was noted in any of these patients. An abnormality in the liver was indicated by a failure of the blood glucose to rise following epinephrine or glucagon. A normal response of blood glucose to galactose administration differentiates the liver response from that seen in glucose-6-phosphatase deficiency.

REFERENCES

1. Swaiman, K. F., and Wright, F. S. *The Practice of Pediatric Neurology.* C. V. Mosby, St. Louis, 1975.
2. Brunberg, J. A., McCormick, W. F., and Schochet, S. S. Type III glycogenosis: an adult with diffuse weakness and muscle wasting. Arch. Neurol. *25:* 171–178, 1971.
3. Murase, T., Ikada, H., Muro, T., Nakao, K., and Sugita, H. Myopathy associated with type 3 glycogenosis. J. Neurol. Sci. *20:* 287–295, 1973.
4. DiMauro, S., Hartwig, G. B., Hays, A., Eastwood, A. B., Franco, R., Olarte, M., Chang, M., Roses, A. D., Fetell, M., Schoenfeldt, R. S., and Stern, L. Z. Debrancher deficiency: neuromuscular disorder in 5 adults. Ann. Neurol. *5:* 422–436, 1979.

Amylo-1,4 to -1,6-Transglucosidase Deficiency (Brancher Enzyme Deficiency, Type 4 Glycogenosis)

This illness generally causes a failure to thrive, hepatosplenomegaly, and liver failure. The inheritance is autosomal recessive. Respiratory muscle and skeletal muscles are affected, but only rarely are muscular symptoms a prominent part of the picture. In one case, a child with this illness was thought to have Werdnig-Hoffmann disease on clinical grounds (1). She was born with hip dislocations, had a poor sucking response, hypotonia, and severe atrophy. Her muscles were scarcely able to move the limbs against gravity, and reflexes were absent. Serum creatine phosphokinase was normal. Hepatosplenomegaly and ascites developed, and the child died in the 2nd year from cardiorespiratory failure. Widespread deposits of amylopectin were found at postmortem.

A 59-year-old man was described who had experienced 25 years of progressive weakness which had been diagnosed as limb-girdle muscular dystrophy. He had marked wasting and weakness of the thighs, some calf hypertrophy, and a waddling gait. He also had some weakness, although less noticeable in the shoulders and arms. Muscle biopsies demonstrated the presence of many vacuoles which were limited to the Type 1 fibers (2). A similar clinical picture was noted in another patient in whom the muscle brancher enzyme was not evaluated.

The enzyme is absent not only in the muscle but also in the peripheral white blood cells. Cultured fibroblasts are also deficient in the enzyme in the patients and their parents.

REFERENCES

1. Zellweger, H., Mueller, S., Ionasescu, V., Schochet, S. S., and McCormick, W. F. Glycogenosis IV: A new cause of infantile hypotonia. J. Pediatr. *80*: 842–844, 1972.
2. Ferguson, I. T., Mahon, M., and Cumming, W. J. K. An adult case of Andersen's disease—type 4 glycogenosis. J. Neurol. Sci. *60*: 337–351, 1983.

Abnormalities of Lipid Metabolism

Carnitine Deficiency

Carnitine (β-hydroxy-α-N-trimethylammonium butyrate) is a molecule which is vital to muscle and heart since it assists in the the the normal metabolism of fatty acids (1). In a normal 70-kg adult, 98% of the approximately 100 mM of carnitine in the body is in skeletal and cardiac muscle. The normal values of "total" carnitine in the serum or plasma are around 60 ± 10 nmol/ml in males and 50 ± 10 nmol/ml in females "total" carnitine includes "free" carnitine as well as all the esters of carnitine with various chain length fatty acids. "Free" carnitine values are 47 ± 10 nmol/ml for males and 40 ± 10 nmol/ml for females. Muscle contains approximately 20 ± 8 nmol/mg of total non-collagen protein and 18 ± 8 nmol/mg of free carnitine. In liver, the values are 10 and 7 nmol/mg (2).

Although important in the normal functioning of muscle and abundant in such tissue, neither cardiac nor skeletal muscle have the ability to synthesize carnitine. The amount of carnitine supplied by the diet (in red meats and dairy products) is not usually sufficient to supply the body's demands and it must, of necessity, be manufactured in other tissues, principally the liver and kidney. In humans, the kidney plays a minor role in synthesis, but there is evidence that both in rats and humans, carnitine is excreted into the tubular lumen and then reabsorbed. The uptake of carnitine into the muscle is by an active transport system.

Carnitine is synthesized from trimethyl-lysine residues which are present in proteins such as actin, myosin, histones, and cytochrome *c*. Four enzymes are involved in this conversion as trimethyl lysine is first hydroxylated and then split between the second and third carbon atoms forming glycine and α-trimethylaminobutyraldehyde. This is then oxidized to α-butyrobetaine which is finally oxidized to carnitine. Although some of these enzymes are present in muscle, the hydroxylase which catalyzes the final step is present only in the liver and kidney.

As mentioned previously, one of the functions of carnitine in fat metabolism is to shuttle the long chain fatty acids across the inner mitochondrial membrane, which action is controlled by the enzyme acylcarnitine translocase.

Were this the only function of carnitine, one would expect the symptoms of carnitine deficiency to be similar to that of carnitine palmityl transferase deficiency. That there is almost nothing in common between the two illnesses must indicate that carnitine has other functions, the disturbance of which is at the root of the illness. Many metabolic processes in the body produce acyl-CoA. These are compounds in which various fatty acid and organic acid moieties are linked to CoA. They may be employed in useful metabolic pathways, degraded by the liver, or excreted by the kidney. The formation of acyl carnitine is often a step in these processes enabling the transport of fatty and organic acids across membranes (such as mitochondrial membranes).

A surplus of acyl-CoA derivatives is deleterious to several biochemical pathways, inhibiting reactions as diverse as the oxidation of pyruvate, steps in the tricarboxylic acid cycle, and gluconeogenesis (see (3) for review). Thus, an adequate amount of carnitine is necessary for the normal function of the organism. The concept of "adequate" is flexible and not absolute. The body's supply of carnitine may be used up in a futile attempt to buffer an excess of abnormal organic acids or other intermediary metabolites. The acylated carnitine may then be excreted and lost to the body. It is also possible that a lack of carnitine may arise from defective steps in the biosynthesis of the compound or in its destruction. Whether carnitine is present in sufficient amounts to fulfill the body's needs can be evaluated by comparing the amount of acylated carnitine with the amount of "free" carnitine. Acylated carnitine is obviously committed to one or other acid and is therefore no longer available. Free (nonacylated) carnitine is obviously the stuff of which the buffer is made. If this is depleted, it matters not how much total carnitine is available, the effects of carnitine deficiency will be apparent. Conversely, if the amount of free carnitine is a major percentage of the total amount of carnitine it is less likely that carnitine deficiency exists, even if the total amount of carnitine is low.

Relative carnitine deficiency may be seen in many of the inborn errors of metabolism with an overproduction of organic acids such as propionic acidemia, branched chain aminoaciduria, and methylmalonic aciduria. It is also present in Reye's syndrome, in Jamacian vomiting sickness, and in abnormalities in fatty acid metabolism and hyperammonemia produced by valproate.

Remember, also, that the percentage of free versus total carnitine varies in relationship to the metabolic state of the patient. Fasting, which throws the body into a dependence on fatty acid metabolism and encourages protein breakdown may cause a fall in the levels of free carnitine to abnormal levels, a situation which may be undetectable in the fed state. Dynamic tests, such as fasting or prolonged gentle exercise, are worth considering in any patient whose condition is perhaps related to an insufficiency of carnitine. There is some risk to these tests and the clinical picture should always be considered before recommending them.

The syndromes of carnitine deficiency most often seen in the muscle clinic seem to have settled out into three different groups; "muscle" carnitine deficiency, "systemic" carnitine deficiency, and carnitine deficiency secondary to other disorders. This classification ignores some patients who sit uneasily astride the boundaries, unwilling to fall neatly into a pigeon hole.

"Muscle" Carnitine Deficiency. The initial report of this illness described a 24-year-old woman who had never been able to sit up from the supine

position without using her hands and who slept with her eyes slightly open (4, 5). At the age of 18, she had a sudden exacerbation and was confined to bed by her weakness. At the same time, she developed a nasal voice and, in addition to the proximal weakness of shoulders and hips, she had weakness of her face, palate, neck, and poor esophageal motility. Most, although not all of the patients, note their first symptoms during childhood and the commonest clinical picture is that of a slowly progressive weakness, superimposed upon which are sudden exacerbations or a fluctuating course. There are exceptions to this as in the case described by Markesberry et al. (6) where a 61-year-old woman had noticed her first symptoms at the age of 38 with both proximal and distal weakness. There may be EKG abnormalities (7) and one patient died at an early age with cardiac failure, but in general, the heart muscle seems to be spared, at least clinically. Although fatigue and exercise-related pains have been noted, they are not usually a prominent part of the picture. Myoglobinuria, the hallmark of the exercise provoked disorders, has been recorded only rarely (8). Exercise capacity was reduced in one patient following a fast. This is not quite as straightforward as it seems because, in addition, the ketone body concentrations rose, metabolic acidosis was noted, and hypoglycemia was present, none of which is conductive to the patient's desire to exercise. The treatment of this patient with oral carnitine maintained the blood glucose levels, but ketonemia was even more marked and the exercise capacity did not improve (9).

The diagnosis is usually made quite simply by muscle biopsy in which a heavy deposition of lipid is noted in the muscle fibers, particularly in the Type 1 or oxidative fibers. Biochemical evaluation of free and total carnitine shows low levels in the muscle, and more normal levels in the serum. The response to fasting is a normal elevation of ketone bodies in the blood and urine, indicating normal liver fat metabolism. The stores of carnitine seem to be sufficient to respond to the fasting stress unless exercise is superimposed.

The disorder, like so many biochemical disorders, is inherited as an autosomal recessive, as indicated by the occurrence of the disease in siblings and moderately reduced carnitine levels in the muscles of the presumably heterozygote parents in other cases (10, 11). There must also be a certain genetic heterogeneity in this group. In the original case, the addition of carnitine to the muscle homogenate restored its ability to oxidize fatty acids normally. Identical studies in a subsequent case, failed to demonstrate this (12).

The routine laboratory studies give results which might be anticipated. The EMG appears to be "myopathic" and the serum levels of CK and the other "muscle" enzymes are variably elevated. Muscle biopsy samples show the fibers to be infiltrated with fat droplets (Figs. 7.28–7.30). Because of the fact that the serum carnitine concentrations are normal and the muscle concentrations are so low, a defect in carnitine transport has been proposed as a cause of the illness. Direct measurements of this aspect in one patient (12) were normal. Since this is the same patient whose biochemical defect was not corrected with carnitine, it may be another indication of genetic heterogeneity.

Treatment of the disorder with L-carnitine appears inescapable. Muscle levels are low, the precise defect has not been identified, and no dangerous side effects are known. Ideally, it would be wise to treat the patient with L-

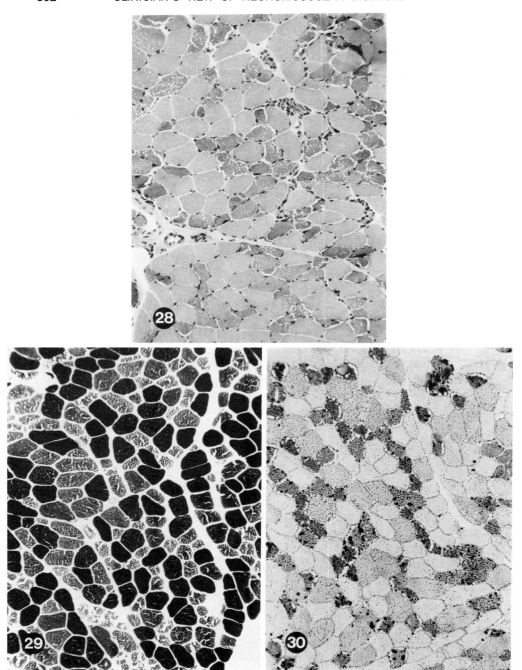

Figure 7.28.   Carnitine deficiency. With the routine hematoxylin and eosin stain there is variation in the size of fibers. Many of the fibers are peppered with small vacuoles.

Figure 7.29.   These vacuoles are particularly well seen with a routine ATPase reaction. They seem to affect the Type 1 (oxidative) fibers more than the Type 2 (glycolytic) fibers but the changes are not limited to one fiber type.

Figure 7.30.   This Sudan black stain demonstrates lipid. There is a population of fibers with a very heavy deposition of lipid, characteristic of carnitine deficiency.

carnitine since the D-form is not used by the tissue. Most studies, however, have used a mixture of D,L-carnitine. Results have been variable with quite dramatic improvement in some cases (8, 10, 13–15) but not in others (9, 12). This may again mirror the genetic heterogeneity and certainly mirrors the variable biochemical response to carnitine. In the first patient described, a beneficial response to prednisone was noted before the diagnosis of carnitine deficiency had been made and prednisone improved the clinical state in other patients with the myopathic effects of carnitine deficiency. One patient, who was nonresponsive to carnitine, showed an increase in her exercise capacity and in her general strength following riboflavin treatment (16). It is often difficult to interpret the effect of medications against a background in which the disease fluctuates spontaneously. An exacerbation of the disease postpartum has been noted in one patient, and the obverse, an improvement in the illness during pregnancy with a normal muscle biopsy was described in one patient.

Nonspecific Lipid Myopathy. Treatment with a diet free of long chain fatty acids was successful in a family in whom 3 members had a lipid myopathy (17). A 36-year-old woman had a long history of slowly progressive proximal muscle weakness and nausea, abdominal cramps and a feeling of weakness after fatty meals. She had 2 sons age 16 and 7, both of whom had fixed proximal weakness and some exercise-related symptoms. The muscle biopsy showed a deposition of lipid droplets. Muscle and serum carnitine levels were normal although only the total carnitine was presented and the level of free carnitine was not described. The patients were given a diet free of long chain fatty acids together with multivitamins and α-tocopherol. All were reported to have a marked improvement in strength and endurance.

"Systemic" Carnitine Deficiency. In this variety the effects of insufficient carnitine are more widespread, even if the disease does not clearly have a different etiology. In the first report (18), a young boy had always been somewhat clumsy with a "floppy" head. The weakness was progressive and, by the age of 11, he was no longer able to walk to school. Superimposed on this were attacks of hepatic encephalopathy resembling those of Reye's syndrome. Since then, there have been several other descriptions of this entity (19–25).

The disorder usually begins in childhood and is sometimes ushered in by episodes of encephalopathy which may precede clinical symptoms of weakness. The weakness is usually greater around the limb-girdle musculature than distally, but there is also involvement of the facial and neck muscles. The initial symptom of the encephalopathy is usually protracted vomiting, followed by changing levels of consciousness, culminating in coma. Hypoglycemia is noted in most of the patients and there is evidence of liver damage, both clinically, with an enlarged tender liver, and chemically, with increased serum levels of the hepatic enzymes. Hypoprothrombinemia, hyperammonemia and excess lipid in the liver are reminiscent of the features of Reye's syndrome. Many of the attacks were apparently provoked by fasting, a not unreasonable association since the fasting state throws the body increasingly into a dependence on fatty acids. Since carnitine may also be involved in branched chain amino acids oxidation, all alternative pathways to glucose and glycogen metabolism seem to be closed off. Metabolic studies of the forearm showed that long chain fatty acids were not utilized by the muscle, although there was excessive glucose uptake (6). The accumulation of abnormal metabolites may play havoc with the remaining metabolic pathways, leading to a spiraling accumulation of lactic acid, keto acids, and dicarboxylic acids (perhaps derived from the abnormal oxidation of fatty acids). Although many of the patients have recovered spontaneously from such episodes, death is a not infrequent complication, with several patients dying from cardiorespiratory failure.

Postmortem studies have shown lipid accumulation not only in the muscle, but also in the liver, heart and kidneys. Biochemical studies show a reduction in the levels of carnitine in muscle, blood and other tissues such as liver and kidney. It should be noted, however, that the carnitine level does not always parallel the severity of the lipid storage.

The cause or causes of systemic carnitine deficiency are no more clear than those of the muscle variety. A defect in biosynthesis would seem to be an obvious possibility, but evaluation of the responsible enzymes in the liver showed nothing untoward. Furthermore, when a labeled precursor was administered intravenously, this was converted to labeled carnitine in a normal fashion (26). Another possibility is that carnitine is lost from the body by an abnormality in renal reabsorption. Although a renal abnormality in carnitine transport has been demonstrated in patients with carnitine deficiency, it was also noted in a normal control, therefore it does not seem to be, by itself, responsible for the problem. Treatment of the illness with carnitine has also been attempted with variable effects; some patients responding quite well and others showing no response. As in muscle carnitine deficiency, the increase in the serum levels of carnitine, following such treatment, was not accompanied by normalization of the tissue levels.

Secondary Carnitine Deficiency. There are many chronic illnesses in which weakness of a rather nonspecific type complicates a disorder which is obviously not primarily of the muscle. On occasion, low levels of carnitine have been found in the muscle and in the serum (2). It is difficult to know whether this has anything to do with the origin of the weakness since there are even larger numbers of chronically ill patients who complain of weakness without any disturbance of tissue carnitine. Patients with renal failure, who have been treated with hemodialysis and those with liver cirrhosis who are in addition severely wasted, may have a secondary carnitine deficiency. Low carnitine has also been described in myxedema, hypopituitarism, and adrenal insufficiency, as well as patients suffering from abnormalities in renal transport function, such as Fanconi syndrome. Patients with other chronic myopathies, such as Duchenne and Becker dystrophy, have also been noted to have low carnitine levels, although here the situation is more complicated since other abnormalities in fatty acid metabolism have been described. Carnitine deficiency has also been described in association with a mitochondrial myopathy (27).

As mentioned, carnitine is a critical substance. If it is not synthesized or transported, is excreted excessively, or is used up in buffering abnormal toxic compounds, the normal function of the body will be disturbed. It is probable that in only a small minority of the cases is there anything wrong with carnitine production itself. Even in the disorders described as muscle and systemic carnitine deficiency, a primary defect in carnitine metabolism is unproven.

REFERENCES

1. Rebouche, C. J., and Engel, A. G. Ċarnitine biosynthesis in humans. In: *Disorders of the Motor Unit*, edited by D. L. Schotland. John Wiley & Sons, New York, 1982, pp. 629–639.
2. Rebouche, C. J., and Engel, A. G. Carnitine metabolism and deficiency syndromes. Mayo Clin. Proc. *58*: 533–540, 1983.
3. Stumpf, D. A., Parker, W. D., and Angelini C. Carnitine deficiency, organic acidemias, and Reye's syndrome. Neurology *35*: 1041–1045, 1985.
4. Engel, A. G., and Siekert, F. G. Lipid storage myopathy response to prednisone. Arch. Neurol. *27*: 174–181, 1972.
5. Engel, A. G., and Angelini, C. Carnitine deficiency of human skeletal muscle with associated lipid storage myopathy: A new syndrome. Science *173*: 899–902, 1973.
6. Markesbery, W. R., McQuillen, M. P., Procopis, E. G., Harrison, A. R., and Engle, A. G. Muscle carnitine deficiency, association with lipid myopathy, vacuolar neuropathy and vacuolated leukocytes. Arch. Neurol. *31*: 320–324, 1974.
7. Van Dyke, D. H., Griggs, R. C., Markesbery, W., and DiMauro, S. Hereditary carnitine deficiency of muscle. Neurology *25*: 154–159, 1975.
8. Prockop, L. D., Engel, W. K., and Shug, A. L. Nearly fatal muscle carnitine deficiency with full recovery after replacement therapy. Neurology *33*: 1629–1631, 1983.
9. Carroll, J. E., Brooke, M. H., DeVivo, D. C., Shumate, J. B., Kratz, R., Ringel, S. P., and Hagberg, J. M. Carnitine "deficiency": lack of response to carnitine therapy. Neurology *30*: 618–626, 1980.
10. Angelini, C., Lucke, S., and Cantarutti, F. Carnitine deficiency of skeletal muscle; report of a treated case. Neurology *26*: 633–637, 1976.
11. Hart, Z. H., Chang, C. H., DiMauro, S., et al. Muscle carnitine deficiency and fatal cardiomyopathy. Neurology *28*: 147–151, 1978.
12. Willner, J. H., DiMauro, S., Eastwood, A., Hays, A., Roohi, F., and Lovelace, R. Muscle carnitine deficiency: genetic heterogeniety. J. Neurol. Sci. *41*: 235–246, 1979.
13. Engel, A. G., and Rebouche, C. J. Pathogenetic mechanisms in human carnitine deficiency syndromes. In: *Disorders of the Motor Unit*, edited by D. L. Schotland. John Wiley & Sons, New York, 1982, pp. 643–655.
14. Angelini, C. Carnitine deficiency. Lancet *2*: 1151, 1975.
15. Smyth, D. P. L., Lake, B. D., MacDermot, J., and Wilson, J. Inborn error of carnitine metabolism (carnitine deficiency) in man. Lancet *1*: 1198–1199, 1975.
16. Carroll, J. E., Shumate, J. B., Brooke, M. H., and Hagberg, J. M. Riboflavin responsive lipid myopathy and carnitine deficiency. Neurology *31*: 1557–1559, 1981.
17. Askanas, V., Engel, W. K., Kwan, H. H., Reddy, N. B., Husainy, T., Carlo, J., Siddique, T., Schwartzman, R. J., and Hanna, C. J. Autosomal dominant syndrome of lipid neuromyopathy with normal carnitine: successful treatment with long chain fatty acid free diet. Neurology *35*: 66–72, 1985.
18. Karpati, G., Carpenter, S., Engel, A. G., Watters, G., Allen, J., Rothmann, S., Klassen, G., and Mamer, O. A. The syndrome of systemic carnitine deficiency. Neurology *25*: 16–24, 1975.
19. Boudin, G., Mikol, J., Guillard, A., and Engel, A. G., Fatal systemic carnitine deficiency with lipid storage in skeletal muscle heart and kidney. J. Neurol. Sci. *30*: 313–315, 1976.
20. Cornelio, F., Didonato, S., Peluchetti, P., Bizzi, A., Bertagnolio, B., D'Angelo, A., and Wiesmann, U. Fatal cases of lipid storage myopathy with carnitine deficiency. J. Neurol. Neurosurg. Psychiatry *40*: 170–178, 1977.
21. Engel, A. G., Banker, B. Q., and Eiben, R. B. Carnitine deficiency: clinical, morphological, and biochemical observations in a fatal case. J. Neurol. Neurosurg. Psychiatry *40*: 313–322, 1977.
22. Scarlato, G., Pellegrini, G., Cerri, C., Meola, G., and Veicsteinas, A. The syndrome of carnitine deficiency: morphological and metabolic correlations in two cases. Can. J. Neurol. Sci. *5*: 205–213, 1978.
23. Ware, A. J., Burton, C. W., and McGarry, J. D. Systemic carnitine deficiency: report of a fatal case with multisystem manifestations. J. Pediatr. *93*: 959–964, 1978.
24. Glasgow, A. M., Eng, G., and Engel, A. G. Systemic carnitine deficiency simulating recurrent Reyes syndrome. J. Pediatr. *96*: 889–891, 1980.
25. Scholte, H. R., Meijer, A. E. F. H., VanWijngaarden, G. K., et al. Familial carnitine deficiency: a fatal case and subclinical state in a sister. J. Neurol. Sci. *42*: 87–101, 1979.
26. Rebouche, C. J., and Engle, A. G. Primary systemic carnitine deficiency; I. Carnitine biosynthesis. Neurology *31*: 813–818, 1981.

27. Didonato, S., Cornelio, F., Balestrini, M. R., Bertagnolio, B., and Peluchetti, D. Mitochondria-lipid-glycogen myopathy, hyperlactic acidemia, and carnitine deficiency. Neurology *28*: 1110–1116, 1978.

Mitochondrial Abnormalities

Disorders of the electron transport chain frequently cause severe neurological deficit rather than neuromuscular problems (see (1) for review). In spite of the fact that most of these illnesses present with neurological disturbances, examination of muscle tissue reveals the usual morphological changes in the mitochondria and the presence of ragged red fibers. This has led to the generic term of "encephalomyopathies" for these illnesses. Delineation of all of these is beyond the scope of this book and I will simply concentrate on those that, because of the involvement of muscle, are often referred to the neuromuscular clinician.

REFERENCE

1. Morgan-Hughes, J. A., Hayes, D. J., Clark, J. B., Landon, D. N., Swash, M., Stark, R. J., and Rudge, P. Encephalomyopathies. Biochemical studies in two cases revealing defects in the respiratory chain. Brain *105*: 553–582, 1982.

Cytochrome-c-Oxidase Deficiency (Complex IV)

There are now many reports of infants with severe hypotonia associated with respiratory weakness, which often has its onset within the first few weeks of life. The disorder is associated with marked lactic acidosis and a urinary abnormality characteristic of De Toni-Fanconi-Debre syndrome in which there is a generalized aminoaciduria, glycosuria, proteinuria, and phosphaturia (1–7). The extraocular muscles may also be involved. In addition, hepatomegaly and macroglossia have been reported. The disorder is usually fatal within the first year of life. The high levels of lactic acid would obviously make one suspect a mitochondrial process and muscle biopsy confirms this. There may, on occasions, be overt ragged red fibers, although often an increase in the stippling of fibers, as visualized with the oxidative enzyme reactions, or subsarcolemmal collections of mitochondrial deposits, is the only change noted. Electron microscopy shows severe degeneration of the mitochondria with loss of cristae, lamellar changes, and other evidence of mitochondrial abnormality. The histochemical reaction for cytochrome oxidase is absent on light microscopy and may be confirmed biochemically. In one family (5), an unusual combination of changes was seen in two cousins. In the first, with the typical illness associated with lactic acidemia, the abnormalities were limited to the muscle. In the second cousin, mitochondria in the liver were abnormal and the child had no systemic lactic acidosis. The muscle was not studied in this second child. An 8-month-old child who died from the illness was noted to have decreased amounts of the enzyme protein when this was assayed by its immunoreactivity (7).

The picture is further complicated by a report of a reversible form of this illness (8). The child was admitted to the hospital at 2 weeks of age because of persistent weakness, which had developed after delivery. He had profound hypotonia and weakness of all muscles, except the extraocular muscles. He also had macroglossia, but the liver, heart, and spleen were normal. Severe metabolic acidosis was noted with a serum lactate concentration of 28 mM. He did not have the De Toni-Fanconi-Debre abnormality. After some time, he started to improve and could hold his head by 4½ months, roll over at 7 months, and was walking by 16 months. The macroglossia had disappeared by 4 months. The blood lactic acid declined steadily and was normal by 14 months. At approximately 3 years of age, he still had a moderate degree of weakness and an associated lumbar lordosis with a waddling gait. In this report, it is interesting that two of his cousins, age 13 and 19, had been diagnosed as having muscular dystrophy.

Three muscle biopsies were obtained and the first one, although appearing superficially normal, demonstrated abnormal mitochondria, as well as an absence of cytochrome *c* oxidase activity. The second biopsy was more abnormal and there was a superimposed accumulation of lipid and glycogen. The third biopsy was taken at 3 years of age. By this time, the cytochrome *c* oxidase activity had returned to normal and the biopsy showed variability in the size of fibers, more resembling a mild dystrophy than a metabolic myopathy. This gives rise to the possibility that some of the patients with undiagnosed fixed weaknesses or the entity originally described under (mitochondrial-lipid-glycogen disease (MLG) might have their origin in cytochrome *c* oxidase deficiency early in life.

REFERENCES

1. Vanbiervliet, J. P. A. M., Bruinvis, L., Ketting, D., Debree, P. K., Van der Heiden, C., Wadman, S. K., Willems, J. L., Bookelman, H., Van Haelst, V., and Monnens, A. H. Hereditary mitochondrial myopathy with lactic acidemia, a De Toni-Fanconi-Debre syndrome and a defective respiratory chain in voluntary striated muscles. Pediatr. Res. *11*: 1088–1093, 1977.
2. DiMauro, S., Mendell, J. R., Sahenk, Z., Bachman, D., Scarpa, A., Scofield, R. M., and Reiner, C. Fatal infantile mitochondrial myopathy and renal dysfunction due to cytochrome *c* oxidase deficiency. Neurology *30*: 795–804, 1980.
3. Heiman-Patterson, T. D., Bonilla, E., DiMauro, S., Foreman, J., and Schotland, D. L. Cytochrome *c* oxidase deficiency in a floppy baby. Neurology *32*: 898–900, 1982.
4. Minchom, P. E., Dormer, R. L., Hughes, I. A., Stansbie, D., Cross, A. R., Hendry, J. A. F., Jones, O. T. G., Johnson, M. A., Scherratt, S. H. A., and Turnbull, B. M. Fatal infantile mitochondrial myopathy due to cytochrome *c* oxidase deficiency. J. Neurol. Sci. *60*: 453–463, 1983.
5. Boustany, R. N., Aprille, J. R., Halperin, J., Levy, H., and Delong, G. R. Mitochondrial cytochrome deficiency presenting as a myopathy with hypotonia, external ophthalmoplegia, and lactic acidosis in an infant and as fatal hepatopathy in a second cousin. Ann. Neurol. *14*: 462–470, 1983.
6. Treijbels, F., Sengers, F., and Monnens, L., A patient with lactic acidemia and cytochrome oxidase deficiency. J. Inherited Metab. Dis. *6*(Suppl 2): 127–128, 1983.
7. Zeviani, M., Nonaka, I., Bonilla, E., Okino, E., Moggio, M., Jones, S., and DiMauro, S. Fatal infantile mitochondrial myopathy and renal dysfunction caused by cytochrome *c* oxidase deficiency; immunological studies in a new patient. Ann. Neurol. *17*: 414–417, 1985.
8. DiMauro, S., Nicholson, J. F., Hays, A. P., Eastwood, A. B., Papadimitriou, A., Koenigsberger, R., and DeVivo, D. C. Benign infantile mitochondrial myopathy due to reversible cytochrome-*c* oxidase deficiency Ann. Neurol. *14*: 226–234, 1983.

"ATP-ase" Deficiency

Just in the same way that an absence of myophosphorylase has been associated with two different clinical syndromes, one clearly exercise related and the other with the late onset of proximal weakness, so it is with mitochondrial abnormalities. An example of a patient with fixed weakness was described by Schotland et al. (1). The patient was a 37-year-old woman who had life-long difficulty with weakness. She had been noted to have difficulty in sitting up from a lying position or standing from squatting since early childhood. She was not able to participate in physical education classes at school, and in adult life, had difficulty with climbing stairs and carrying bags of groceries. In addition to moderate proximal weakness of the arms and legs, she had a pes cavus and thoracic scoliosis. The cranial muscles were not involved. EMG revealed an increased number of small polyphasic potentials and EKG showed biventricular hypertrophy with strain.

The muscle fibers were abnormal with an increase in subsarcolemmal staining and increased stippling with the modified Gomori trichrome and the oxidative enzyme reactions. Electron microscopy demonstrated large numbers of subsarcolemmal mitochondria containing paracrystalline inclusions and round osmiophilic inclusions. Other mitochondria showed an electron lucid matrix with decreased number of cristae. The biochemistry of this condition was different from the preceding ones. Neither NAD-linked substrates, such as pyruvate and malate nor the flavoprotein-linked succinic dehydrogenase produced any change in oxidation when ADP and inorganic phosphate were added. Since DNP, which uncouples oxidative phosphorylation restored respiration to normal levels, it was suggested that this defect was of the phosphorylation pathway common to all three parts of the electron chain. An analysis of mitochondrial ATPase showed this to be decreased and the authors suggested that the basis of the patient's illness was a deficient production of ATP. Fatigue was not, apparently, a part of this patient's clinical picture, although the absence of exercise studies makes it difficult to draw exact comparisons between this patient and the other adults with defects in the electron transport chain. Perhaps the biventricular hypertrophy could be explained on the basis of a hyperkinetic circulation.

REFERENCE

1. Schotland, D. L., DiMauro, S., Bonilla, E., Scarpa, A., and Lee, C. P. Neuromuscular disorder associated with a defect in mitochondrial energy supply. Arch. Neurol. *33:* 475–479, 1976.

Kearns-Sayre Syndrome (Oculocraniosomatic Neuromuscular Disease with Ragged Red Fibers)

Chronic progressive weakness of the extraocular muscles may occur as part of a complex and varied picture of dysfunction (1–3) (Figs. 7.31–7.33). It may be associated with neurological, cardiac, and other deficits. Many of these different syndromes have seemed to coalesce into one entity.

Most cases are sporadic but familial cases have been described perhaps on the basis of a dominant gene with variable penetrance or an autosomal recessive gene (4). The symptoms may appear at any time in life, but most often during childhood or adolescence. In some, there is a history of a flu-like illness associated with drowsiness and confusion at the onset. An early sign is the development of weakness of the extraocular muscles and ptosis. Muscle fatigue during exercise is also a common symptom. In two patients in our clinic, the fatigue has been severe enough that the patients are unable to walk more than 60 or 70 yards. The illness is progressive and there may be any or all of the following abnormalities: pigmentary degeneration of the retina, sensorineural deafness, pyramidal tract disease, cerebellar incoordination, endocrine abnormalities (such as amenorrhea or hypoparathyroidism) cardiac conduction defects, and, when the illness begins early in life, mental

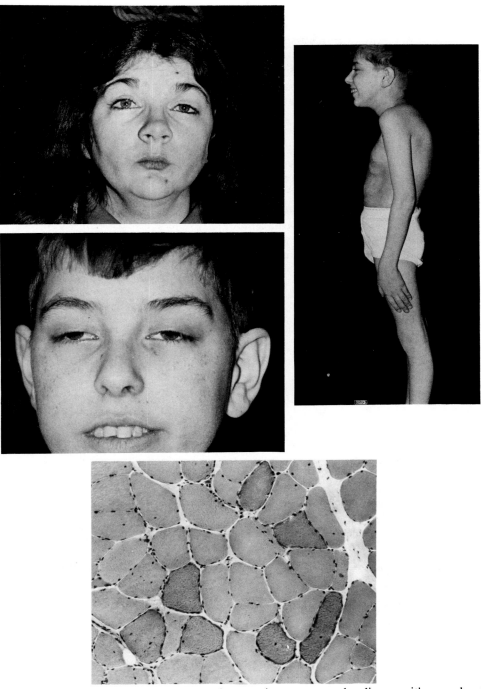

Figures 7.31 through 7.34. Oculo-cranio-somatic neuromuscular disease with ragged red fibers. Ptosis and extraocular palsies are a prominent part of this syndrome (Fig. 7.31, *top, left,* and Fig. 7.32, *center, left*). Minor degrees of axial muscle weakness are found and occasionally a mild kyphosis is noted (Fig. 7.33, *right*). The muscle biopsy shows a large number of "ragged red" fibers, these are fibers with an abnormal granular appearance and a bright red stain with modified trichrome stains (Fig. 7.34, *bottom*). The red staining material is frequently around the periphery fibers and is due to large numbers of abnormal mitochondria.

and growth retardation. There is also a defect in ventilatory drive, the patient's respiration responding poorly to increasing hypoxia, or hypercapnia (5). This may have been the cause of an episode of confusion and lethargy which one patient experienced when traveling at an altitude of 10,000 ft. It is also important to bear such respiratory abnormality in mind if anesthesia is being contemplated since patients may be abnormally sensitive to drugs which are respiratory depressants. There may be sudden deterioration of the neurological state, with the onset of vomiting, headache, and coma. The autopsy findings in two such patients showed a spongy degeneration of the brainstem and cerebral white matter. Evidence of this may be seen pre-mortem on tomography with lucencies in the white matter and calcification of the basal ganglia (4, 6). Almost all patients with the illness have a moderate increase in cerebrospinal fluid (CSF) protein. One report indicated that the IgA and the IgG fractions were all increased, but that the albumin was normal (6). These authors suggested that the increased CSF immunoglobins and other proteins

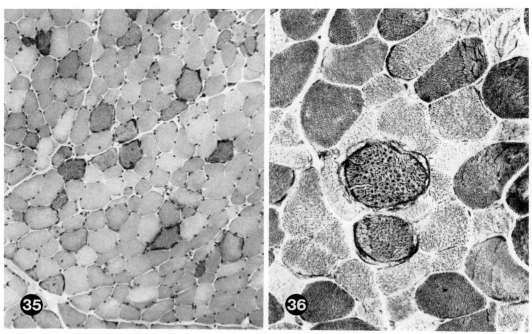

Figure 7.35.   Kearns-Sayre syndrome. The characteristic feature of the Kearns-Sayre syndrome is the presence of numerous "ragged red" fibers. The ragged red fiber itself is not pathognomonic of this disease but when it occurs in profusion and is not associated with other major changes in the biopsy it may be reliably employed to make the diagnosis. The ragged red fibers can be seen scattered throughout these routine hematoxylin and eosin stain preparations. They are a rather granular appearing fiber often rimmed with intense basophilic material. Were this photograph in color the fibers would appear to be blue, they are red only with the modified Gomori trichrome stain. There is also a variation in the size of fibers and occasional internal nuclei but no other major change.

Figure 7.36.   With the oxidative enzyme reaction the ragged red fiber has a characteristic appearance with the edges of the fiber ballooned out. The material which is basophilic with the hematoxylin and eosin stain may be indicated only by a rim of stain with the oxidative enzyme reaction. Electron microscopic preparation shows these areas to be full of abnormal mitochondria. In addition, there may be an increased dark stippling of the ragged red fibers which is due to small lipid-filled vacuoles.

were due to an alteration of the blood CSF barrier. Serum CK is often mildly elevated, but the marked elevations seen in florid myopathies is not to be expected. EMG is usually not helpful in substantiating the diagnosis, although there may be some "myopathic" changes.

The muscle biopsy is diagnostic in this illness. Even when the general abnormalities (variation of fiber size, internal nuclei, etc.) are not striking, there are characteristic "ragged red" fibers scattered through the biopsy (Figs. 7.34–7.38) (7). Under the electron microscope, the mitochondria are increased in number and share features common to the other mitochondrial myopathies with crystalloid inclusions (7) and a lack of cristae (8). These abnormalities are not limited to the muscle. Systemic involvement is evidenced by abnormal mitochondria in the cerebellum (9), the liver (10), and also in the sweat glands (11). There may also be an increase in glycogen deposition in the fibers as well as lipid (11, 12).

As might be expected with a mitochondrial disorder, high resting lactate and pyruvate levels have been described (2, 13). In one patient, the response to exercise was also abnormal with a high production of both pyruvate and lactate. An elevation of the lactate to pyruvate ratio, and the hydroxybutyrate to aceto-acetate ratio followed exercise, which also suggested difficulty in oxygen transport. Reduced plasma and cerebrospinal fluid folate levels were noted with a reversal of the normal ratio of CSF/plasma folate to less than 1. Folate absorption studies were normal (14, 15).

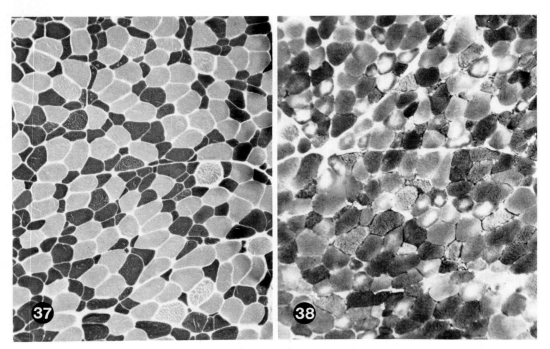

Figure 7.37.   The ATPase stains show the ragged red fibers with the associated mini vacuoles. Both Type 1 and Type 2 fibers are affected and appear to be peppered with small vacuoles.
Figure 7.38.   PAS stains often show abnormal fibers and demonstrate a form of glycogen depletion similar to that seen in other metabolic myopathies causing myoglobinuria.

The morphological change in mitochondria may be produced experimentally by the administration of compounds such as 2,4-dinitrophenol (DNP) which are known to uncouple oxidative phosphorylation (16). Experimental thiamine deficiency has also been associated with the same mitochondrial abnormalities (16). The biochemical evaluation of mitochondrial function showed a decrease in respiration with both NAD and FAD linked substrates, although the control with ADP was still maintained. There was no measurable difference in the cytochrome content between the patients and controls (8).

In the medical management of the patient it is important to monitor the EKG. The conduction defect can become severe enough, on occasion, so that the implantation of a pacemaker becomes necessary. Some patients have died suddenly, presumably because of the conduction defect.

Thiamine, in large doses, has been used in the treatment of patients but is by no means always successful (17). Because of the abnormality in folate levels and a decrease in muscle carnitine levels in one patient (14), therapy with 15 mg folate 10g DL-carnitine and 500 mg of the folate precursor methionine was instituted on a daily basis with some clinical improvement.

REFERENCES

1. Kearns, T. P. External ophthalmoplegia, pigmentary degeneration of the retina and cardio-myopathy: a newly recognized syndrome. Trans. Am. Ophthalmol. Soc. *63*: 559–625, 1965.
2. Shy, G. M., Silberberg, A. H., Appel, S. H., Mishkin, M. M., and Godfrey, E. H. A generalized disorder of nervous system, skeletal muscle and heart resembling Refsum's disease and Hurler's syndrome. Part I. Am. J. Med. *42*: 163–178, 1967.
3. Drachman, D. A. Ophthalmoplegia plus. Arch. Neurol. *18*: 654–674, 1968.
4. Okamoto, T., Mizuno, K., Iida, M., Sobue, I., and Mukoyama, M. Ophthalmoplegia plus: its occurrence with periventricular diffuse low density on computed tomography scan. Arch. Neurol. *38*: 423–426, 1981.
5. Carroll, J. E., Zwillich, C., Weil, J. V., and Brooke, M. H. Depressed ventilatory response in oculocraniosomatic neuromuscular disease. Neurology *26*: 140–146, 1976.
6. Coulter, D. L., and Allen, R. J. Abrupt neurological deterioration on children with Kearns-Sayre syndrome. Arch. Neurol. *38*: 247–250, 1981.
7. Olson, W., Engel, W. K., Walsh, G. O., and Einaugler, R. Oculocraniosomatic neuromuscular disease with ragged red fibers. Arch. Neurol. *26*: 193–211, 1972.
8. Mitsumoto, H., Aprille, J. R., Ray, S. H., Nemni, R., and Bradley, W. G. Chronic progressive external ophthalmoplegia (CPEO); clinical morphological and biochemical studies. Neurology *33*: 452–462, 1983.
9. Schneck, L., Adachi, M., Brite, P., Wolintz, A., and Volk, B. W. Ophthalmoplegia plus with morphological and chemical studies of cerebellar and muscle tissue. J. Neurol. Sci. *19*: 37–44, 1973.
10. Okamura, K., Santa, T., Nagae, K., and Omae, T. Congenital oculoskeletal myopathy with abnormal muscle and liver mitochondria. J. Neurol. Sci. *27*: 79–91, 1976.
11. Karpati, G., Carpenter, S., Larbrisseau, A., and Lafontaine, R. The Kearns-Shy syndrome: a multisystem disease with mitochondrial abnormality demonstrated in skeletal muscle and skin. J. Neurol. Sci. *19*: 133–151, 1973.
12. DiMauro, S., Schotland, D. L., Bonilla, E., Lee, C. P., Gambetti, P., and Rowland, L. P. Progressive ophthalmoplegia, glycogen storage and abnormal mitochondria. Arch. Neurol. *29*: 170–179, 1973.
13. Sulaiman, W. R., Doyle, D., Johnson, R. H., and Jennett, S. Myopathy with mitochondrial inclusion bodies; histological and metabolic studies. J. Neurol. Neurosurg. Psychiatry *37*: 1236–1246, 1974.
14. Allen, R. J., DiMauro, S., Coulter, D. L., Papadimitrion, A., and Rothenberg, S. P. Kearns Sayre syndrome with reduced plasma and cerebrospinal fluid folate. Ann. Neurol. *13*: 679–682, 1983.
15. Dougados, M., Zittoun, J., Laplane, D., and Castaigne, P. Folate metabolism in Kearns-Sayre syndrome. Ann. Neurol. *13*: 687, 1983.
16. Melmed, C., Karpati, G., and Carpenter, S. Experimental mitochondrial myopathy produced by in vivo uncoupling of oxidative phosphorylation. J. Neurol. Sci. *26*: 305–318, 1975.
17. Lou, H. C. Correction of increased plasma pyruvate and lactate levels using large doses of thiamine in patients with Kearns Sayre syndrome. Arch. Neurol. *38*: 469, 1981.

Myoclonus Epilepsy with Ragged Red Fibers

This entity shares many features in common with Kearns-Sayre syndrome (1), but the ophthalmoplegia, retinal degeneration and heart block, which are such constant accompaniments to Kearns-Sayre syndrome are lacking in this entity. The illness often begins with myoclonus, usually in childhood. The disease is progressive and ataxia, weakness, dementia, nerve deafness and lactic acidosis are features common to this disease and to Kearns-Sayre syndrome. Epilepsy is common and the EEG shows generalized paroxysmal discharges. The disorder is differentiated from the Ramsey-Hunt syndrome by the presence of the typical changes on muscle biopsy of mitochondrial abnormalities. Ragged red fibers are profuse and the electron microscope reveals the abnormal structure of the mitochondria. A further differentiating point is that the illness has often occurred in families. In one large pedigree (2), maternal inheritance was demonstrated consistent with a mutation in the mitochondrial DNA. Mitochondrial DNA is responsible for several of the polypeptides located on the inner mitochondrial membrane and associated with the respiratory chain. Thus, although nuclear DNA codes for most of the mitochondrial structure, a critical part of the biochemical apparatus is coded for by the mitochrondrial DNA. Since, at the time of fertilization, the ovum contributes most of the mitochondria, mitochondrial DNA is handed down from mother to child and not along the more familiar lines of inheritance.

REFERENCES

1. Fukuhara, N., Tokiguchi, S., Shirakawa, S., and Tsubaki, T. Myoclonus epilepsy associated with ragged red fibers (mitochondrial abnormalities); disease entity or syndrome? Light and electron microscopic studies of two cases and review of the literature. J. Neurol. Sci. *47*: 117–133, 1980.
2. Rosing, H. S., Hopkins, L. C., Wallace, D. C., Epstein, C. M., and Weidemheim, K. Maternally inherited mitochondrial myopathy and myoclonic epilepsy. Ann. Neurol. *17*: 228–237, 1985.

Mitochondrial Myopathy, Encephalopathy, Lactic Acidosis and Stroke-like Episodes

This syndrome which has become known as the "Melas" syndrome occurs during childhood when the patient has periodic vomiting and encephalopathic symptoms, such as seizures and stroke-like episodes. The patient's stature is small, and they may have sensorineural hearing loss, dementia, and lactic acidosis as in the two preceding syndromes. Nonenhancing lucencies may be seen with the head CT scan. The muscle biopsy again demonstrates mitochondrial abnormalities. The inheritance may again be maternally determined (1).

REFERENCE

1. Pavlakis, S. G., Phillips, P. C., DiMauro, G., DiVivo, D. C., and Rowland, L. P. Mitochondrial myopathy, encephalopathy, lactic adicosis and stroke-like episodes. A distinctive clinical syndrome. Ann. Neurol. *16*: 481–488, 1984.

OTHER BIOCHEMICAL ABNORMALITIES

Myoadenylate Deaminase Deficiency

The enzyme myoadenylate deaminase (AMPDA) is normally found in high concentration in muscle. It catalyzes the deamination of AMP with the resulting production of ammonia and IMP. It is suspected of playing a part in maintaining the energy charge of the muscle cell by removing AMP (see p. 244). It would be logical, though it is unproven, for AMPDA to be most important in the situation of an acute drain on the energy supply. Consequently the report of an absence of this enzyme in patients suffering from muscular aches and pains was of great interest (1). Since nonspecific muscle pain, with and without relationship to exercise, is a very common presentation in the Muscle Clinic, there seemed a real possibility that here was a key to unlocking the door to a major clinical problem. We screened over 250 consecutive biopsies in our clinic to try and found out how often we had missed the diagnosis. We did, indeed, find two patients with exercise related fatigue and pains who had a total deficiency of the enzyme. Curiously, we also found a larger number of patients in whom the enzyme was absent, who not only did not suffer from aches, cramps, and pains, but whose illnesses fell into various other categories. We have seen AMPDA deficiency in spinal muscular atrophies, ALS, facioscapulohumeral dystrophy, myasthenia gravis, and congenital hypotonia (2, 3). We suggested that AMPDA deficiency might be a common and inconsequential enzyme defect with an incidence of around 1% in the general population. Subsequent papers have added more fuel to the debate. Keleman et al. (4) described 14 members of 4 families in which there was an hereditary syndrome of exertional myalgia associated with AMPDA deficiency. They pointed out that the incidence of AMPDA deficiency in patients with myalgia was much higher than in the general population or in patients with other neuromuscular diseases and concluded that it must have some relationship to the production of myalgia. The argument was strengthened by the description of the familial incidence of both AMPDA deficiency and exertional myalgia. Even so, there was no clear explanation for why two of the family members with symptoms of muscle pain and exercise had normal AMPDA levels and did not seem to differ clinically from those in whom AMPDA was absent. Furthermore, one of the sporadic cases of AMPDA deficiency described by the authors was a competitive swimmer and had never experienced muscle pains.

Two brothers developed muscle pain during their teenage years and again the same situation was noted. One had a deficiency of the enzyme and in the other the levels were 60% of normal which should have been adequate for normal functioning (5).

The deficiency may be inherited as an autosomal recessive since reduced levels of the enzyme have been found in other family members and in parents. As in the case of phosphorylase deficiency, the enzyme "reappears" in cultured fibroblasts and in muscle cultures (6). Levels of the enzyme in the red blood cell are normal.

What, then, is one to conclude from these conflicting opinions? The most honest answer is probably that we do not yet know the significance of AMPDA deficiency. My own view is that it is possible for someone with the enzyme deficiency to go through life totally unaware of the problem at all. The relatively large number of patients with aches, cramps, and pains who have been described with this anomaly may simply be due to the fact that exertional myalgia is one of the commonest disorders to be seen in the Muscle Clinic and therefore represents a large proportion of anybody's biopsy material. A finding which may pass unnoticed in a severely necrotic biopsy from a patient say with acute polymyositis becomes much more striking when it occurs in a biopsy which is morphologically normal or in a patient whose disorder is otherwise inexplicable. On the other hand, the enzyme must be doing something! Perhaps if we were to biopsy 500 Olympic class weight lifters, we would find the incidence of the enzyme defect to be nil! I would suggest that an absence of the enzyme must reduce the muscle's reserve for exercise. Perhaps symptoms appear only when another factor, such as an additional biochemical defect or the demand for an excessive work load such as may occur in competitive sports or in manual labor, is superimposed on the original anomaly. The disorder is not difficult to diagnose. Not only is it revealed by the histochemical stain for AMPDA when the muscle is biopsied, but forearm exercise may also make the diagnosis. In the normal individual, following forearm exercise, both ammonia and hypoxanthine appear in the venous blood. These are both ultimately derived from the reaction catalyzed by AMPDA. In the enzyme deficiency, although lactate production is normally brisk, ammonia and hypoxanthine fail to make an appearance. One word of caution should be noted. In the 1-min ischemic exercise test, the exercise load may not be sufficient in all patients to elevate the levels of ammonia and hypoxanthine. However, if the exhaustive forearm is used (see p. 257), in my experience, an absence of ammonia and hypoxathine always indicates AMPDA deficiency (7).

REFERENCES

1. Fischbein, W. N., Armbrustmacher, V. W., and Griffin, J. L. Myoadenylate deaminase deficiency: a new disease of muscle. Science 200: 545–548, 1978.
2. Shumate, J. B., Katnik, R., Ruiz, M., Kaiser, K. K., Frieden, C., Brooke, M. H., and Carroll, J. E. Myoadenylate deaminase deficiency. Muscle Nerve 2: 213–216, 1979.
3. Shumate, J. B., Kaiser, K. K., Carroll, J. E., and Brooke, M. H. Adenylate deaminase deficiency in hypotonic infant. J. Pediatr. 96: 885–887, 1980.
4. Kelemen, J., Rice, D. R., Bradley, W. G., Munsat, T. L., DiMauro, S., and Hogan, E. L. Familial myoadenylate deaminase deficiency and exertional myalgia. Neurology 32: 857–863, 1982.
5. Hayes, D. J., Summers, B. A., and Morgan-Hughes, J. A. Myoadenylate deaminase deficiency or not? Observations on two brothers with exercise induced muscle pain. J. Neurol. Sci. 53: 125–136, 1982.
6. DiMauro, S., Miranda, A. F., Hays, A. P., Franck, W. A., Hoffman, G. S., Schoenfeldt, R. S., and Singh, N. Myoadenylate deaminase deficiency—muscle biopsy and muscle culture in a patient with gout. J. Neurol. Sci. 47: 191–202, 1980.
7. Patterson, V. H., Kaiser, K. K., and Brooke, M. H. Exercising muscle does not produce hypoxanthine in adenylate deaminase deficiency. Neurology 33: 784–786, 1983.

Glycerol Kinase Deficiency

A deficiency of glycerol kinase, which catalyzes a necessary step in the utilization of glycerol, results in high levels of glycerol in both the blood and the urine of patients with this illness. The disorder is a systemic one rather than a specific myopathy and patients will probably not find their way into the Muscle Clinic. There is, however, a definite myopathy associated with high levels of CK and a biopsy which demonstrates necrotic changes reminiscent of those of the early stages of Duchenne dystrophy. Since the gene for glycerol kinase is close to that for Duchenne muscular dystrophy, this may be more than coincidental. Clinically, the disease presents as psychomotor retardation, spasticity, growth failure, multiple fractures due to osteoporosis and adrenal insufficiency. Esotropia was also noted. The disorder was described in two brothers. The elevation of serum glycerol gave rise to a spurious elevation of the levels of serum triglycerides since these are usually measured without accounting for the free glycerol present in the serum. CK levels were noted up to 6,000. One of the brothers died during childhood following an illness with vomiting and dehydration, an episode which the other child also experienced but survived.

REFERENCE

1. Guggenheim, M. A., McCabe, E. R. B., Rogi, M., Goodman, S. I., Lum, G. M., Bullen, W. W., and Ringle, S. P. Glycerol kinase deficiency with neuromusculoskeletal and adrenal abnormalities. Ann. Neurol. *7*: 441–449, 1980.

PERIODIC PARALYSES

Episodic bouts of weakness which occur with varying severity and frequency are common to all the periodic paralyses. Such paralyses are classified according to whether the serum potassium is increased, decreased, or unchanged during an attack. Hence, there are two major categories: hypokalemic and hyperkalemic. There may also be a third variety in which the potassium is unchanged although this "normokalemic" variety is poorly defined. The distinction into separate categories based on the age of onset, the severity and duration of the attack, and the nature of the provocative factors seems quite clear as one reads the literature. Unfortunately these lines of distinction become blurred by a number of features which all three varieties share in common, and the clarity of the textbook definition may become obscure at bedside.

Familial Hypokalemic Periodic Paralysis

Clinical Aspects. This illness occurs as an autosomal dominant, but it is often not expressed in the female and may appear to be an autosomal recessive if an asymptomatic mother has affected children. Similarly, there are 3 times as many men with the illness as there are women. Although the disease may begin at any time, it commonly does so in the second decade, when the patient complains of episodes of severe weakness. The weakness often starts in the legs with a feeling of heaviness and aching in the back and thighs and gradually, over a period of an hour or so, spreads to other muscle groups. Muscles of the shoulders and hips are usually more affected than distal muscles. The attack may be severe enough to paralyze the patient's arms and legs completely and prevent him from raising his head from the pillow. Weakness of the eye muscles occurs rarely, if at all, and the facial muscles are seldom involved. Mild disturbance of breathing may be seen in a severe attack, but respiratory paralysis of a severity to threaten the patient's life is rare. At the height of the weakness, the muscle is electrically and mechanically inexcitable and the reflexes are lost. The muscles feel swollen, and an increased circumference of the limb has been noted (1). Usually an attack will last from a half a day to a day. The patient's strength will return as suddenly as it disappeared; the last muscles to become weak are usually the first to recover. Even after recovery from an attack, there may be a residual weakness for 2–3 days before completely normal strength returns.

The frequency of these attacks varies from several times a week to isolated attacks separated by intervals of years. The severity ranges from mild focal weakness of a few muscles to a total flaccid paralysis of all limbs. During and preceding an attack there is often an increased thirst and, not uncommonly, oliguria. The patient may also differentiate between "light" and "heavy" attacks. The latter is an episode of paralysis, and the former, a transient sense of weakness lasting for an hour or two.

Provocative factors are fairly stereotyped. Heavy exercise (or exercise to which a patient is not accustomed) followed by a period of sleep or rest, a heavy meal, particularly one rich in carbohydrates and salt, emotional stress, alcohol, trauma, and cold may all precipitate the weakness. Thus, the man who mows the lawn in the afternoon prior to playing a game of touch football, later going out with the team to slake a ravenous appetite with beer, pizza, and popcorn, and arrives back home late enough to become embroiled in a domestic argument may wake up with considerable weakness the next morning.

Although an attack commonly develops in the early hours of the morning, it may occur at other times during the day. It may be warded off by gentle exercise in the early stages, although less commonly than in the hyperkalemic variety. Some drugs, such as epinephrine, norepinephrine, and corticosteroids, may have a provocative effect on the disease. In patients who have frequent attacks, particularly if these attacks are severe, a permanent weakness may develop which is usually proximal and which involves the hips more than the shoulders (2–4). Eyelid myotonia, originally described in hyperkalemic periodic paralysis, may be prominent in the hypokalemic disease (5). The disease is usually at its worst during the third and fourth decades and may improve spontaneously thereafter.

Laboratory Studies. Studies during an attack are essential to make the diagnosis. There is a fall in the serum potassium. This may be as low as 1.5 meq/liter during an attack, but the patient's weakness may commence with levels of 3 meq and become quite marked by the time they have dropped to 2–2.5 meq, levels which are better tolerated by the normal person. There are concomitant EKG changes. Bradycardia is often seen, the T waves are flattened, and there are prominent U waves with prolongation of the PR and QT interval. The heart size has been observed to increase during an attack. The serum CK may be elevated during or after an attack.

Since patients do not always present themselves conveniently at the height of their weakness, it is necessary on occasion to use provocative measures so that the change in potassium can be monitored while the paralysis is present. In patients with hypokalemic periodic paralysis, the usual method is to administer glucose with or without insulin. As an initial test, glucose can be given orally 1.5 g/kg to a total dose of 100 g. If this is unsuccessful, an intravenous regimen can be adopted with the administration of up to 3.0 g/kg in over a period of 1 hour. Insulin may be given intravenously during this infusion (up to 0.1 U/kg at the 30-minute and 60 minute time point) (6). The EKG should be monitored throughout the procedure and potassium levels drawn at regular intervals (15–30 minutes). Maximum change in the potassium levels is seen within 3 hours. A clinical attack of weakness can occur at any time, but it may be delayed for as long as 6–7 hours after the administration of glucose. A clear-cut attack of paralysis is indicative of hypokalemic periodic paralysis. If no weakness develops, it is important to make sure the serum potassium level has fallen to at least 2.5 meq. Even then it may be difficult to interpret a negative test. In any patient given large amounts of glucose and insulin, hypoglycemia may occur and should, of course, be treated appropriately.

The muscle biopsy is sometimes, but not always, abnormal. On occasion, some atrophic fibers are present and vacuoles may be found in the central part of muscle fibers. These vacuoles may be numerous and are often reactive with the PAS stains for glycogen. Collections of tubular structures (tubular aggregates), although more common in hyperkalemic paralysis, are also to be found (Figs. 7.39–7.41). Such structural changes are not the invariable accompaniment to an acute attack. They may be florid in the interictal period and absent during the attack itself. Electron microscopic studies show that the vacuoles arise from local dilatation of the T tubules and sarcoplasmic reticular vesicles (7), but whether these changes are associated with the primary abnormality or whether they represent a secondary change is not yet certain.

A disease in which the pathophysiology is associated with fluxes in electrolytes must surely be amenable to investigative research. Unhappily the basic defect is still elusive. That the inexcitability of the muscle during an attack was not due to the contractile mechanism but was due to dysfunction of the membrane was shown by Engel and Lambert (8). The muscle from patients during the paralytic phase of the disease is inexcitable either upon stimulation or when calcium is applied locally to the intact muscle. If the sarcolemmal membrane is stripped from the muscle, the fiber regains its contractile response to the local application of calcium.

During the early stages of the acute attack there is a movement of potassium into muscle cells. This is probably associated with a similar movement of water and sodium ions. The reason for this flux is not known and various theories such as changes in the membrane permeability, the accumulation of abnormal negatively charged intermediates of carbohydrate metabolism, and the abnormal production of aldosterone have all been proposed as underlying mechanisms; however, all have received rather substantial challenges.

Hofmann and Smith (9) studied single muscle fibers in vitro and found that the fibers were not able to withstand the isolation procedure as well as those from normal individuals. There was a significant degree of depolarization regardless of the patient's clinical condition at the time of the biopsy (none of the patients was studied during the time of an attack, although one had weakness). There was also an anomalous response to insulin, which caused repolarization of fibers when the external potassium levels were markedly reduced.

Studies on intercostal muscle fibers (which have the advantage of being intact from end to end) from patients with hypokalemic periodic paralysis have provided additional clues (10). The resting membrane potentials of the muscle fibers were slightly depolarized by about 5–15 mv and the membrane potential was less stable. Reducing the external potassium concentration in the medium rendered the fibers inexcitable and depolarized them to about −50 mv. The effect was directly due to the reduction in potassium concentration externally and not secondary to some other factor. This low concentration has an effect on the sodium potassium pump and would be expected to decrease the conductance of potassium and increase that of sodium. Although a low potassium conductance was suggested as a possible etiology (11), it was

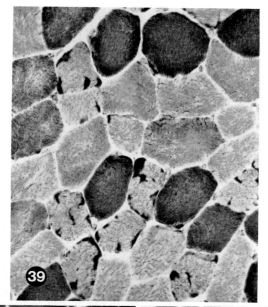

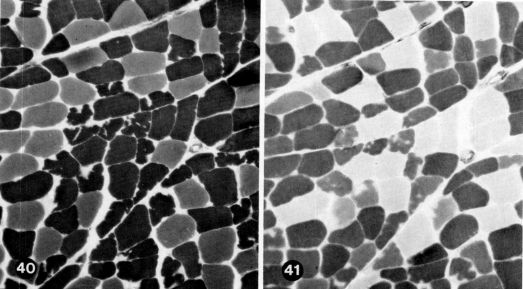

Figure 7.39. Tubular aggregates. The tubular aggregates can be recognized with the oxidative enzyme reaction, in which there is an intense blue staining area in many of the fibers.

Figures 7.40 and 7.41. The tubular aggregates always seem to occur in Type 2B fibers. The photographs are of serial sections from a biopsy stained with a routine ATPase stain (Fig. 7.40) and the ATPase stain modified by preincubation at pH 4.6 (Fig. 7.41). In the regular stain the Type 1 fibers are light and the Type 2 fibers are dark. Notice that the tubular aggregates, which are the negatively stained areas causing a ragged appearance in many of the small fibers, occur only in the dark Type 2 fibers. With the pH 4.6 modified ATPase reaction Type 1 fibers are darkly stained the Type 2A fibers are very lightly stained and the Type 2B fibers are intermediate in stain. Notice that the fibers which can be identified in the other photograph as containing tubular aggregates are all Type 2B fibers.

a suggestion that was not well received and Rudel et al. (10) were unable to demonstrate any decrease in potassium conductance. On the contrary, they suggested that the disorder was due to an increased conductance of sodium. There was an increased concentration of sodium in the resting fibers of patients with the illness, and removal of 90% of the external sodium restored the membrane potential to its normal level and stability. Since the sodium conductance was not blocked by tetrodotoxin, presumably it was mediated by mechanisms other than the normal sodium channels. Such an abnormality would throw particular responsibility on the sodium potassium pump for maintaining the muscle fibers in the interictal period. If the pump is operating at too high a level, then the external potassium will be reduced leading to attacks of paralysis. If the pump operates at too low a level, the internal sodium is increased leading to the same effect. There would, therefore, be a critical level for the sodium potassium pump and its optimal operation. The effect of carbohydrates and insulin may be due to their influence on the sodium potassium pump.

Treatment. The treatment of the disease is not always easy. A clear-cut episode of paralysis is best treated by oral potassium, between 5 and 10 g being an average dose. This may be repeated in 1 hour if no response is seen. It is, of course, important to evaluate renal function before administering potassium to a patient.

The long-term treatment of the disease to prevent attacks may be less successful. The prophylactic administration of potassium chloride has been recommended, but is often without effect in aborting the attacks when given over a long period of time. Spironolactone has also been found effective, but there are some disturbing side effects such as gynecomastia. The use of a carbonic anhydrase inhibitor such as acetazolamide (Diamox) (12) or dichlorphenamide (13) has been the subject of some enthusiastic reports. These compounds are diuretics and, since they further the loss of potassium, the effect seems paradoxical, but it is probable that the benefit pertains more to changes in membrane function than to changes in the potassium content of the body. Experimentally acetazolamide reduces the movement of potassium into red blood cells. It also diminishes the hypokalemic effect of glucose insulin provocation in patients with periodic paralysis. Part of its effect may be mediated through the production of metabolic acidosis (14). Acetazolamide works well for some patients, but there are others for whom the drug is of no value. If it is going to help, it does so within 24 hours of starting treatment. It is used in doses of 250 mg b.i.d. up to 500 mg t.i.d. Sometimes it may be effective in doses as low as 125 mg daily. Side effects include tingling in the extremities, anorexia, and renal calculi.

Secondary Hypokalemic Paralysis

Probably the best known form of this is the periodic paralysis associated with thyrotoxicosis. There is a high incidence in the oriental population, but it also occurs in other races. The reason for this close association is unknown. Usually the disease is sporadic and affects men more commonly than women. It is seldom seen before the second decade, and the illness disappears when the thyroid function returns to normal. The attacks are usually not as disabling as in the familial variety, and residual weakness is unusual.

Episodic weakness is also seen in many of the illnesses in which potassium is depleted. Attacks of weakness may occur in hyperaldosteronism, with chronic diarrhea or vomiting, as well as in the chronic administration of potassium depleting diuretics. An interesting, although rare, example occurs after the chronic ingestion of licorice (15). The compound responsible is glycyrrhizate, which is a potent mineralocorticoid.

REFERENCES

1. McArdle, B. Metabolic myopathies. Am. J. Med. *35:* 661–672, 1963.
2. Engel, A. G., Lambert, E. H., Rosevear, J. W., and Tauxe, M. N. Clinical and electromyographic studies in a patient with primary hypokalemia periodic paralysis. Am. J. Med. *38:* 626, 1965.
3. Pearson, C. M. The periodic paralyses; differential features and pathological observations in permanent myopathic weakness. Brain *87:* 341, 1963.
4. Dyken, M., Zeman, W., and Rusch, T. Hypokalemic periodic paralysis. Neurology *19:* 691–699, 1969.
5. Resnick, J. S. and Engel, W. K. Myotonic lid lag in hypokalemic periodic paralysis. J. Neurol. Neurosurg. Psychiatry *30:* 47–51, 1967.
6. Riggs, J. E., and Griggs, R. C. Diagnosis and treatment of the periodic paralyses. Clin. Neuropharmacol. *4:* 123–138, 1979.
7. Engel, A. G. Evolution and content of vacuoles in primary hypokalemic periodic paralysis. Mayo Clin. Proc. *45:* 774–814, 1970.
8. Engel, A. G. and Lambert, E. H. Calcium activation of electrically inexcitable muscle fibers in primary hypokalemic periodic paralysis. Neurology *19:* 851–858, 1969.
9. Hofmann, W. W. and Smith, R. A. Hypokalemic periodic paralysis studied in vitro. Brain *93:* 445–474, 1970.
10. Rudel, R., Lehmann-Horn, F., Ricker, K., and Kuther, G. Hypokalemic periodic paralysis: in vitro investigation of muscle fiber membrane parameters. Muscle Nerve *7:* 110–120, 1984.
11. Layzer, R. B. Periodic paralysis and the sodium potassium pump. Ann. Neurol. *11:* 547–552, 1982.
12. Griggs, R. C., Engel, W. K., and Resnick, J. S. Acetazolamide treatment of hypokalemic periodic paralysis. Ann. Intern. Med. *73:* 39–48, 1970.
13. McArdle, B. Metabolic and endocrine myopathies. In: *Disorders of Voluntary Muscle,* edited by J. N. Walton. Churchill-Livingstone, London, 1974.
14. Vroom, F. Q., Jarrell, M. A., and Maren, T. H. Acetazolamide treatment of hypokalemic periodic paralysis. Arch. Neurol. *32:* 385–392, 1975.
15. Conn, J. W., Rovner, D. R., and Cohen, E. L. Licorice induced pseudoaldosteronism. J.A.M.A. *205:* 492–496, 1968.

Hyperkalemic Periodic Paralysis (Adynamia Episodica Hereditaria (1)

If in one variety of periodic paralysis the serum potassium was always abnormally reduced and in the other abnormally increased, it would be a good deal easier to write about hyperkalemic periodic paralysis. However, the matter is not so straightforward, and perhaps it is safer merely to state that the electrolyte changes are different from those seen in hypokalemic paralysis.

Clinical Aspects. Clinically, the disease is inherited as an autosomal dominant with strong penetrance and an equal involvement of the two sexes. The disease begins early in childhood and often in infancy. Such children have spells during which they become unusually floppy and move poorly. In some, the sound of the child's crying changes. The parents may notice a staring appearance which the child develops either spontaneously or on exposure to cold. This is probably due to the eyelid myotonia which exposes the sclera on downward gaze.

The attacks are usually provoked by rest after exercise but, unlike the hypokalemic form, the weakness develops in a shorter time interval. In one patient, sitting in a chair after carrying out her household chores would cause a feeling of tiredness in the back and legs and within 30 minutes it would be difficult for her to arise from a chair. The onset of the weakness while sitting at a desk at school or while sitting in the theater has been described. The patient may be able to "walk off" the symptoms early in an attack. This postponement of an attack seems to be only temporary, and the maneuver is sometimes associated with the development of painful "knots" in the muscles (2). Many patients also prefer to allow an attack to develop because it will be followed by a period of relative freedom from weakness. At times, eating candy or taking a light meal postpones an attack.

There may be odd sensory complaints that vary from a full, heavy feeling in the legs to the occurrence of a "musty" odor preceding an attack (3). The wife of one patient commented that her husband's skin had a peculiar taste just before an attack. Others have noted that patients smell of ketone bodies during induced paralysis (4). The duration of the paralysis is said to be much briefer than in the hypokalemic form, and it usually lasts less than an hour. However, more prolonged attacks have also been described which are clinically indistinguishable from those in hypokalemic periodic paralysis. In my experience patients complain of two types of attack, "light" and "heavy." It is not uncommon for mild weakness to be present several days after an episode of paralysis. The frequency varies from two or three mild attacks a day to attacks which are separated by intervals of months.

Although it has been emphasized that hyperkalemic periodic paralysis is the milder form, the literature does not always bear this out. Permanent weakness is often found; it affects the abdominal muscles, the hip flexors, and then spreads to the other muscles of the legs and shoulders. In some this has been severe enough to keep the patient confined to a wheelchair. Some patients tell the story of a very slow but steady progress in weakness, upon which are superimposed briefer and more dramatic attacks of paralysis. In addition to rest after exercise, other provocative factors include exposure to cold, anesthesia, and sleep. The illness may also worsen during pregnancy.

The association of a form of myotonia with hyperkalemic paralysis is well recognized. Symptomatic myotonia suggests the diagnosis of hyperkalemic paralysis, but it is not exclusive to this disease and has been noted in the eyelids of patients with hypokalemic paralysis. The myotonia often involves the muscle of the face, eyes, and tongue as well as the hands. In order to demonstrate eyelid myotonia, the patient is asked to gaze upwards for a short period of time and then to look swiftly downwards. The eyelids "hang up" exposing the sclera and then slowly descend to their proper level as the myotonia relaxes. The stiffness is made worse by cold, and immersion of a limb in cool water can be used as a provocative test for this as well as for exacerbation of the paralysis. For the demonstration of eyelid myotonia it is helpful to lay a towel soaked in ice water across the eyes for a few minutes before carrying out the test. Symptomatically the patient may feel his face stiffen when he walks out in cold weather and the ocular myotonia may make it difficult to look from side to side. The similarity between this and paramyotonia congenita together with the episodic weakness which patients with paramyotonia congenita experience upon exposure to cold has led some to suggest that paramyotonia and hyperkalemic paralysis may be two aspects of the same disease. Families in which both types of illness are found lend credence to this view (5).

When a patient is examined during an attack, the muscles are inexcitable as in the hypokalemic form. Some evidence of nerve hyperexcitability may be seen in the presence of a Chvostek sign (1) in a minority of cases.

Laboratory Studies. The diagnosis may be established in hyperkalemic periodic paralysis by finding an elevated serum potassium during an attack of weakness. As in the hypokalemic form, patients become paralyzed with levels of serum potassium which would not be sufficient to affect the normal individual. Attacks are associated with the exit of potassium from muscle into the serum. This may be a local phenomenon and limited to the blood supply from paralyzed muscles, perhaps explaining why some patients with leg weakness may have a normal serum potassium when blood is drawn from the arm (3). It is not a complete explanation, however, since there are undoubtedly some who suffer from the disease with a normal potassium level in the face of generalized weakness. Pearson (6) found that 80% of a patient's attacks were associated with increased potassium, in 15% there was no change, and in 5% the potassium was actually decreased in the serum. Hourly monitoring of patients in the interictal period showed persistent elevation of the serum potassium levels. Over a period of 36 hours, at least 80% of the values were abnormal and wide swings in the levels were noted in the patients but not in controls (7).

The EKG may show the changes of hyperkalemia. The creatine kinase may also be elevated during an attack or in the interictal period. In the advanced case, muscle biopsy shows changes with variability in the size of fibers, internal nuclei, vacuoles, tubular aggregates, and bizarre distortions of the internal architecture. In milder cases, the biopsy may be normal or may demonstrate scattered tubular aggregates (Figs. 7.42–7.48). Physiological studies during an attack show slight depolarization of the muscle fibers (3, 8, 9). Decreased potassium levels in the muscle and an increase in the sodium, water, and chloride contents have been reported. Provocative testing for hyperkalemic periodic paralysis should be done with some caution. Potassium may only be given orally starting with a relatively small dose. The EKG should be monitored during the course of this test. An initial test should be done using approximately 0.05 g per kg body weight of potassium. This may be increased to 0.10 g per kg body weight on a subsequent occasion if there is no positive response and a maximum test of 0.15 g per kg body weight should be carried out only if preceding tests give no indication of weakness and the diagnosis of hyperkalemic periodic paralysis seems to be indicated on clinical grounds. The maximum rise in potassium occurs within 90–180 minutes after administration of the compound. Obviously, this test is not carried out in people with renal disease.

EMG may show myotonic runs or other irritable phenomena. During an attack, the muscle is inexcitable.

An in vitro evaluation of muscle fibers from patients was performed on intact muscle fibers obtained from the intercostal muscle (10). Two patients were studied, each with slightly different results. In one patient, there was a high level of spontaneous muscle activity even in the normal solution, increasing the external concentration of potassium gradually depolarized the cells but was associated with a paradoxical increase in the sodium conductance which was reversed by tetrodotoxin. The other patient's fibers failed to show any abnormal spontaneous activity. They were also paralyzed when the

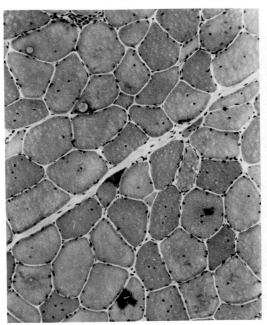 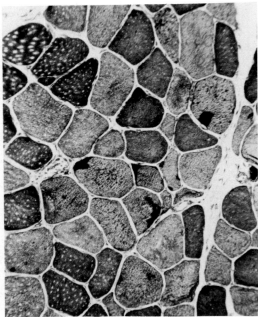

Figure 7.42 (*left*). Hyperkalemicperiodic periodic paralysis, biceps muscle. There is marked variation in the size of fibers with increased fibrosis and many internal nuclei. The darkly staining areas in the muscle fibers are tubular aggregates which are basophilic in this hematoxylin and eosin stain.

Figure 7.43 (*right*). This histochemical reaction for NADH-tetrazolium reductase highlights the tubular aggregates which are intensely dark areas in the muscle fibers. The small holes in the fibers are due to ice crystal artifact.

external potassium concentration was increased, but the mechanism was uncertain.

Treatment. Treatment of an acute attack is seldom necessary since many of them are mild and brief. Often patients themselves learn to drink a sweet drink (preferably not fruit juice) or to eat a candy bar. In the event of a more severe attack of weakness, intravenous calcium gluconate has been recommended. Intravenous sodium chloride may rarely abort an attack. Maintenance therapy on acetazolamide (Diamox) or chlorthiazide is helpful in decreasing the frequency of attacks. Acetazolamide has been shown to lessen the changes in serum potassium following provocative maneuvers (4), as well as to decrease the levels of serum potassium on a continuing basis (11). The combination of hydrochlorthiazide with potassium may be even more effective although the reason is unclear. Since acetazolamide is a sulfonamide, it should not be used in combination with other sulfonamides because of the dangers of renal damage. There are other possible side effects including tingling, nausea, and renal calculi. Dichlorphenamide, another carbonic anhydrase inhibitor, has been used in daily doses of 50–100 mg (12). Bendrofluazide, 5 mg daily, is also reported to be beneficial. None of these medicines improves the permanent fixed weakness which may develop.

Secondary Hyperkalemic Paralysis

Retention of potassium in the body is associated with many different symptoms, one of which is weakness. This weakness is seen only with

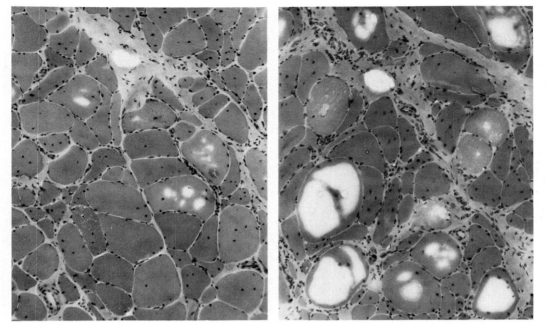

Figures 7.44 (*left*) and 7.45 (*right*). Hyperkalemic periodic paralysis. This is from the patient shown in Figure 7.42. This biopsy was from the quadriceps muscle which is more severely affected and shows variation in the size of fibers, fibrosis, and internal nuclei. Vacuoles are obvious and in some fibers replace most of the substance of the fiber.

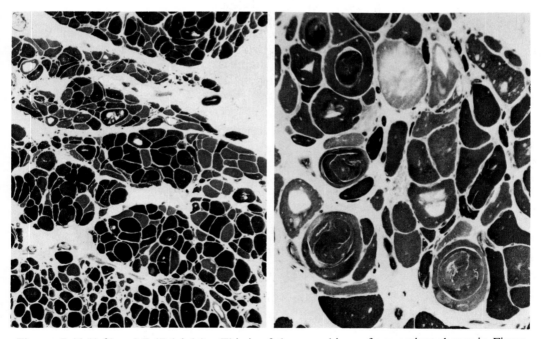

Figures 7.46 (*left*) and 7.47 (*right*). This is of the same biopsy from patient shown in Figure 7.42. The stain is a histochemical reaction for ATPase. Notice the marked variation in the size of the fibers and the vacuoles within the fibers. Bizarre distortions of the muscle fibers are occurring in addition to the vacuoles.

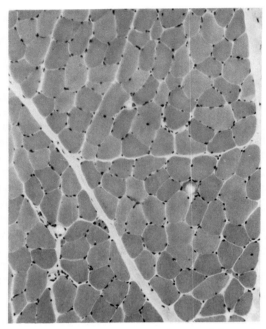

Figure 7.48.   A biopsy taken from the 11-year-old son of the patient shown in Figure 7.42. This boy also had periodic spells of weakness secondary to hyperkalemia. The changes in this biopsy are very mild. One fiber is undergoing vacuolar degeneration and in the lower right hand corner a small angulated fiber can be seen. Several other small fibers are scattered in the biopsy.

extremely high levels of potassium, and usually cardiac abnormalities take precedence over weakness. Causes include renal failure (when the associated uremia may mask the symptoms of hyperkalemia), adrenal failure, or the administration of potassium retaining diuretics. Possibly due to the potassium abnormality or to the associated metabolic abnormalities, muscle twitching and facial myokymia are not uncommon. The muscle is also unduly irritable to percussion.

REFERENCES

1. Gamstorp, I. Adynamia episodica hereditaria. Acta Paediatr. Scand. *45*(Suppl. 108): 1–126, 1956.
2. McArdle, B. Adynamia episodica hereditaria and its treatment. Brain *85:* 121–148, 1962.
3. Bradley, W. G. Adynamia episodica hereditaria: clinical, pathological and electrophysiological studies in an affected family. Brain *92:* 345–378, 1969.
4. Hoskins, B. and Vroom, F. Q. Hyperkalemic periodic paralysis: effects of potassium, exercise, glucose and acetazolamide on blood chemistry. Arch. Neurol. *32:* 519–523, 1975.
5. Layzer, R. B., Lovelace, R. E., and Rowland, L. P. Hyperkalemic periodic paralysis. Arch. Neurol. *16:* 455–472, 1967.
6. Pearson, C. M. Periodic paralysis: differential features and pathological observations in permanent myopathic weakness. Brain *87:* 341–353, 1964.
7. Lewis, E. D., Griggs, R. C., and Moxley, R. T. Regulation of plasma potassium in hyperkalemic periodic paralysis. Neurology *29:* 1131–1137, 1979.
8. Creutzfeldt, O. D., Abbott, B. C., Fowler, W. M., and Pearson, C. M. Muscle membrane potentials in episodic adynamia. Electroencephalogr. Clin. Neurophysiol. *15:* 508–519, 1963.
9. Brooks, J. E. Hyperkalemic periodic paralysis: intracellular electromyographic studies. Arch. Neurol. *20:* 13–18, 1969.
10. Lemann-Horn, F., Rudel, R., Ricker, K., Lorkovic, H., Dengler, R., and Hopf, H. C. Two cases of adynamia episodica hereditaria: in vitro investigation of muscle cell membrane and contraction parameters. Muscle Nerve *6:* 113–121, 1983.

11. Riggs, J. E., Griggs, R. C., Moxley, R. T., and Lewis, E. D. Acute effects of acetazolamide in hyperkalemic periodic paralysis. Neurology *31:* 725–729, 1981.
12. McArdle, B. Metabolic and endocrine myopathies. In: *Disorders of Voluntary Muscle,* edited by J. N. Walton. Churchill-Livingstone, London, 1974.

Normokalemic Periodic Paralysis

It is difficult to know whether this is an entity in its own right or whether the reports cited are of slightly atypical varieties of hyperkalemic paralysis, a disease to which it bears a suspicious resemblance. At all events, it must be a rare disease as there have been very few reports following the description by Poskanzer and Kerr (1) of a type of episodic paralysis which had its onset in childhood, was associated with normal serum levels of potassium, and responded to treatment with 9-fluorohydrocortisone and acetazolamide. The weakness was exacerbated by potassium and relieved by sodium chloride.

In 1951 Tyler et al. (2) described a large kindred with a variety of periodic paralysis which differed from the previously recognized hypokalemic variety not only in the clinical picture but also in the response to provocative stimulation with glucose and insulin. It was noted that the potassium in the serum was not reduced during the attacks. The administration of potassium, although it did not cause an attack, was unpopular with the patients, who felt worse on receiving this medication. The provocative effect of rest after exercise was noted, as well as the ability of the patients to "fight off" an attack by continued activity. The initial attacks occurred during the first year of life and were easily recognized by affected parents. The comment was made that the episodes were more frequent during childhood and then decreased in severity with advancing age. The presence or absence of myotonia was not commented on, but no symptoms of myotonia were elicited.

I have seen four members of this kindred not included in the original report. They were a father and son and a mother and son from two separate branches of the family. Interestingly, neither knew of the others' existence although they were both aware that the illness ran in the family. All four had symptoms of myotonia and periodic bouts of weakness. The attacks of paralysis were associated with elevation of potassium, and the administration of potassium to one patient produced unequivocal weakness. Electrical myotonia was present at rest and was exacerbated on exposure to cold. The oldest patient was confined to a wheelchair, whereas the youngest one merely has slight difficulty arising from the floor. The disease appears to be the hyperkalemic variety although the poor response to treatment exhibited by one patient is noteworthy.

Another report detailed the occurrence of episodic weakness in a mother and son (3). Serum potassium levels were normal and the muscle biopsy showed tubular aggregates. The authors commented on the similarity between their patients and those in the report of Tyler et al.

REFERENCES

1. Poskanzer, D. C., and Kerr, D. N. S. A third type of periodic paralysis, with normokalemia and a favorable response to sodium chloride. Am. J. Med. *31:* 328–342, 1961.
2. Tyler, F. H., Stephens, F. E., Gunn, F. D., and Perkoff, G. T. Studies in disorders of muscle; VII. Clinical manifestations and inheritance of a type of periodic paralysis without hypopotassemia. J. Clin. Invest. *30:* 492–502, 1951.
3. Meyers, K. R., Gilden, D. H., Rinaldi, C. F., and Hansen, J. L. Periodic muscle weakness, normokalemia and tubular aggregates. Neurology *22:* 269–279, 1972.

"ENDOCRINE" MYOPATHIES

Hyperthyroidism

Disorders of thyroid function cause a multitude of different symptoms, and muscle involvement is often minor and overlooked by the patient. On rare occasions the neuromuscular symptoms predominate, but even then other signs of thyroid disorder are usually to be found. Patients with thyrotoxicosis may develop proximal weakness with some muscular wasting. The shoulders are often more affected than the hips. The reflexes may be preserved. The majority of patients with thyrotoxicosis probably have some muscle involvement (1). Although this usually occurs in the adult, it may also be seen in children (2). The older literature describes the spontaneous occurrence of muscle twitching, the so-called "fasciculating myopathy of thyrotoxicosis." However, this entity may be largely mythical since electromyography does not typically reveal fasciculations. In one case in which obvious twitching was noted, myokymia was found to be the cause (3). Neither the muscle biopsy nor the EMG give any further clues as to the underlying etiology; although abnormalities are seen in both studies, these are nonspecific. The serum creatine kinase may be normal. Treatment of the thyrotoxicosis usually alleviates the muscle symptoms. Biochemical studies of mitochondrial function have been carried out, but again fail to give precise information on the way in which the disease occurs (4).

A common complication of thyrotoxicosis is exophthalmic ophthalmoplegia with associated abnormalities in the extraocular muscles. Standard texts should be consulted for further description of this illness.

Hypothyroidism

Patients with hypothyroidism also have signs of muscular abnormality. The best known is a peculiar change in contractility of the muscles. When a deep tendon reflex is elicited, instead of prompt relaxation after the initial contraction, the relaxation phase is slowed. Thus, when an ankle jerk is obtained, the prompt return of the foot to its resting position is replaced by a slow drift. In patients whose muscular symptoms are marked, not only may there be delay in relaxation but stiffness and cramps may be found and the muscle may hypertrophy. Myedema is found, but percussion myotonia is not part of the picture. Electromyography may demonstrate increased insertional activity with trains of repetitive activity, but true myotonia is not found.

In children, the disease is associated with an impressive hypertrophy and seems to occur more often in boys than in girls (Kocher-Debre-Semelaigne syndrome) (5). Some authors have been impressed by the fact that these children are unusually strong (6). The development of the illness may be related to the duration and the severity of the hypothyroid state; after treatment the muscle bulk returns to normal, although the strength does not change. In adults, the symptoms are similar although the occurrence of painful cramps is more noticeable, and there is an impressive elevation of serum CK. Again, the disease usually responds to appropriate treatment of the hypothyroid condition.

Associated Disorders

Thyroid dysfunction has as adverse an effect on the strength of patients with muscle disease as on that of normal patients. It is not surprising that patients with various forms of weakness may become worse if their thyroid function is abnormal. There are two diseases which are more commonly associated with thyroid disturbance than can be explained purely by chance. Exacerbations of myasthenia gravis are sometimes associated with the onset of dysthyroid states, and the onset of the one should be sufficient grounds to consider the possibility of the other.

Hypokalemic periodic paralysis may also be seen with thyrotoxicosis. Males suffer from the illness more than females and almost 85% of the cases occur in the third and fourth decades. Ninety-five per cent of cases are sporadic, and the vacuolar myopathy which is often noted in the other varieties is uncommon in thyrotoxic periodic paralysis. Pharmacologically the disease has a different reaction to intra-arterial epinephrine. In familial periodic paralysis the intra-arterial injection of minute amounts of epinephrine is said to cause a prompt paralysis of the arm, even in the absence of attacks, whereas in thyrotoxic periodic paralysis, patients tolerate epinephrine without such paralysis (7).

Parathyroid Dysfunction

Tetany is the only neuromuscular complication of hypoparathyroidism, but neuromuscular symptoms in hyperparathyroidism have been described frequently (8–10). Cystic bone disease, kidney stones, renal failure, peptic ulceration, pancreatitis, and mental disturbances are most often thought of as the presenting complaints of patients with hyperparathyroidism, but a significant number of patients also have muscular weakness. The incidence of this weakness in hyperparathyroidism is difficult to ascertain, but it may be as high as 75–80%, although it may be overshadowed by the more dramatic effects of the disease. Patients experience fatigue as well as aching in the muscles and may have overt weakness and wasting of the proximal muscles. The hips are usually more involved than the shoulders. The deep tendon reflexes are not only preserved but may be hyperactive. At least two reports stress that the illness may simulate a primary neuromuscular disorder (8, 10). Some patients have bulbar findings, with hoarseness, fasciculations of the tongue, and dysarthria. These when combined with axial weakness, hyperreflexia, and, in some patients, extensor plantar responses simulate motor neuron disease. In some patients these symptoms respond to correction of the hyperparathyroidism. The possibility that the patients actually had motor neuron disease as well as hyperparathyroidism is not totally excluded. In addition to primary hyperparathyroidism, patients with other forms of osteomalacia may experience similar weakness. The administration of vitamin D seems to help such patients considerably. The severity of the disease does not seem to be correlated with the calcium or phosphate levels in the blood, and the exact mechanism whereby weakness occurs is again unknown. The most helpful laboratory tests are those designed to uncover the hyperparathyroid abnormalities. Changes seen on the muscle biopsy suggest some denervation, but Type 2 atrophy is prominent.

Adrenal and Pituitary Dysfunction

Muscle weakness is part of the clinical picture of acromegaly and Cushing's syndrome. It is also present in Addison's disease and is seen with the administration of steroids, particularly the halogenated compounds. All of these situations are associated with a rather nonspecific muscle weakness which is usually proximal and which responds to the correction of the underlying abnormality. The muscle biopsy in these conditions usually reveals Type 2 fiber atrophy, another nonspecific change (11).

REFERENCES

1. Ramsay, I. D. Muscle dysfunction in hyperthyroidism. Lancet *2:* 931–934, 1966.
2. Johnston, D. M. Thyrotoxic myopathy. Arch. Dis. Child. *49:* 968–969, 1974.
3. Harman, J. B. and Richardson, A. T. Generalized myokymia in thyrotoxicosis. Lancet *2:* 473–474, 1954.
4. Peter, J. B. In "Hyperthyroidism," Solomon, D. H. (moderator). Ann. Intern Med. *69:* 1015–1035, 1968.
5. Najjar, S. S. Muscular hypertrophy in hypothyroid children; the Kocher-Debre-Semelaigne syndrome. J. Pediatr. *85:* 236–239, 1974.
6. Hopwood, N. J., Lockhart, L. H., and Bryan, G. T. Acquired hypothyroidism with muscular hypertrophy and precocious testicular enlargement. J. Pediatr. *85:* 233–236, 1974.
7. Engel, A. G. Neuromuscular manifestations of Graves' disease. Mayo Clin. Proc. *47:* 919–925, 1972.
8. Smith, R., and Stern, G. Myopathy osteomalacia and hyperparathyroidism. Brain *90:* 593–602, 1967.
9. Cholod, D. J., Haust, M. D., Hudson, A. J., and Lewis, F. N. Myopathy in primary familial hyperparathyroidism. Am. J. Med. *48:* 700–707, 1970.
10. Patten, B. M., Bilezikian, J. P., Mallette, L. E., Prince, A., Engel, W. K., and Aurbach, G. D. Neuromuscular disease in primary hyperparathyroidism. Ann. Intern. Med. *80:* 182–193, 1974.
11. Pleasure, D. E., Walsh, G. O., and Engel, W. K. Atrophy of skeletal muscle in patients with Cushing's syndrome. Arch. Neurol. *22:* 118–125, 1970.

NUTRITIONAL AND TOXIC MYOPATHIES

Man is spared some of the muscle diseases which affect other animals as a result of nutritional deficiencies. Thus the presence or absence of vitamin E, selenium, and other compounds is not recognized as a clinical problem. There are, of course, nutritional deficiencies such as are seen with protein deprivation and starvation, but these are not selectively muscle diseases. The nutritional myopathies of man seem to be a result not so much of what is missing from the diet as of what is added. Alcohol remains one of the commonest, and alcoholic myopathy is now well recognized and well described (1, 2). The typical illness takes one of two forms: either an acute attack of muscle pain, swelling, and weakness after "binge" drinking or a more chronic, rather slowly progressive proximal weakness in alcoholics who maintain a steady intake. In some patients there is evidence of muscle destruction resulting in elevation of serum creatine kinase levels without any overt signs or symptoms.

In the acute alcoholic myopathy, after a bout of enthusiastic drinking the patient may experience the sudden onset of pain and swelling in the muscles. This usually affects the thigh muscles, but other large muscle groups may be involved. The muscle is tense, swollen, and exquisitely tender. Weakness can be profound and there may be associated myoglobinuria. Renal failure may ensue, and the disease should be treated the same way as any acute myoglobinuria. Such an attack may resolve completely, or there may be residual weakness.

In patients with chronic alcoholic myopathy, the weakness is usually of the legs, although occasionally additional weakness of the shoulders is seen. This picture is sometimes superimposed on a preceding history of acute alcoholic myopathy, although it may be difficult to obtain such a story from the patient. In some chronic alcoholics whose acute myopathy has been documented, a later visit to the clinic with the chronic syndrome has revealed no memory of the acute attacks. In addition to the rather typical clinical picture, the muscle biopsy may show a variety of changes, all of them unfortunately nonspecific. There may be muscle breakdown in the same fashion as in other patients with myoglobinuria, and there may be more peculiar alterations such as the tubular aggregates described by Chui et al. (3). An unexplained chemical abnormality is the failure to develop a normal rise of lactate with ischemic exercise and a deficiency in the activity of phosphorylase in the muscle.

Other chemicals have been associated with muscle breakdown. Chloroquine and vincristine may be associated with a myopathy. The myotonia associated with the administration of diazacholesterol is known in both experimental and therapeutic situations. Clofibrate may produce muscle cramps, although the mechanism is not known, and toxins such as plasmocid and ε-aminocaproate are also associated with muscle breakdown. Such patients, however, rarely present to a muscle clinic and usually the etiology is obvious.

REFERENCES

1. Ekbom, K. Hed, R., Kirstein, L., and Astrom, K. E. Muscular affections in chronic alcoholism. Arch. Neurol. *10:* 449–458, 1964.
2. Perkoff, G. T. Alcoholic myopathy. Ann. Rev. Med. *22:* 125–132, 1971.
3. Chui, L. A., Neustein, H., and Munsat, T. L. Tubular aggregates in subclinical alcoholic myopathy. Neurology *25:* 405–412, 1975.

8   abnormal muscle activity

Abnormal and repetitive muscle activity occurs as part of many different diseases. Myokymia is not infrequently seen in abnormal metabolic states. Carpopedal spasms are a part of calcium deficiency, and myotonia may occur in acid maltase deficiency. There are two clinical syndromes in which abnormal muscle activity in the muscle is the dominant part of the illness. The first of these has come to be known as the stiff-man syndrome, and the second as continuous muscle fiber activity. In both of these conditions there is sustained repetitive activity of muscle fibers.

STIFF-MAN SYNDROME

A muscle cramp is a not uncommon experience in normal people. The physiology of this phenomenon is unclear, but it seems to be associated with an unduly powerful, voluntary contraction of a muscle, especially when it is held in a shortened position. The muscle then sustains an excruciatingly painful contraction of its own volition. Fortunately for most of us the threshold to produce such an unpleasant phenomenon is high. In the stiff-man syndrome it is as if this threshold were lowered, and extraordinary and disabling cramps are produced in many muscle groups under slight, or even no, provocation. It is not known whether the normal physiological cramp and the abnormal muscle activity in the stiff-man syndrome have the same origin, but it is perhaps a useful way to remember the clinical stigmata of the disease.

Clinical Aspects

The illness was first described by Moersch and Woltman (1). Since then, many reports have appeared in the literature, and a review of these has presented a composite and rather typical picture (2–4). The disease is usually one of adult life and affects both men and women. There may be some preceding aching and tightness of the back and chest muscles before the full manifestation of the illness. Firm and uncontrollable contractions of the muscles, particularly of the hips, thighs, and shoulders then ensue, and these may spread to all the muscles of the body. Facial grimacing, difficulty with swallowing, and difficulty with breathing may be noted. The contractions themselves are unlike any produced voluntarily. The limbs are held rigid and immobile, the bellies of the muscles stand out in sharp relief and feel as if carved out from wood. The limb is usually held in a distorted position since the most powerful muscles in the limb overcome the antagonistic action of other muscles. The foot, for example, is often held in a position of inversion and plantar flexion since the slender muscles in the anterior compartment are no match for the bulky gastrocnemius and soleus group.

The spasms are extremely painful and may cause the patient to cry out aloud. During the worst of them, voluntary movements are not possible and the patient is totally immobilized. Some idea of the force which the contracting muscle exerts is illustrated by the fact that fractures of the long bones have occurred during such spasm. Stiffness disappears entirely during sleep and during general anesthesia but reoccurs following many different stimuli. These include voluntary movement, passive movement of the limb, emotional stress, and even the sudden appearance of visitors in the room. Although the symptoms disappear during sleep, the patient may wake frequently during the night, and when he does so the spasms return promptly.

The physical examination reveals no neurological abnormalities other than occasional increase in the reflexes and, rarely, extensor plantar responses. The latter should not be accepted automatically as part of the syndrome and may indicate other pathology.

A condition in which the abnormalities resemble the cramps which the patient can produce by voluntary movement, which disappear during sleep, and which are associated with normal electromyographic (EMG) pattern may make the examiner suspect that hysteria is the basis for this disease. It is unlikely, however, that the hysteric would have the fortitude to produce contractions strong enough to break long bones, and these titanic contractions take the disease out of the realm of the more gentle symptoms which the average hysteric manifests. Another intriguing question which is not yet answered about this illness is whether it exists in a subclinical form. Many patients who have aches, cramps, and pains of their limbs also have some degree of stiffness. Although there has been a tendency in the past to dismiss these patients as having functional disease, it is possible that they represent subclinical variety of the stiff man syndrome. It is wise to remember that strychnine and tetanus may also produce abnormal muscle spasms.

Laboratory Studies

EMG examination shows a sustained interference pattern that persists in spite of all attempts to relax the muscle. Electroencephalographic investigation has shown an abnormality in the sleep pattern with less REM sleep than usual. These patients rarely attain stage three or stage four sleep (5).

The spasms are easily abolished by curarization, block of the peripheral nerve with local anesthetic, or spinal anesthesia. In some patients, excretion of an abnormal metabolite perhaps derived from norepinephrine has been reported (6). The origin of the disease is not clear. It has been ascribed to an overactivity of the gamma (γ) efferent system. A selective block of the γ system by Xylocaine, which was not sufficient to cause paralysis of the limb, abolished the spasms. This possible abnormality of γ motor neurons was said to be due to a persistent drive from suprasegmental areas. The block of the γ efferent system produced by Xylocaine would remove the tonic "driving" of the intrafusal fibers and might be expected to decrease the reflex evoked activity of the alpha (α) motor neurons. Others have felt that the disease is caused by some loss of the inhibitory influence from interneurons or by a deficiency in Renshaw cell function preventing the normal inhibitory feedback on anterior horn cells. An imbalance between a catecholaminergic and γ-aminobutyric acid (GABA) system has also been proposed (5). Defective activity of the interneuronal inhibitory pool might impair the release of

GABA and cause overactivity of the catecholaminergic neurons. A tentative beneficial effect of baclofen, a derivative of GABA, gives some slight support to this view.

Treatment

This is one neuromuscular disease for which an effective form of treatment is known. The use of high doses of diazepam is recommended (7). The dose necessary to give relief of the symptoms may be 300 mg a day or even higher. For some patients the side effects of this dose are too great to allow the drug to be used. Others tolerate enormous doses without any side effects. The drug takes some days before it exerts its maximum effect. Clonazepam has also been shown to be of use in the treatment of this illness (8).

REFERENCES

1. Moersch, F. P., and Woltman, H. W.: Progressive fluctuating muscular rigidity and spasm (stiff man syndrome). Proc. Staff Meet. Mayo Clin. *31*: 421–427, 1956.
2. Gordon, E. E., Januszko, D. M., and Kaufman, L. A critical survey of the stiff man syndrome. Am. J. Med. *42*: 582–599, 1967.
3. Franck, G., Cornett, M., Grisar, T., Moonen, G., and Gerebtzoff, M. A. Le syndrome de l'homme raide. Acta Neurol. Belg. *74*: 221–240, 1974.
4. Spehlman, R., and Norcross, K. Stiff-man syndrome. Clin. Pharmacol. *4*: 109–121, 1979.
5. Guilleminault, C., Sigwald, J., and Castaigne, E. Sleep studies and therapeutic trial with L-dopa in a case of stiff-man syndrome. Eur. Neurol. *10*: 89–96, 1973.
6. Schmidt, R. T., Stahl, S. M., and Spehlmann, R. A pharmacologic study of the stiff-man syndrome. Neurology *25*: 622–626, 1975.
7. Howard, F. M. A new and effective drug in the treatment of stiff-man syndrome. Mayo Clin. Proc. *38*: 203–212, 1963.
8. Mamoli, B., Heiss, W. D., Maida, E., and Podreska, I. Electrophysiological studies on the "stiff-man" syndrome. J. Neurol. *217*: 111–121, 1979.

CONTINUOUS MUSCLE FIBER ACTIVITY (NEUROMYOTONIA)

Another condition in which the motor unit has a tendency to discharge spontaneously is known as continuous muscle fiber activity (1, 2). This entity has been known under many different names and may be present with varying degrees of severity. Perhaps in the same way that the stiff-man syndrome may be thought of as an extension of the sometimes normal phenomenon of muscle cramping, continuous muscle fiber activity may be an extension of the normal phenomenon of fasciculations or at least an extension of the tendency of the motor unit to discharge spontaneously. In its mildest forms, it occurs as myokymia. This is a brief contraction of parts of the muscle, a phenomenon which is difficult to distinguish from fasciculations, and indeed the words in the past have been used interchangeably. There is, however, an important point of distinction when electrical studies are carried out. A fasciculation is an isolated motor unit discharge and, although it may be repetitive, the interval between individual fasciculations of the same motor unit are quite prolonged. In myokymia, one or more motor units discharge in rapid sequence. Thus, short bursts of action potentials are seen on the EMG and are associated with brief tetanic contractions of the muscle fibers. The frequency of these trains of motor units varies from roughly 10 to 100 Hz. The length of the trains also varies from doublets and triplets to sustained bursts lasting several seconds. The appearance of the muscle during these times is of a quivering, undulating "bag of worms." When the myokymic trains are prolonged, they are easy to differentiate from fasciculations because the strip of muscle that is contracting does so over a longer period of time and does not resemble the brief twitch of a fasciculation. On the other hand, brief myokymic trains are impossible to distinguish with the naked eye from the contraction seen with a fasciculations.

Clinical Aspects

In the mild form of the disease the patient suffers no particular handicap. The movements may be disturbing since the patient is aware of them and they may keep him awake at night. The myokymia does not disappear during sleep. There may be difficulty relaxing the muscle after a voluntary contraction. In the most severe form, stiffness is present at rest and impedes movement. When walking, the patient may give the impression of wading through a sea of molasses. The disease occurs at any age, even during the neonatal period (3). There is usually no precipitating cause and most of the cases occur sporadically.

The symptoms often start gradually with a period of increasing stiffness, frequently in the legs. In one or two cases muscle pains have been noted (4). The patient notices the twitching movements in the legs and may also complain of excessive sweating. This is perhaps related to the necessary dissipation of heat generated by the constant muscle activity, but its exact cause is unclear. With increasing symptoms, the body becomes stiff and the wrists are flexed with the fingers extended. The feet turn into an equinus position. The patient may have a stooped posture because of the rigidity. When the patient tries to move, the stiffness is quite variable. Initially it may increase and then decrease again, waxing and waning throughout the course of movement. Laryngeal stridor has been noted in one patient (5).

The abnormal tone and myokymia do not disappear during sleep. The fact that they are not altered during spinal block, during Pentothal anesthesia, or by proximal nerve block has suggested that the defect was in the distal part of the motor unit. Subsequent reports, in fact, showed that both epidural and periheral nerve block markedly decreased the abnormal activity (6). A motor point infiltration with Xylocaine reduces the activity although it does not abolish it completely. Curarization is associated with abolition of the spontaneous activity. Sometimes the muscle fiber activity is also absent for a few seconds after voluntary contraction. In several patients, peripheral wasting has been noted, perhaps further evidence of a neuropathic problem in this illness. An increased level of GABA was found in the spinal fluid of one patient (6). A possibly related condition has been described in two families with sustained muscle stiffness and myokymia without evidence of damage to the peripheral nerves. There was repetitive after discharges in the muscle following a single shock to the nerve or percussing the nerve and the disorder seemed to originate in the peripheral nerve since it could not be altered by proximal nerve block (7).

Laboratory Studies

The EMG abnormalities are characteristic and have already been described. The pathology is obscure, but most of the cases have shown not only physiological evidence of damage to the peripheral nerves but pathological evidence with signs of deneration and reinnervation in the muscle as well as anatomical changes in the peripheral nerve. In two cases, abnormal chemicals have been incriminated. In a severe case in an infant, a derivative of DDT was found in the serum and in another case (4) exposure to the herbicide 2,4-D was noted. These two cases may closely resemble myotonia which can be produced experimentally by 2,4-D.

Treatment

The treatment of the disease with diphenylhydantoin has been remarkably successful and in patients with myokymia alone as well as those with fully developed syndrome, the administration of diphenylhydantoin has removed the symptoms. Carbamazepine (Tegretol) and dantrolene sodium have been reported to help (6, 8).

REFERENCES

1. Issacs, H. A syndrome of continuous muscle fiber activity. J. Neurol. Neurosurg. Psychiatry *24*: 319–325, 1961.
2. Mertens, H. G., and Zschocke, S. Neuromyotonie. Klin. Wochenschr. *17*: 917–925, 1965.
3. Black, J. T., Garcia-Mullin, R., Good, R., and Brown, S. Muscle rigidity in a newborn due to continuous peripheral nerve hyperactivity. Arch. Neurol. *27*: 413–425, 1972.
4. Wallis, W. E., Van Poznak, A., and Plum, F. Generalized muscular stiffness, fasciculations and myokymia of peripheral nerve origin. Arch. Neurol. *22*: 430–439, 1970.
5. Levinson, S., Canalis, R. F., and Kaplan, H. J. Laryngeal spasm complicating pseudomyotonia. Arch. Otolaryngol. *102*: 185–187, 1976.
6. Sakai, T., Hosokawa, S., Shibasaki, H., Goto, I., Kuroiwa, Y., Sonoda, H., and Murai, Y. Syndrome of continuous muscle fiber activity: increased CSF GABA and effect of dantrolene. Neurology *33*: 495–498, 1983.
7. Auger, R. G., Daube, J. R., Gamez, M. R., and Lambert, E. H. Hereditary form of sustained muscle activity of peripheral nerve origin causing generalized myokymia and muscle stiffness. Ann. Neurol. *15*: 13–21, 1984.
8. Issacs, H., and Heffron, J. J. A. The syndrome of "continuous muscle fiber activity cured: further studies. J. Neurol. Neurosurg. Psychiatry *37*: 1231–1235, 1974.

Neurological Causes of Increased Muscle Tone

There are obviously many causes of muscular rigidity and increased tone. In most cases, the central origin of this rigidity is obvious. It is difficult to mistake Parkinson's disease for disorders of the peripheral nerves, for example. On the other hand, there are disorders of the central nervous system which give very prominent peripheral manifestations. One of these is exemplified by Leigh et al. (1) of a man with a reflex myoclonic jerks which occurred every few seconds for periods up to 5 hours and in bouts which occurred every day. Superimposed upon this was severe rigidity of the abdominal, paraspinal, and leg muscles sufficient to alter the posture of the patient and cause difficulty in walking. As in the stiff-man syndrome, the disorder was markedly helped by diazepam. The disorder appeared to be secondary to central nervous system involvement since the radiologic studies showed severe cerebellar atrophy and an enlarged fourth ventricle.

REFERENCE

1. Leigh, P. N., Rothwell, J. C., Traub, M., and Marsden, C. D. A patient with reflex myoclonus and muscle rigidity: "jerking stiff-man" syndrome. J. Neurol. Neurosrug. Psychiatry *43*: 1125–1131, 1980.

SCHWARTZ-JAMPEL SYNDROME
(CHONDRODYSTROPHIC MYOTONIA)

This syndrome is easier to recognize than it is to describe (Figs. 8.1–8.3). It is a congenital disorder in which chondrodystrophy and epiphyseal dysplasia is superimposed on an abnormality of muscle activity, which superficially resembles myotonia. The children are short statured with short necks. Pectus carinatum is characteristic with the sternum shaped like the prow of a boat. There is marked facial dysmorphism with micrognathia, narrowed papebral fissures, low set ears, dental abnormalities, and double rows of eyelashes. Some intellectual impairment may be noted. The muscles are often enlarged and firm. Myotonia-like contraction can be noted in the face causing dimpling of the chin and blepharospasm. Often the lips are pursed. The children move somewhat stiffly. Accompanying the muscle abnormalities, there may contractures of joints such as the elbows. Careful electromyography with both the concentric needle and with single fiber recordings, differentiates the spontaneous activity from myotonia (1). The abnormal activity takes the form of runs of complex potentials which do not have the waxing and waning characteristic of myotonia. During complete relaxation (which is seldom possible given the age of which these children are usually studied) there is electrical silence, although the least voluntary movement again kindles the repetitive discharges. Curare abolishes these trains and the activity of the nerve clearly has something to do with the phenomenon. Jablecki and Schultz (1) suggested that the discharges arise by ephaptic transmission from adjacent muscle fibers which sets up reverberating impulses instead of one "clean" action potential. Little is known of the origin of this illness. Occasional reports of immunologic abnormalities have not been confirmed (2, 3). Treatment with growth hormone has been unavailing and no other treatment has proved useful (4).

REFERENCES

1. Jableki, C., and Schultz, P. Single muscle fiber recordings in Schwartz-Jampel syndrome. Muscle Nerve 5: S64–69, 1982.
2. Stewart, S. R., Gershwim, M. E., Fowler, W. M., and Taylor, R. Immunologic profile of the Schwartz-Jampel (osteochondromuscular dystrophy) syndrome. J. Pediatr. 96: 958–959, 1980.
3. Mollica, F., Messina, A., Stivala, F., and Pavone, L. Immunodeficiency in Schwartz-Jampel syndrome. Acta Pediatr. Scand. 68: 133–135, 1979.
4. Edwards, W. C., and Root, A. W. Chondrodystrophic myotonia (Schwartz-Jampel syndrome): report of a new case and follow-up with patients initially reported in 1969. Am. J. Med. Genet. 13: 51–56, 1982.

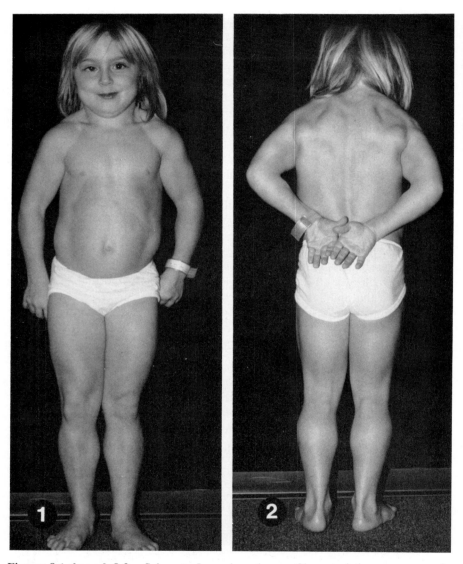

Figures 8.1 through 8.3. Schwartz-Jampel syndrome. Characteristic appearance of a patient with Schwartz-Jampel syndrome. Notice the overdevelopment of many of the muscles.

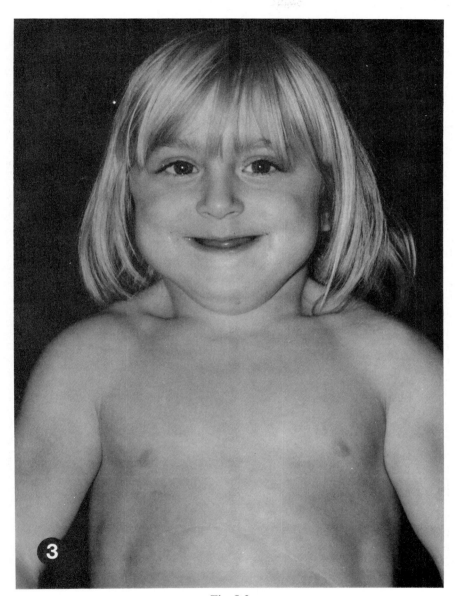

Fig. 8.3

9

congenital (more or less) muscle diseases

The ungainly title to the chapter is a measure of the uncertainty associated with diseases described herein. Originally the chapter was to be entitled, "Congenital Nonprogressive Myopathies," but although most are congenital many are in fact progressive, and the evidence that these illnesses are primarily of the muscle itself is shaky. "Morphologically Distinct Myopathies" was equally inexact since the morphology by which they are distinguished may, in fact, represent epiphenomena in the muscle rather than any fundamental part of the disease. The ideal solution, a chapter entitled "Other," seemed somehow escapist. In some of these illnesses, such as the congenital hypotonias, the pathology is uncertain although the clinical picture is better described. In others, the abnormalities in the muscle are so striking thay they are embodied in the name of the disease. In yet others, such as the congenital dystrophies, we are certain neither of the clinical picture nor of the pathological changes, although certain patterns are beginning to emerge. The first section will deal with floppy infants, excluding children such as those with infantile spinal muscular atrophy, whose diseases have been described in preceding chapters. This will be followed by discussion of the various illnesses characterized by peculiar structural alterations, such as central core disease and nemaline myopathy.

CONGENITAL HYPOTONIA

Observation of the way in which a baby moves and the postures adopted by its limbs, together with an evaluation of the passive tone, are the most useful tests of muscle function in the newborn period. Poverty of movement, the assumption of abnormal postures, and a reduction in the baby's tone are the characteristics of the floppy infant. Such infants may have respiratory difficulties at birth and shortly afterwards are noted to be lying with the limbs externally rotated and abducted, the so-called "frog leg" position. The hypotonia is expressed in various ways. When the child is pulled by his hands from the supine position the head falls backwards in extreme extension. When supported under the abdomen and lifted from the bed (ventral suspension) the hypotonia causes the child to droop in an inverted "U." A more precise description is given elsewhere (1). Hypotonia may be due to causes other than abnormalities of the neuromuscular system; mental retardation and other forms of cerebral damage being among the commonest. Myasthenia, either congenital or neonatal, as well as infantile botulism are abnormalities of the neuromuscular junction which cause hypotonia in the newborn child. Obviously any disorder of muscle, such as the infantile metabolic disorders, may be associated with marked floppiness. These are all discussed in preceding sections. A substantial number of floppy babies have no clear weakness. In some this is due to abnormalities of cerebral function, the cause in others can be categorized in to one of three main groups: benign congenital hypotonia, the Prader-Willi syndrome, and congenital hypotonia associated with Type 1 fiber predominance.

Hypotonia Due to Suprasegmental Factors

Abnormalities of the brain and of those higher centers which control muscle function would be expected to have a profound effect on muscle tone. Probably the majority of floppy infants have a suprasegmental cause of their illness. Often a history of perinatal hypoxia will be found. The older these infants become, the more apparent it is that their mental function lags behind the normal and their delay in motor abilities is simply one aspect of much more global damage. These babies demonstrate the nonparalytic hypotonia described by Dubowitz (1). Thus although the child may appear weak and floppy when carried by his mother or picked up by the examining physician, spontaneous movements of the arms and legs occur readily enough against gravity. The deep tendon reflexes are sometimes absent, but the presence of brisk tendon jerks in a hypotonic child almost clinches the impression of "cerebral hypotonia." A muscle biopsy in these children shows selective atrophy of Type 2 fibers but little else (Fig 9.1).

Benign Congenital Hypotonia

In 1900 it was recognized that there were floppy children who differed from the patients described by Werdnig and Hoffmann and by Brandt by a clinical course which was more benign and did not terminate in death. Oppenheim

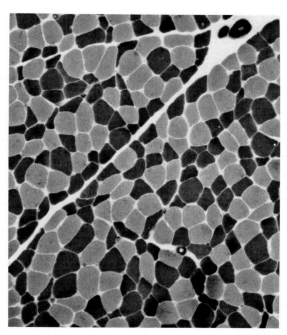

Figure 9.1. Selective atrophy of Type 2 fibers. This photograph is of a routine ATPase stain and demonstrates that most of the small fibers are dark or Type 2.

suggested the name "myatonia" for this type of illness and, for the next 50 years, such children were variously termed as having myatonia congenita or amyotonia congenita (the latter name was also used for children with Werdnig-Hoffmann disease).

The term benign congenital hypotonia was coined by Walton (2) in a report on the fate of 109 cases of "amyotonia congenita." In a sense, this article ushered in the modern period in neuromuscular diseases. Walton began with the comment, "For more than half a century our approach to these disorders has been dominated by terms and concepts which by continued use have come to be regarded as valid explanations rather than tentative labels." Even though the title of his article was "Amyotonia Congenita," Walton suggested that the term be abandoned.

Seventeen of the cases Walton described seemed to have a relatively benign disease resembling Oppenheim's original description. Recognizing the confusion which existed in the literature, Walton suggested the use of the term benign congenital hypotonia. In a subsequent article the 17 patients were presented in more detail (3). About half of them recovered completely, whereas the others remained moderately disabled. The symptoms which were characteristic of the illness were the onset of hypotonia in the infantile period, hypermobility of the joints, and a uniform delay in the attainment of motor milestones. A quarter of the patients developed kyphoscoliosis. Contractures of muscles were seen only rarely. The deep tendon reflexes were often depressed or absent, but sometimes in the group of patients who experienced complete recovery the reflexes were normal. No abnormality was found in the muscle biopsy although histochemical stains were not used. Although the outcome in these two groups of patients was different, Walton felt that the early history was so similar that they must certainly have the same disease. He also suggested that perhaps those whose illness was mildest might be looked upon as those with the best prognosis.

The concept of benign congenital hypotonia is a very useful one, although in our clinic it is used in a more stringent sense than was originally proposed. We make the diagnosis in those children whose physical examination reveals only abnormal tone. The deep tendon reflexes are normal. There is neither weakness nor wasting. Occasionally strabismus is noted but this may be merely incidental rather than part of the illness. The laboratory tests including the serum muscle enzymes, electromyography (EMG), and even more importantly muscle biopsy are all normal. Children in this group have a uniformly good prognosis and the parents can be reassured that eventually the child will develop normally. It is possible that some children with additional findings, such as decreased deep tendon reflexes, or with mild abnormalities of muscle histochemistry may do equally well. However, if the category of benign congenital hypotonia is broadened to include these patients, a small percentage will be shown later to have some other illness and an excellent prognosis cannot be given with such certainty.

Congenital Hypotonia with Type 1 Fiber Predominance

Muscle fibers can be differentiated into two basic types using the appropriate histochemical reactions. These have been termed Type 1 (slow, red) and Type 2 (fast, white). In normal muscle the Type 2 fibers usually outnumber the Type 1 fibers by about 2:1. Type 1 fiber predominance refers to a change in which the Type 1 fibers comprise more than 60% of the fibers in the biopsy.

Since Type 1 fiber predominance is a common connecting link that joins many of the illnesses described in this chapter, it is not surprising that in some instances it is the only change to be found. Such is the case in children who present with congenital hypotonia (Figs. 9.2 and 9.3). There may be some decrease in the deep tendon reflexes and a higher incidence of skeletal anomalies such as flat feet or pes cavus, congenital hip dislocation, or kyphoscoliosis. Mild weakness of the limbs may persist into adult life, but most of these children improve. They may remain ungainly and somewhat clumsy, but a normal life is possible. Type 1 fiber predominance is the only abnormality in the biopsy, and the presence of fibrosis, internal nuclei, phagocytosis and necrosis, or variability in the size of fibers is probably a reason to exclude the diagnosis.

Prader-Willi Syndrome

A cause of hypotonia which is not uncommon in a muscle clinic is the Prader-Willi syndrome (4). The incidence in the general population lies between 1:10,000 and 1:30,000 (5). The children are floppy at birth. Very frequently they have a low birth weight and experience considerable feeding difficulties in the neonatal period, with a poor suck response and some difficulty swallowing. The reason for the hypotonia is often not detected until about the age of 3 years, when the children gain weight in a striking and characteristic fashion. They become enormously obese and their appetite is legendary. It is not uncommon for the parents to have to padlock the refrigerator or for the children to be found rummaging in the garbage cans of their neighbors in search of food.

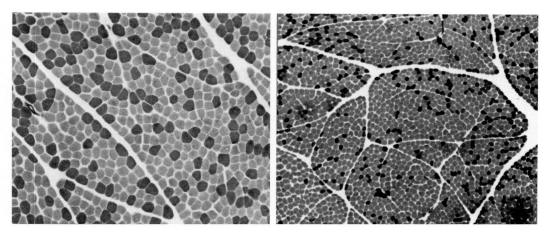

Figure 9.2 (*left*). In an 18-month-old boy who had a history of congenital hypotonia and some delay in the attainment of motor milestones, the muscle biopsy from the biceps showed the majority of fibers to be Type 1 (light). This is an example of congenital hypotonia with Type 1 fiber predominance (ATPase, pH 9.4).

Figure 9.3 (*right*). A similar patient with congenital hypotonia, in whom there was mild weakness of the legs and decreased reflexes, showed Type 1 fiber predominance in a biopsy from the biceps muscle (ATPase, pH 9.4).

The hands and feet are small. The face is rather characteristic with almond-shaped eyes, often there is a strabismus (Figs. 9.4 and 9.5). Boys are more often affected with the illness than girls. Hypogonadism with a small penis and small, often undescended, testicles is commonly found.

The symptoms all point towards a defect in hypothalamic function, but none has yet been found. An abnormality in growth hormone has been reported (6) with a less than normal increase following insulin administration. The levels of estradiol, testosterone, luteinizing hormone and follicle-stimulating hormone (FSH) were found to be decreased in some patients but no primary cause was discovered (5). Mental retardation is the rule and may be quite severe although it is masked by the personality of these children. They combine pleasant outgoing behavior with a flow of speech which is unusual. The questions they ask are often repetitive and trivial. The voice is high pitched and they may suffer from problems with pronunciation. All in all their friendliness, although charming, can be a little wearing. Personality problems become evident as the patients mature.The children are frequently short statured and the bone age may be retarded. Scoliosis and occasionally convulsions may be noted.

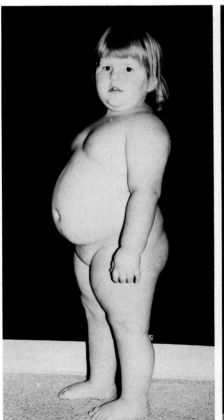 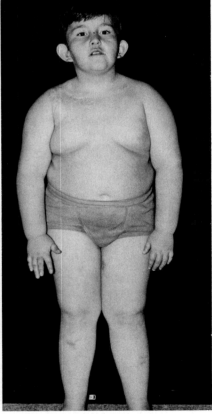

Figures 9.4 and 9.5.   Prader-Willi Syndrome.

Laboratory studies reveal little evidence of muscle abnormality. Serum muscle enzymes are usually normal. EMG reveals no abnormality and light microscopy shows normal muscle biopsy. Some changes have been described following electron microscopic studies (7) but are rather unconvincing.

In about 15% of the patients, abnormalities on chromosome 15 are present. The genetic abnormality is not identical in all cases: some have a deletion or other abnormality of a region on the short arm, in others there is a translocation between the short arm of 15 and another autosomal chromosome (8–11).

There is no specific treatment for this disease. The obesity, complications of which present the major threat to the patient's life, responds poorly to dietary management. Although harsh restriction of diet is of value, it is seldom attained.

CONGENITAL MUSCULAR DYSTROPHY

In a previous edition of this book, I confessed that I reserved the diagnosis of congenital muscular dystrophy for those children who were undoubtedly suffering from a malign muscle disease but whose diagnosis, in my ignorance, I was not able to ascertain. I also had the temerity to suggest that there were others who shared by confusion. To judge from the number of articles appearing on congenital muscular dystrophy in recent years, I must be alone in my confusion. I am not entirely repentant. Although it is true that certain clinical pictures are emerging from the large numbers of children born with hypotonia, contractures and other evidence of muscle involvement, just when I think I have the entities clearly in mind, a new patient comes along with features common to more than one of these entities. What is badly needed is some irrefutable biochemical test which will separate the diseases one from another. This, of course, is too much to hope for and at present the differentiation is based on clinical grounds with some help from laboratory studies. Contrary to common belief, many of these congenital muscular dystrophies are either nonprogressive or worsen only very slowly.

The designation of congenital muscular dystrophy was used earlier to denote children who were born weak and floppy, frequently with contractures of various muscles, and who attained normal motor milestones with difficulty. There was no clear pattern of inheritance, although cases of affected relatives were described. Muscle biopsies were interpreted as myopathic, which distinguished these children from others with weakness in early childhood. There was fibrosis, variation in the size of fibers and internal nuclei. In 1965 the situation seemed clear enough that Wharton (12) felt that there were two types. One of these was rapidly progressive, terminating in death, and the other was more slowly progressive or even static. Modern techniques for the investigation of these children were not available. Nevertheless, there were some intriguing comments (12). One report involved a brother and sister with arthrogryposis and a progressive weakness that ended in the childrens' death (13). There were large numbers of "fetal" fibers in the muscle biopsy characterized by internal nuclei and it is possible that this disease represented the severe infantile form of myotubular myopathy. The same comment was made in the description of two brothers with a similar clinical picture dying in the first year of life (14). Other reports from the mid-1960s suggested that the typical patient with congenital muscular dystrophy was born hypotonic and very often had either respiratory or feeding difficulties early in life and had such associated anomalies as congenital hip dislocation, club feet or contractures (15–17). Often there was a family history of a similar illness in a sibling but the parents were in general normal. There was rather diffuse involvement of the muscles, although poor head control was often commented on as an early finding. Kyphoscoliosis was frequently noted. The patients reported by Zellweger et al. (17) as having congenital muscular dystrophy had prominent facial weakness. Indeed, the authors discussed the possibility of this being due to facioscapulohumeral dystrophy. They mentioned as a differentiating feature that facioscapulohumeral dystrophy was always inherited in an autosomal dominant fashion and that it had never occurred in infancy. Recent experience with this disease would not confirm this and the patients may well have had the infantile FSH picture. Reports originating in the 1970s categorized congenital muscular dystrophy not according to the severity of the progression but rather according to the association with cerebral malformations. Two earlier reports by Fukuyama et al. (18) and Fowler and Manson (19) described children who were born hypotonic with contractures and mental retardation and who had marked abnormalities of the central nervous system at autopsy. Other children without mental retardation or evidence of neurological damage have also been classified as having congenital muscular dystrophy. There seem to be four common types of clinical presentation in this illness, although it is again to be emphasized that differentiations are not clear.

Congenital Muscular Dystrophy with Central Nervous System Disease (Fukuyama Type) (20)

The disorder is inherited as an autosomal recessive (Figs. 9.6–9.11). All of the reported cases have had their onset at less than 9 months of age. The children are often born floppy. Joint contractures may not be noted in early infancy but are present in 70% of patients by age 3 with the hip and knee commonly involved. Funnel chest may be an early finding. The suck reflex is decreased and feeding may be difficult. Hip dislocations are not uncommon. The children are often severely mentally retarded, the development of speech is affected and some children have convulsions, either major motor seizures or petit mal. Plagycephaly or asymmetry of the skull is commonly noted, either clinically or on x-ray. Few of the children learn to walk and most lead a passive existence, being cared for by their family. The muscle weakness is quite diffuse but often difficult to test because of lack of cooperation from the children. Weakness of the face and neck has been noted. There may be weakness of the extraocular muscles and some difficulty with gaze. After the age of 8 none of the patients attained any new motor skills and in several cases there was a decline in previously attained skills. Laboratory studies demonstrate elevation of the creatine kinase (CK), often to quite high levels, and a myopathic EMG. The muscle biopsy shows marked variation in the size of the fibers, most of which are round, and all are embedded in fibrous tissue. There is no remarkable change in the fiber types, although occasional

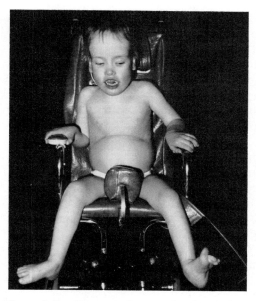

Figure 9.6. Congenital muscular dystrophy with central nervous system involvement. This child was severely retarded, had seizures and muscular weakness with contractures. CAT scan of the head showed no abnormal lucencies.

Type 1 predominance and numberous Type 2C fibers are noted (21). About one half of the patients demonstrate an abnormality with CAT scan of the head. There are areas of increased lucency in the white matter which seem to be particularly prominent in the frontal areas (Figs. 9.11 and 9.12) (22). There was associated ventricular dilatation in about two-thirds of the cases. Oddly, these changes often improved over time (23). The capillary endothelium has been found abnormal in some patients with an accumulation of tubular structures within the cell. These tubular formations are not specific for the disease, however (24). The eye is often involved with high myopia and optic atrophy as well as an occasional case with choroidal atrophy of the retina and a paucity of vessels in the retina (25). Autopsy studies show marked abnormalities in the central nervous system. In a girl dying at the age of 7½ months there was a disorganized cerebral cortex which was thicker than normal. The border between the gray and white matter was blurred. Heterotopias were frequent and the central white matter was poorly myelinated and reduced in quantity (19). The pathologic findings were reviewed by Kamoshita et al. (26). In many cases there was micropolygyria and agyria with distortion of the architecture of both the cerebral and cerebellar cortices. The changes were, in general, dysplastic. Meningeal thickening over the temporal and occipital lobes was noted in some patients.

The illness seems to be very common in Japan. My own experience is limited to eight cases, five of which were reported elsewhere (27). Of these cases, three were very typical, occurring in siblings with severe mental

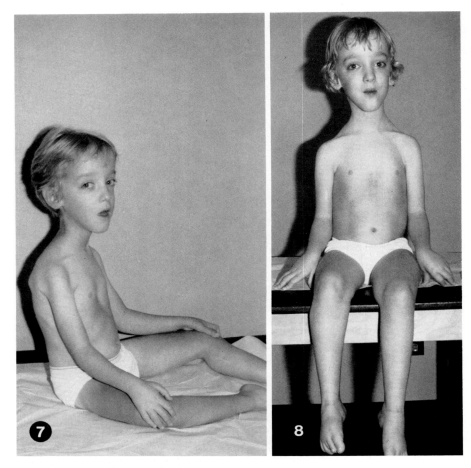

Figures 9.7 and 9.8. Congenital muscular dystrophy with central nervous system disease. Notice the facial appearance of this patient who had weakness and contractures but who had neither seizures nor mental retardation. The facial features should be compared with the next two patients (Figs. 9.9 and 9.10). A CAT scan showed markedly abnormal lucencies in the white matter.

retardation. In the other five, all of which were sporadic, one demonstrated mental retardation but two were of relatively normal intelligence, although other features including the cerebral hypomyelination were present.

Because of the occurrence of some inflammatory changes in the muscle as well as the suggestion that the brain pathology might have an inflammatory cause, steroids were tried in some patients. The serum CK was reduced but this is a nonspecific response seen in other illness. The muscle weakness was only "slightly" responsive to this treatment but there was said to be improvement in the mental status. Further studies are needed to investigate this (28).

Congenital Muscular Dystrophy without Central Nervous System Damage (Undifferentiated Type)

There are many children who demonstrate similar characteristics to those described above in whom there are no signs or symptoms of central nervous

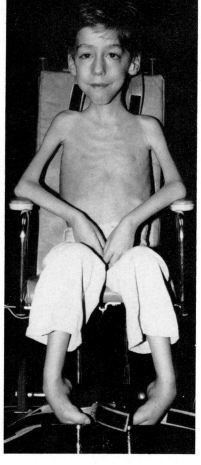

Figure 9.9. Congenital muscular dystrophy with central nervous system disease. This patient had muscle weakness and contractures as evidenced by the position of the feet. His IQ was below average and the CAT scan demonstrated abnormal lucencies.

system disorder. The hypotonia and weakness is often noted at birth or during the first year of life; contractures of the joints occur, particularly of the elbows, knees and hips. Once again, even though the illness can be disabling, only in the rare case is it rapidly progressive. Serum CK is elevated. The EMG is myopathic and the muscle biopsy shows increased fibrosis with random variability in the size of fibers. There is often Type 1 fiber predominance in this illness as there is in many of congenital muscle diseases. Because the intellectual function is preserved, medical management is easier than in the Fukuyama type. These children may adapt quite well to braces or devices such as "stand in" tables which will allow them to stand. The development of a kyphoscoliosis can be a troublesome problem as the child grows older.

Congenital Muscular Dystrophy (Atonic Sclerotic Type)

This very rare type of congenital muscular dystrophy was first recognized by Ullrich (29). Once again, the children are born floppy. There are contractures of the proximal joints, the hips, knees, shoulders and elbows. The joints of the hands, however, are extremely lax and the fingers are hyperextensible. The children also demonstrate excessive sweating over the trunk and over the

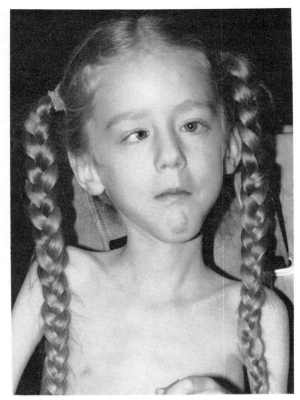

Figure 9.10. The sister of the patient in Figure 9.9. She had an identical clinical picture. Abnormalities of the extraocular muscles were seen in several of the patients and are well demonstrated in this photograph.

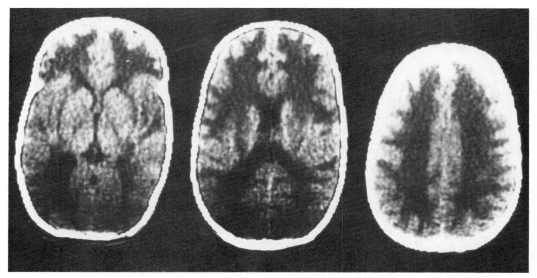

Figure 9.11. A CAT scan of the patient illustrated in Figure 9.6. This CAT scan was obtained in 1977 and demonstrates widespread lucencies in the white matter.

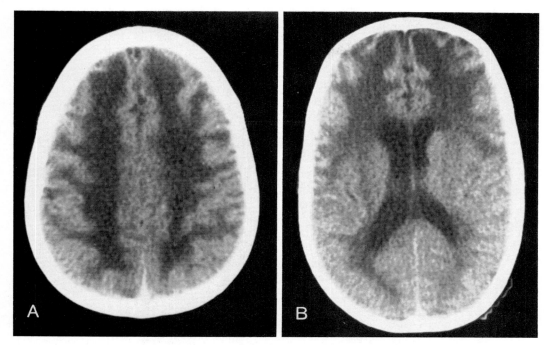

Figure 9.12 (*A* and *B*). CAT scan obtained 7 years later of patient shown in Figure 9.11 demonstrating similar changes.

palms of the hands and soles of the feet. Dysmorphic features such as a high arched palate and deformities of the chest and spine have been noted. A curious feature is a prosterior displacement of the calcaneum (Figs. 9.13 and 9.14). Respiratory infections are common and the weakness can be quite severe. Far from demonstrating any mental retardation, these children are unusually bright. The muscle biopsy shows nonspecific myopathic changes and the EMG is also myopathic. CK is variably elevated, but not to the extent seen in some of the other cases of Duchenne muscular dystrophy (30).

Congenital Muscular Dystrophy (Stick Man Type)

A relatively common form of neuromuscular disease of childhood which appears to have a dystrophic basis may be much milder than the varieties above. In my own clinic this is colloquially called the "Stick Man" dystrophy because the patients limbs are extremely thin, almost skeletal, resembling children's drawings of stick men (Figs. 9.15–9.18). In spite of muscles which are almost vanishingly small, the patients retain a moderate amount of strength. Some of the cases reported by Goebel et al. (31) resemble these patients. A comment made by these authors "in spite of considerable muscle atrophy, there was almost no deteriation of gross motor function" reflects a similarity with our own experience. Our patients, when followed for more than 10 years, have shown little deterioration in function as opposed to most of the patients with congenital muscular dystrophy who show a very slow progression (31). Typically some abnormality is noted during the first year of life. Often the children are weak and floppy. They are very thin and sometimes there are unusual contractures of the feet which may be everted and flat

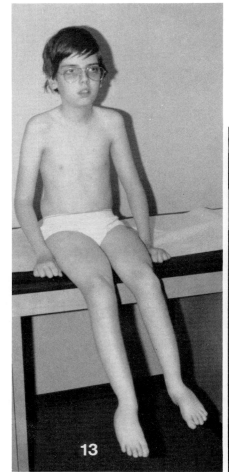
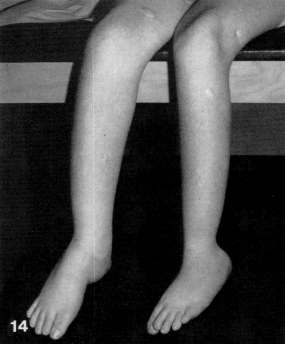

Figure 9.13. Congenital muscular dystrophy, atonic sclerotic type. This patient had weakness from birth associated with contractures. The contractures were unusual in their distribution. For example, his knees could bend no further than illustrated in the photograph due to contractures of the quadricep muscle.

Figure 9.14. Congenital muscular dystrophy, atonic sclerotic type. There is posterior displacement of the calcaneum as illustrated.

footed shortly after birth. The motor milestones are often delayed although some of our patients developed normally. Usually within the first 5 years the children begin to walk on their toes and are unable to get their heels on the ground. Contractures may remain limited to the heel cords or may develop in other joints such as the knees, hips, elbows and the posterior cervical region. On examination there is a rather generalized weakness. Perhaps it is slightly more severe proximally than distally but this is difficult to judge. The muscles are extremely thin and deep tendon reflexes are diminished to absent. The strength although not normal is always suprisingly good for the amount of palpable muscle tissue. The children we have followed have been uniformly bright and many of them have been "straight A" students. Laboratory tests

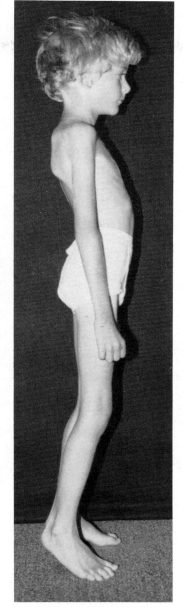

Figure 9.15. Congenital muscular dystrophy, stick-man type. Notice, in addition to the asthenic build, that heel cord contractures are associated with toe walking.

show mild elevation of CK and a myopathic EMG with normal conduction velocities. The muscle biopsy is unusual (Figs. 9.19–9.25). It certainly shows the typical myopathic or even dystrophic features with fibrosis, variability in the size of fibers, occasional internal nuclei, and often Type 1 predominance. In addition, there is a change which is puzzling and almost unique to this disease. This is a "nonrandom" distribution in the variously sized fibers. Some fascicles will contain fibers which are, on the whole, smaller than others. This does not, however, look like the large group atrophy of denervation

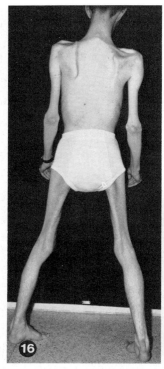
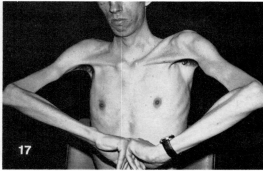

Figures 9.16 and 9.17.   Congenital muscular dystrophy, stickman type. This again illustrates the skeletal appearance of this patient who has a life-long nonprogressive weakness. In Figure 9.17 he is pushing his fist together to accentuate the pectoralis muscle.

although it is difficult to set down on paper the ways in which it differs. Figures 9.22–9.25 demonstrate this change. Treatment of this illness is uncertain. There are often marked heel cord contractures and toe walking may be the patients only major concern. However, in those patients on whom we have performed a heel cord release the dynamics of walking were disturbed enough that the patient had some difficulty adjusting to the reconstructed ankles. In one extreme case a young girl whose hobby as a teenager was ballet was no longer able to dance "on point"!

Rigid Spine Syndrome

An interesting condition which is probably related to the previous ones is the rigid spine syndrome (32). In this condition there is a marked limitation of flexion of the whole spine from the cervical to the lumbar region. Extension is not impaired and the power of the extensor muscles is normal. A mild amount of weakness in the limb musculature has been noted and in some patients there were associated contractures of the tendo achillis. The CK was moderately elevated. An EMG of the spinal muscles showed a myopathic pattern with a muscle biopsy revealing fibrosis and replacement of the muscle by connective tissue (33).

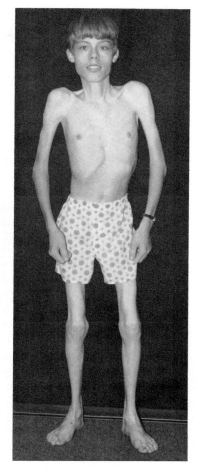

Figure 9.18. Congenital muscular dystrophy stickman type. This patient has also developed a scoliosis. The heel cord contractures are not evident because the Achilles tendons were lengthened surgically.

CONGENITAL FIBER TYPE DISPROPORTION

The first description of this illness had its origin in an attempt to analyze children's biopsies (34). The original aim of the analysis was to study a series of patients with a specific disease and then to describe the changes seen in their muscle biopsies. This attempt floundered when it became apparent that there were almost as many diagnoses as there were biopsies. Consequently, the procedure was reversed, and the biopsies were grouped simply according to the changes in fiber size. Of the five groups outlined, four are irrelevant to this discussion, but the fifth was a group of biopsies in which the Type 1 fibers were smaller than the Type 2 fibers. In some of these cases, diagnoses such as myotonic dystrophy or cerebellar disease were well established, but in others the illness was obscure.

Twelve additional cases presented in a later report (35) fulfilled the criteria of having Type 1 fibers with an average diameter 15% smaller than that of the Type 2 fibers and a normal degree of variability in the larger fiber type. Because this type of biopsy was originally associated with a rather stereotyped

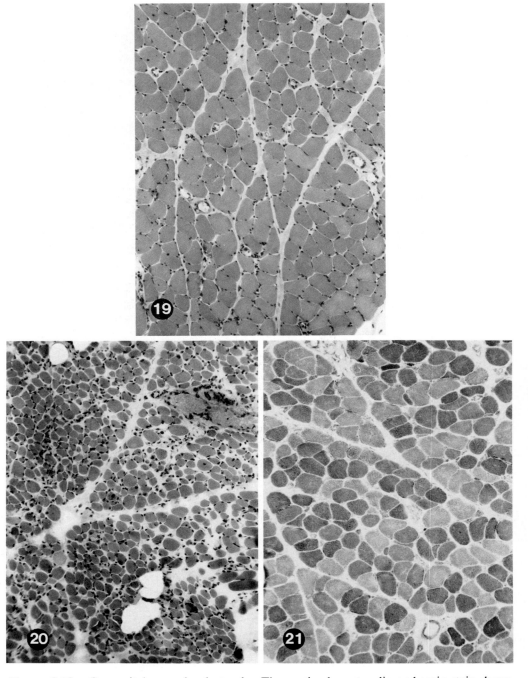

Figures 9.19.   Congenital muscular dystrophy. The routine hematoxylin and eosin stain shows an abnormal variation the size of fibers with some increase in fibrous tissue between the individual fibers. There are also a few internal nuclei.

Figure 9.20.   "Stickman" muscular dystrophy. A similar biopsy but showing more severe changes with a greater variability in the size of fibers and more fibrosis.

Figure 9.21.   Oxidative enzyme reactions, such as this NADH-tetrazolium reductase preparation, show no special changes in the intermyofibrillar network pattern but merely confirm the changes seen with the routine hematoxylin and eosin stain.

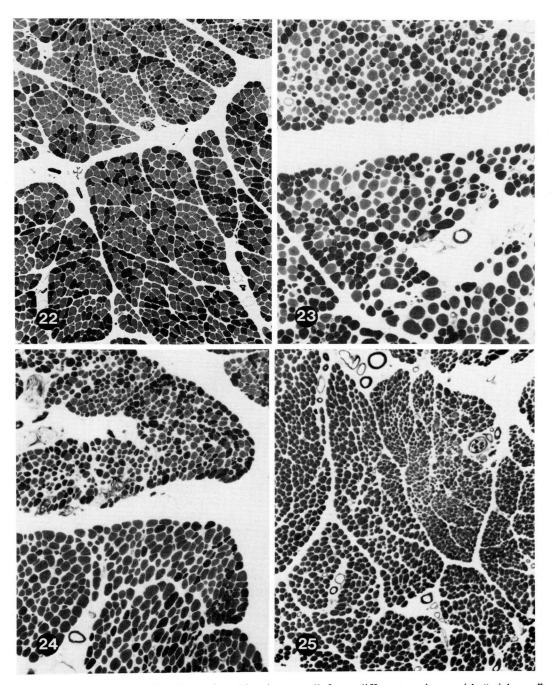

Figures 9.22 through 9.25. These four biopsies are all from different patients with "stickman" dystrophy. In addition to a general increase in the variability of the size of fibers, there are more specific changes. All show an increase in the number of Type 1 fibers, including a total predominance of Type 1 fibers seen in Figure 9.25. Notice that no Type 2 fibers are present in this biopsy. In addition, there is another peculiar change which we have called the "nonrandom" size change. In all of the pictures the size of the fibers in the fascicles towards the top of the photograph is less than those in the fascicles towards the bottom part of the photograph. The change is a subtle one but is most noticable in Figure 9.24. This is different from the large groups of atrophic fibers which characterize denervation. In large group atrophy the fibers are relatively (although not completely) uniform in size, whereas within the individual fascicles illustrated here there is still an abnormal variation in the size of fibers.

clinical picture, it was suggested that it constituted a clinical syndrome and this was named congenital fiber type disproportion. The illness showed no preference for either sex. The children were floppy at birth and had varying degrees of weakness. On occasion the disease was so severe that respiratory compromise and recurrent respiratory infections were seen in the first year of life. In over half of the cases, contractures of various muscles were noted, often involving the hands or feet, although one patient had a torticollis. Congenital hip dislocation was noted in one-half of the patients, which may represent no more than the secondary effect of intrauterine weakness and hypotonia. The weakness often seemed to be at its most severe during the first 2 years of life. After this, the disease either improved or became relatively stable. Attainment of motor milestones was uniformly delayed. It should be emphasized that residual weakness is the rule in these patients. In only 3 out of the 12 original patients did muscle strength attain the normal. As the children grew older, their weight fell below the third percentile, and frequently the patients were also short. Other skeletal abnormalities included a high arched palate and kyphoscoliosis, which were seen in over half. Valgus or varus deformities of the feet were noted. There was no disturbance of intellectual function. Clinical examination showed decreased to absent deep tendon reflexes with mild to moderate weakness of the arms and legs. The proximal muscles around the shoulders and hips were slightly more involved than the distal muscles. Mild facial weakness has been seen on occasions.

There have been several subsequent reports of similar patients (26, 36–42). The disease has been described in some families with autosomal dominant inheritance. The father of two patients had biopsy changes characteristic of congenital fiber types disproportion without being aware of any weakness himself. He did, however, have a long, thin face, some proximal muscle wasting, and an absence of tendon reflexes in the arms (39).

All of the patients in these reports had a similar clinical picture. Congenital hypotonia was common to all, and there was a tendency for slow improvement to occur. One patient (37) had severe respiratory difficulties. Contractures, scoliosis, short stature, high arched feet, and a high arched palate were noted in some of the patients.

There are obvious pitfalls in making a diagnosis mathematically rather than clinically. For example, one of the patients in the original report (35) (case 4) was subsequently found to have the infantile variety of facioscapulohumeral dystrophy. Since large Type 2 fibers are associated with facioscapulohumeral dystrophy, this was perhaps not surprising.

Two reports emphasized abnormalities of the spine, and the patients conformed to the rigid spine syndrome (43, 44). In these patients, the onset of symptoms was slightly later. In one, the patient developed difficulty in flexing the neck at the age of 7. This was progressive and was accompanied by increasing difficulty with flexion of the back. On examination, the patient was found to have weak neck muscles and mild weakness of the arms and legs, with absent tendon reflexes. Flexion contractures of the knees were noted. The other patient was first noted to have a waddling gait at 4 years of age. On examination, there was limitation of flexion of the spine, flexion contractures of the elbows, and mild atrophy of the muscles of the shoulder and pelvic girdles. Deep tendon reflexes were absent. In retrospect, case 11 in the earlier report (35) also had a stiff spine, although this was not noted at the time of examination.

Laboratory studies, other than the biopsy, are not very helpful. The serum muscle enzyme may be slightly elevated. The EMG shows a combination of small, short potentials together with large amplitude potentials. Conduction velocities are normal. The muscle biopsy shows the disproportion in the number and size of the fiber types (Fig. 9.26), sometimes with additional features such as scattered internal nuclei or occasional fibers with rods.

Some comment should be made with regard to the relationship between this illness and some of the other morphologically distinct myopathies. The illness closely resembles nemaline myopathy, in which the Type 1 fibers are also smaller than the Type 2 fibers, and there is frequently Type 1 fiber predominance. The profusion of rod-like structures in the muscles of patients with nemaline myopathy not only has given the name to the disease but also has been considered a necessary part of the illness. The existence of rods in the muscle, however, is a nonspecific finding. Furthermore, patients with nemaline myopathy have been described in whom the rods are present in only one of several biopsies or in one part of the biopsy. The relationship between this entity and others is a problem which will be discussed later. It is important to emphasize, however, that the change in fiber size which characterizes congenital fiber type disproportion is not unique in infants. It may also occur in myotonic dystrophy, in some cerebellar disorders (34, 44) and in globoid cell leukodystrophy (39). There is reason to believe that the list will grow further.

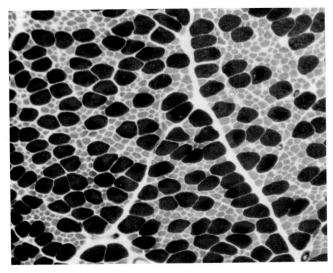

Figure 9.26. A biopsy from the biceps of a patient with congenital fiber type disproportion. Notice the discrepancy between the size of the Type 2 (dark) fibers and the Type 1 (light). In addition, there is a discrepancy in the numbers of fibers, the Type 1 fibers being far more numerous than usual (ATPase, pH 9.4).

CENTRAL CORE DISEASE

In 1959 Shy and Magee (45) observed a pathological change that was so striking that they embodied it in the name they gave the illness. This was central core disease and it was the forerunner of a number of myopathies whose descriptive titles reflect the predominant change on the muscle biopsy. Some of these have stood the test of time. As in the original case report, the disease is often inherited as an autosomal dominant. However, sporadic instances have been described and it is possible that we should think not of central core disease but of central core diseases.

The clinical picture of central core disease can be synthesized from a number of reports (46–61). In most patients the onset is noted at or shortly after birth, when the patient is floppy and attains the motor milestones only slowly. In a number of patients, congenital hip dislocation is noted. As the child grows older he finds that he cannot run as smoothly as other children and jumping is often impossible. Often the family expresses little concern over these symptoms since it is recognized in some of the other members as a mild abnormality and is regarded more as an annoyance than an illness. In only 2 of the 12 families we have seen with central core disease did the patients come to the muscle clinic because of their complaint of weakness. Others arrived for reasons as various as needing a letter in order to be excused from military duty or, in the case of one patient, simply because he worked in the next laboratory to my own.

In adult life the patients are often slender and short statured, but without any focal muscle atrophy (Fig. 9.27). The weakness may be diffuse although some reports have stressed a proximal distribution, particularly of the hips. Mild weakness of the face and neck muscles may also be seen. The deep tendon reflexes are often surprisingly normal. Skeletal deformities are not uncommon, perhaps a reflection of the early onset of this illness. In addition to congenital hip dislocation, lordosis and kyphoscoliosis may be seen. Either high arched feet or flat feet are also relatively common findings. In some, only fragments of the disease are expressed and patients whose only complaint was pes cavus or tight heel cords have been recorded (46).

Malignant hyperthermia has been reported in patients with central core disease, as with other neuromuscular illnesses and this possibility should always be considered in a patient about to undergo surgery (62, 63). As mentioned before, most reported cases are inherited as an autosomal dominant. An exception to this was an instance of the disease in only one of two identical twins. The case was complicated by the fact that the biopsy on which the diagnosis was based was taken from the thigh muscle in a baby who had a below-knee cast for treatment of talipes equinovarus. It is possible that the immobility of the limb played a part in the changes seen in the biopsy, in a fashion similar to the experimental production of cores in animals (64).

Laboratory tests other than the muscle biopsy are usually unhelpful, serum enzymes are normal, and the EMG is rather nonspecific. The muscle biopsy is strikingly abnormal. Mild variability in the size of the fibers is seen. On occasion, extremely small atrophic fibers have been noted. There is often marked Type 1 fiber predominance (Fig. 9.28), and there exists in the center of most of the fibers an area which is unreactive with the oxidative enzyme

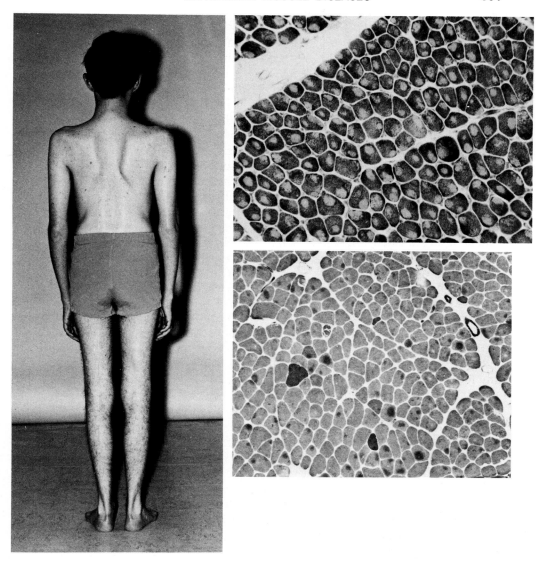

Figures 9.27 through 9.29. Central core disease. In general, the patients with central core disease have a rather diffuse weakness and are slender without any focal muscle wasting (Fig. 9.27, *left*). With the NADH-tetrazolium reductase reaction there are unstained areas within each muscle fiber which give the disease its name (Fig. 9.28, *upper right*). The ATPase reaction (pH 9.4) shows Type 1 fiber predominance (Fig. 9.29, *lower right*). Only two or three Type 2 (dark) fibers are present in the entire biopsy.

histochemistry (Fig. 9.29). With the ATPase reaction the reactivity of the central areas is either decreased or on occasion increased. If the diagnosis is restricted to those patient's demonstrating the changes shown above, then the clinical picture is usually as described. Electron microscopy shows an absence of mitochondria in the core zone, as well as an alteration of the myofibrillar architecture varying from smearing of the Z lines to a total disruption of the cross-striational pattern. It is difficult to distinguish the latter change from that of the target fiber, and only the setting in which the change occurs allows this differentiation to be made. This led to use of the term "core-targetoid fiber" in describing the pathological abnormality (65).

Slightly different changes are seen in some patients with central core disease. These changes have been termed "structured cores" to indicate the maintenance of a very precise pattern of cross striation with clear retention of A, I, and Z banding (48). In the unstructured core, the A, I, and Z bands can still be traced across the cores, but they are markedly disrupted. This differentiation is probably unnecessary, since a combination of structured and unstructured cores can occur in the same patients (46, 61, 66).

The number of cores in the biopsies varies widely, from changes affecting 100% of the fibers to those affecting fewer than 20%. In the report by Morgan-Hughes et al. (47) on central core disease occurring in a mother and her two children, the "core" fibers were found in the mothers biopsy, leading the authors to suggest that the cores were merely an epiphenomenon and were not significant to the illness. As the other end of the scale, central cores have been found in a muscle which was completely normal clinically (46).

Evidence of frank denervation is lacking in patients with central core disease, and no extrajunctional acetylcholine receptor can be visualized using an α-bungarotoxin immunoperoxidase method (67). However, abnormalities in the intramuscular nerve fibers have been described, including increased branching and simplification of the motor endplates (46, 68). The terminal innervation ratio was found to be increased in one patient.

Biochemical abnormalities have been described but may be nonspecific. Phosphorylase activity is reduced (49, 70), a finding which might be expected in view of the paucity of Type 2 (glycolytic) fibers. The calcium-dependent ATPase and the uptake of calcium by the sarcoplasmic reticulum is also reduced (61), which might correlate with the absence of this membrane from the core regions. Fructose-1:6-diphosphatase was deficient in one biopsy but may again represent the paucity of Type 2 fibers (69).

The treatment of central core disease is usually supportive. Genetic counseling should be given on the basis of an autosomal dominant disease unless the family history indicates clearly that this is a sporadic case. Most (although not all) of the patients are so mildly handicapped that no specific treatment is necessary.

NEMALINE MYOPATHY (ROD BODY DISEASE)

Nemaline myopathy is characterized by the presence of small, rod-like particles in the muscle (Fig. 9.31) (71, 72). Based on the electron microscopic findings, A. G. Engel (73) proposed the following criteria as common to all rod bodies:

1. Origin in the Z disc
2. Tetragonal filamentous array when cut transversely
3. Structural continuity with thin filaments
4. Periodic lines perpendicular to the long axis
5. Periodic lines parallel to the long axis.

Since 1963, there have been numerous reports describing patients with these morphological changes (74–92).

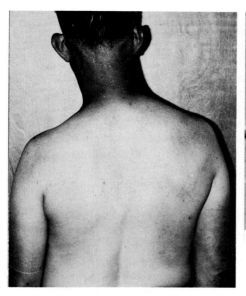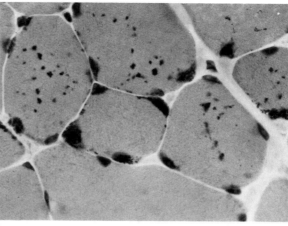

Figures 9.30 and 9.31. Nemaline myopathy. This patient presented to the hospital with a kyphoscoliosis. He was found to have scapular weakness and weakness of the anterior tibial muscles. The muscle biopsy from the biceps showed large numbers of rods scattered throughout the fibers. The small particles are seen at the corners of the muscle fibers and are also scattered throughout the centers of many of them.

The disease has a genetic basis; in some familes it is inherited as an autosomal dominant, whereas in others it occurs as an autosomal recessive. The lack of transmission from father to son has been emphasized, and the possibility of an X-linked dominant inheritance has been raised (81, 87). After reviewing the literature and finding only 5 of 31 reported cases to be male, one report suggested that the illness might be semilethal in males (80). However, of the cases now reported in the literature which are reasonably well documented, there has been a more even distribution between male and female. Arts et al. (78) proposed that, in addition to an autosomal dominant mode of inheritance, there were cases inherited in an autosomal recessive manner in which both parents demonstrated pathological abnormalities even though no symptoms were apparent. A muscle biopsy from the mother of one patient with nemaline myopathy revealed abnormal Type 1 fiber predominance, even though the mother had neither rods nor any clinical weakness (80). Sporadic cases have also been reported.

There are three clinical syndromes associated with nemaline myopathy. The most commonly recognized is of hypotonia and a rather diffuse weakness of the limbs and trunk beginning at a very early age. In addition to weakness of the arms and legs, some mild weakness of the face and other bulbar muscles has been noted (74), but the eye muscles are usually spared. The reflexes are decreased to absent. These children are often dysmorphic with a long narrow face, high arched palate, and slender musculature. High arched feet and kyphoscoliosis are not uncommon, particularly in the older patients. There may be malformation of the jaw which may be either prognathous or abnormally short. For the most part, the disease is not progressive and the patient learns to live with the moderate degree of weakness.

A much more severe form of the illness is occasionally seen. Usually this is noted at birth. The children have marked weakness and hypotonia. In particular, the respiratory muscles are weak and death often occurs in the first few years of life secondary to respiratory failure. Postmortem and muscle biopsy studies in these children show a profusion of rods, and the diaphragm is also involved which may account for some of the respiratory symptoms. Occasionally children with the severe form will survive until teenage life but recurrent respiratory crises are the rule (74, 78, 93–96). In reviewing the congenital fatal cases of nemaline myopathy, Kondo and Yuasa (96) suggested that the inheritance was best described on a basis of an autosomal dominant gene with variable penetrance.

Other patients present with a scapuloperoneal distribution of weakness, and a foot-drop is one of the earliest symptoms (75–77). Sometimes this begins later in adolescence or even adult life. The hip muscles are involved in this type of illness, but this occurs later, and the most severe weakness is of the muscles of the anterior tibial compartment and of the shoulders. I have observed patients with kyphoscoliosis (Fig. 9.30). and this may differentiate the illness from some of the other varieties of the scapuloperoneal syndrome.

As in many of the congenital myopathies, serum enzyme studies and EMG are really not helpful in making the diagnosis. There may be mild elevation of serum creatine kinase and the EMG may show short polyphasic potentials. The muscle biopsy is paramount in arriving at the diagnosis. Most patients show Type 1 fiber predominance which may at times comprise over 90% of the fibers in the biopsy. There is often Type 1 fiber atrophy, particularly in the diffuse childhood form of the disease. The Type 1 fiber predominance has led some to propose an abnormalitiy of innervation as a cause for this illness (97). Coers et al. (68) found minor changes in the terminal nerve endings with the methylene blue stain, but they believed that the significance of such changes was uncertain. They were not able to detect any abnormalities of the neuromuscular junction or of the terminal innervation ratio. No extrajunctional acetylcholine receptor was present in biopsy material to suggest evidence of altered innervation (67). Investigation at autopsy has not led to any real confirmation of a possible cause. Dahl and Klutzow (81) found a reduced number of cell bodies in one anterior horn and in the spinal accessory nuclei at midcervical cord level, as well as geographic large groups of atrophic muscle fibers in the sternocleidomastoid muscle. Whether this is related to the disease is not certain. Patchy demyelination and fibrillary gliosis in the dorsal columns, with a reduction in the number of anterior horn cells in the midcervical cord, were described in an elderly patient with a subluxation of the fifth and sixth cervical vertebrae and cord compression (87). One study showed a reduction in size of the motor neurons in the fifth lumbar ventral root, which was believed to be secondary to the muscle disease (98). Another interpretation might be a lack of development of the large, Type 2-determining motor neurons.

Two of the autopsy reports in patients with nemaline myopathy have stressed the presence of "central cores" in the muscle fibers of the diaphragm

(74, 99). Afifi et al. (49) noted the coexistence, in one family, of rods and central cores in the skeletal muscle. Cardiac muscle and intrafusal fibers may be resistant to rod formation, and this has led Karpati et al. (99) to suggest that the illness is a consequence of an abnormality of the α-motor neurons. At the opposite end of the scales, rods have been found in normal eye muscles in patients with no neuromuscular disease (100).

Rods are believed to be derived from the Z line with which they share certain characteristics. α-Actinin normally functions as one of the structural proteins associated with the Z line. Experiments in which electron microscopic studies were combined with biochemical techniques suggested that a major component of the rod bodies was α-actinin (101, 102). Desmin, another structural protein of muscle, accumulates at the periphery of the Z disc as well as of the nemaline bodies. In patients in whom the occurrence of rods was unusually profuse it was shown that the total amount of α-actinin in the patient's muscle was increased 2–3-fold (103). Other biochemical changes which have been described may reflect the difference in the composition of fiber types in nemaline myopathy. Thus Sreter et al. (92) have shown decreased calcium uptake in the sarcoplasmic reticulum as well as decreased calcium and potassium EDTA activated ATPase acitvity. Abnormalities in the light chain composition of the myosin from the muscle of patients with this illness have also indicated a change in the fiber type composition. Although there are some differences in the results, the majority view seems to indicate an absence of LC3F and markedly decreased levels of LC2F and LC1F. All of these are light chains characteristic of fast muscle.

The problem of nemaline myopathy is further compounded by the undoubted presence of nemaline rods in other diseases which are far removed in their clinical appearance from nemaline myopathy. I have seen rods in patients with Parkinson's disease, rheumatoid arthritis, and polymyositis, and they have been recorded in equally unrelated conditions (104–106). If, in fact, they are relatively nonspecific, perhaps the most significance change in nemaline myopathy is the Type 1 fiber atrophy and/or Type 1 fiber predominance, as has been suggested by Dahl and Klutzow (81). If one disregards the rods then the entity becomes very similar to that described under congenital fiber type disproportion. Two of our patients with this latter entity had a few scattered rods, and another report records a similar family (37).

MYOTUBULAR MYOPATHY (CENTRONUCLEAR MYOPATHY)

In 1966 Spiro and others (107) described an illness in which structures resembling fetal myotubes persisted into adult life. They christened this myotubular myopathy. Others, noting that the resemblance may be superficial and that there are important differences between true myotubes and the changes seen in the disease, have suggested the name of centronuclear myopathy (108). However, the term "myotubular" has established its precedence and is picturesque enough to warrant retention until the basic cause of the disease is uncovered.

Since the disease has been characterized by the muscle biopsy, it is appropriate to describe this first. The most typical cases of myotubular myopathy have a combination of internal nuclei (Fig. 9.32), a characteristic increase in

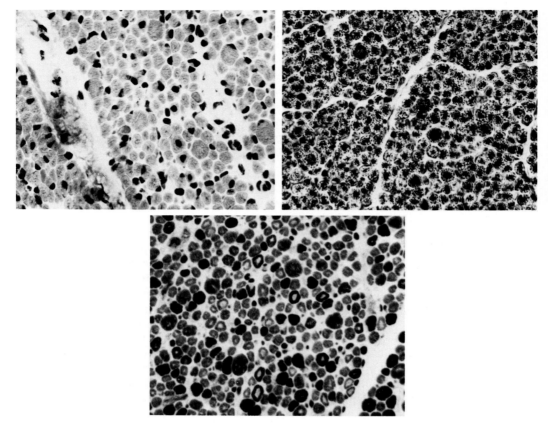

Figures 9.32 through 9.34.   A 3-month-old boy was born with severe weakness and floppiness and had considerable respiratory difficulty, dying from pulmonary complications at the age of 3 months. The hematoxylin and eosin stain showed occasional fibers with large central nuclei (Fig. 9.32, *upper left*). Oxidative enzyme reaction showed an alteration of the normal staining pattern. Instead of a diffuse stain of the intermyofibrillar network, there were increased areas of central staining in most of the fibers (Fig. 9.33, *upper right*). Notice that many more of the fibers have this area of increased staining than demonstrate internal nuclei. The ATPase reaction (pH 9.4) shows these central areas to be nonreactive, giving the appearance of doughnuts (Fig. 9.34, *lower*).

the central staining of the muscle fibers with the oxidative enzyme reactions (Fig. 9.33), and a central pale area with the ATPase reactions (Fig. 9.34). The last two changes are far more frequent than the presence of internal nuclei, since the "myotube" represents rows of plump nuclei separated by spaces and the chances of a section cutting through a space are greater than of cutting through a nucleus. Most of the biopsies reveal Type 1 fiber predominance. The presence of Type 1 fiber atrophy has also been recorded, but this is not necessarily a part of the picture.

A heterogeneous collection of clinical pictures is described under the title of myotubular or centronuclear myopathy. This is partly due to the inclusion of patients whose sole abnormality on the muscle biopsy is internal nuclei. If these patients are excluded, and only those whose biopsies include all the changes above are considered, then the clinical findings are not quite so variegate. The original case was that of a 12-year-old boy whose abnormality was noted in infancy when he was unable to lift his head. He walked at 17 months, never ran well, and suffered from an insidiously progressive weakness affecting almost all of his muscles. There was no familial muscle disease. He was described as having a long, thin face. There was ptosis, severe weakness of the ocular muscles, and facial diplegia. Although the weakness was described as diffuse, particular note was made of weakness of the neck flexors and foot-drop with inversion of the feet. In general, the weakness was slightly more distal than proximal. Areflexia was found. The history was complicated by the occurrence of bilateral subdural hematomas and cerebral atrophy occurring in infancy. Whether associated with this or with the disease itself, the child had motor seizures beginning at the age of 5, which were treated by phenobarbital and diphenylhydantoin. The muscle biopsy showed internal nuclei in a large number of fibers.

Within 3 years, several more cases were described whose clinical pictures and muscle biopsy findings were similar (109–114). A 7-year-old girl had slowly progressive difficulties since birth. She had diffuse weakness with ptosis, extraocular weakness, and facial weakness. She also had areflexia and was of normal intelligenece. A marked equinovarus deformity of the left foot was noted. Since infancy, she had suffered from motor seizures and apneic spells. The biopsy showed Type 1 fiber predominance and a tendency toward Type 1 fiber atrophy, in addition to the internal nuclei (111).

Two teenage sisters had a clinical picture which was almost identical to the latter case, except that there was no weakness of the face (114). Both had an abnormal EEG. The mother of these girls was felt to have a mild ptosis. Muscle biopsy showed the same findings as had been reported in previous cases, although the situation with regard to fiber types was ambiguous. The case reported from Holland was identical (110), with the patient confined to a wheelchair at the age of 27. A 7½-year-old black boy was reported with a similar history (113). The child had a myopathic facies, ptosis, extraocular weakness, facial weakness, and blackout spells with an abnormal EEG. Since all of these patients were clinically identical to the patient described in the original report, they should probably be considered the archetype of this disease. Almost all had ptosis, extraocular palsies, facial weakness, and weakness of the limbs and trunk (Figs. 9.35–9.37). Foot-drop was often found, and sometimes there was an equinovarus deformity of the foot. All except one of these patients were of average intelligence, and all had areflexia. The course of the illness was usually progressive, although in several patients it was very slow. Laboratory studies showed normal or slightly elevated serum CK levels, and EMG studies in three of the reports were "myopathic." Muscle biopsies were very similar in all the patients, with internal nuclei, Type 1 fiber predominance, and an often Type 1 fiber atrophy.

The inheritance of this disorder is not firmly established, many cases seem to be sporadic but an autosomal recessive pattern of inheritance has also been suggested.

Another variety of this illness, if indeed it be the same illness, includes patients whose symptoms are milder and whose weakness is distributed more in the pattern of a limb-girdle dystrophy (112, 115–124). Almost none of

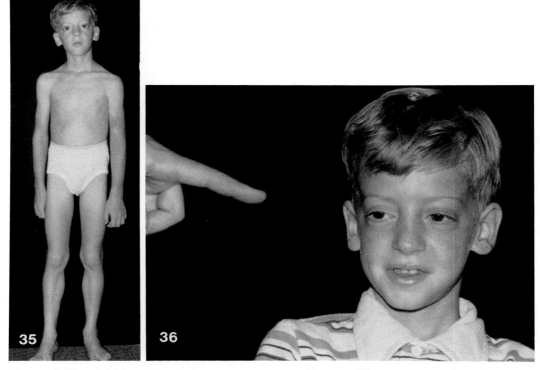

Figures 9.35 and 9.36.   Myotubular myopathy. In addition to diffuse weakness this patient has a defect in ocular movements. In this photograph he is attempting to look at the examiner's finger.

these patients had ptosis or external ophthalmoplegia, and facial weakness was noted in only a few. The disease began at variable times from childhood to middle adult life. Four of the reports indicate an autosomal dominant pattern of inheritance and in one family 16 people were affected (120, 121, 123, 124). I must confess I have never actually seen any of this type of patient although I have seen patients with the pattern of weakness of the limb-girdle musculature whose muscle biopsies demonstated internal nuclei, but lacked the additional findings of Type 1 fiber predominance and Type 1 fiber atrophy which characterize the myotubular myopathy patients.

A third variety of this disorder is inherited as an X-linked recessive. This disorder has been uniformly fatal and the boys die with respiratory failure during the first few months. The symptoms are noted shortly after birth with respiratory difficulty as well as weakness of the extraocular, facial, and neck muscles (125).

TYPE 1 FIBER HYPOTROPHY WITH INTERNAL NUCLEI

This condition may be identical to the infantile form of myotubular myopathy. It also has features in common with congenital fiber type disproportion differing pathologically in the presence of internal nuclei. The original description stressed the association of internal nuclei with small Type 1 fibers in a boy who was born in respiratory distress with diffuse weakness and

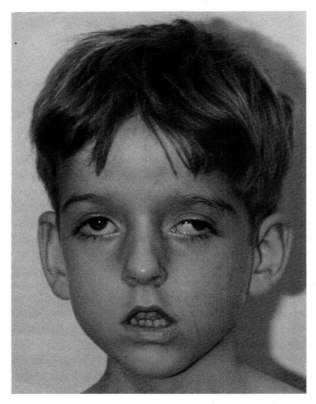

Figure 9.37. Myotubular myopathy. Again notice the defect in extraocular muscles as evidenced by ptosis and divergent gaze.

hypotonia (126). The extraocular muscles and the facial muscles were not involved and there was no ptosis. The child died at the age of 18 months from respiratory complications. Clinically the disorder resembled Werdnig-Hoffmann's disease. A second report documented a similar illness in the patient's brother who died at the age of 7 months (127). The authors suggested that the pattern of inheritance was again that of an X-linked recessive disease.

OTHER MORPHOLOGICAL MYOPATHIES

There are a number of patients reported in the literature whose illnesses are so rare (or possibly their muscle biopsies are so rare) that it is not possible to draw any conclusion about the typical clinical picture. A number of these cases have been characterized on purely morphological grounds. Often these pathological features are to some extent nonspecific and seen in other illness.

Multicore Disease

Two cases of a benign, congenital and nonprogressive muscle disease were described by Engel et al. (128). Several muscle biopsies were obtained and revealed small focal areas of degeneration within the fibers. These bore some resemblance to the change seen in central core disease, but the abnormaliity extended over only a few sarcomeres rather than occupying large parts of the length of the fiber. As in central core disease, the abnormal areas showed a decrease in the number of mitochondria and some disorganization of sarcomere structure beginning in the Z disc.

The patients, who were unrelated, had a life-long history of weakness and their early motor development was retarded. The weakness affected the limbs and trunk, in one patient it was diffuse, whereas in the other the proximal muscles were more severely involved than distal and the shoulders were weaker than the legs. Deep tendon reflexes were decreased and the remainder of the laboratory results were not remarkable. In addition to the "multicores" the biopsy also demonstrated Type 1 fiber predominance, a common finding in congenital hypotonic patients. Subsequent reports have documented similar changes in 6-year-old twins with delayed motor milestones and mild proximal weakness and who were improving (129). Another patient, a 46-year-old man with a progressive history of weakness beginning in middle adult life, was also found to have similar biopsy abnormalities (130). The entity termed "focal loss of cross striations" is also similar in its pathological findings (131).

Sarcotubular Myopathy

Another nonprogressive form of weakness was characterized by Jerusalem et al. (132). Two sons of consanguinous parents suffered from this illness. In both, the attainment of motor milestones was slightly delayed and, when the patients walked or ran, they were noted to be clumsy and awkward. Both demonstrated mild weakness of the neck flexors and of the proximal muscles of all the extremities. There was some weakness of the facial muscles in one patient, and the other was noted to have anterior tibial muscle weakness. Mental development was normal in both cases. The routine laboratory studies showed no specific abnormality; only the muscle biopsy was unusual. Abnormal spaces were found in the fibers. Ultrastructural studies including the use of markers for the membranes of the T system and of the sarcoplasmic reticulum showed that the spaces were probably derived from the membranes of the sarcotubular system (sarcoplasmic reticulum (SR) and T system). The limiting membranes of these spaces were reactive for the SR associated ATPase, and the peroxidase-labeled T tubules were also closely associated with these spaces.

Fingerprint Myopathy

Another nonprogressive, congenital disease characterized by generalized weakness and hypotonia since infancy occurred in a 5-year-old girl. The bulbar muscles and the extraocular muscles were spared, and there was no muscle wasting. Deep tendon reflexes were decreased and a static tremor of the arms was noticed. Intelligence was slightly below the normal level. Most of the laboratory tests were within normal limits. The muscle biopsy showed abnormal inclusions within the muscle fibers which were often subsarcolemmal. With electron microscopy, their structure appeared to be a series of concentric lamellae arranged in spiral fashion and bearing a remarkable resemblance to the pattern of a fingerprint (133). The muscle biopsy also revealed small Type 1 fibers and hypertrophied Type 2 fibers, showing some similarity to congenital fiber type disproportion. A second report described a 1-year-old boy with hypotonia and retarded motor development. Since this description, fingerprint bodies have also been found in myotonic dystrophy, dermatomyositis, and various other conditions (134–136).

A Word of Caution

The clinical descriptions of these last three entities show some noteworthy similarities if they are considered as if they were all one disease. There were 12 in all, 2 of whom were identical twins. With one exception, all were 15 years of age or younger. Three were girls. The disease was noted at birth or in infancy with only two exceptions and in one of these exceptions the illness began in early childhood. Hypotonia was often noted as was a delay of the early motor milestones. Although the weakness was diffuse the trunk and proximal muscles were involved more than the distal muscles. The neck flexors were often noted to be weak. Deep tendon reflexes were decreased in most of the patients. Kyphosis or scoliosis was noted in 3 and muscle contractors were seen in 2 others. In 9 cases the illness was either nonprogressive or only very slowly progressive. A family history of the illness was noted in 8 patients which was compatible with an autosomal recessive inheritance.

The case of multicore disease describd by Bonnette et al. (130) is responsible for many of these exceptions. The patient was said to have the onset of his illness at the age of 33 years, although this is in fact the age at which he retired from his job because of the weakness. He had had a progressive illness with no family history. The CK level was usually normal in this group of diseases although slight elevation was seen in some instances. The EMG, when abnormal, showed changes of a myopathic type. With the exception of pathologic changes which gave the three illnesses their names, the muscle biopsy findings in all of the patients were very similar.

One might even extend such iconoclastic thinking to review the whole range of morphologically characterized myopathies described in this chapter. The morphological changes which seemed so clear-cut in the original descriptions are increasingly being viewed as epiphenomena. Many of the clinical syndromes overlap and, indeed, may be indistinguishable on any grounds other than morphological. It is perhaps too idealistic to believe that, if a morphological change is used to characterize an illness, it should obey some pathologic equivalent of Koch's postulates. Nevertheless, it is worthwhile examining the relationship.

Looking back over the preceding sections there are some very disturbing aspects. The individual pathological changes are often seen in situations in which the patient does not have the illness. It is true that some of these patients may be subclinical cases or carriers, but others have totally unrelated illnesses. Nemaline rods have been found in collagen vascular disease, schizophrenia, parkinsonism, and many other illnesses. They can also be produced experimentally in association with central cores. In addition, central cores are impossible to differentiate from the core targetoid change, which is seen in a wide variety of illnesses. The Type 1 fiber atrophy which characterizes congenital fiber type disproportion has also been noted in myotonic dystrophy, in cerebellar disease, and in rheumatoid arthritis. Fingerprint bodies have been found in myotonic dystrophy, and comments on the nonspecificity of the changes found in multicore myopathy have already been mentioned. In both central core disease and nemaline myopathy, clinically affected relatives have been described in whom cores or rods are lacking. The severity of the change also seems to be unrelated to the clinical weakness in the muscle. Thus, clinically weak muscles have been found without the pathognomonic change; and, on the other hand, clinically normal muscles have been described with the pathological change. The coexistence of central cores and rods is now commonplace enough scarcely to warrant a mention. Scattered rods have also been seen in patients with congenital fiber type disproportion, and I have seen a patient whose biopsy contained rods, cores, and myotubes.

The muscle biopsies of all are characterized by type 1 fiber predominance, with or without Type 1 fiber atrophy. This would include not only central core disease, nemaline myopathy, myotubular myopathy, congenital fiber type disproportion, and the other morphologically distinct myopathies, but also benign congenital hypotonia with Type 1 fiber predominance and some of the patients with congenital muscular dystrophy.

What, then, remains in this group of illnesses if the pathological changes are downgraded? They all share a number of common features. Indeed, if one compares the clinical photographs of patients with centronuclear myopathy (113, 114), congenital fiber type disproportion (37), and nemaline myopathy (87, 88), the similarities are so great that one has the eerie feeling of looking at a family album, even though at least three races are represented. The most common clinical picture is an illness which begins shortly after birth with hypotonia. Hip dislocations or muscle contractures are often found. The attainment of motor milestones is delayed, and the disease is either slowly progressive or static. Typically, there is a rather diffuse weakness of the limbs, although the proximal muscles tend to be slightly weaker than the distal ones. The muscles of the face and neck are affected. The ocular muscles are usually spared, although a ptosis is commented on in several of the patients. Bony deformities with kyphoscoliosis, a long, thin face, a high arched palate, and deformities of the feet (either pes cavus or pes planus) are also common.

Some patients have a much more severe form of illness, although the same distribution of weakness are present. They may develop fatal respiratory difficulties.

Many of the patients inherit the illness according to an autosomal dominant pattern. In others, autosomal recessive inheritance is noted. This should imply at least two types of disease genetically.

The laboratory studies show that the serum muscle enzymes are either normal or slightly elevated. The EMG most often shows a "myopathic" picture, although the abnormalities found may be only minor.

"ODDITIES"

Reducing Body Myopathy

Two unrelated patients with a progressive and fatal disease were described whose muscle biopsies were characterized by the presence of numerous inclusion bodies within the fibers. These had a unique characteristic in that they could be demonstrated by histochemical reactions for sulfhydryl groups (137). Both of these children showed hypotonia very early in life and the motor milestones were retarded. The weakness was progressive and involved both proximal and distal muscles. In one patient, ptosis and facial weakness were noted. Both children died of cardiorespiratory failure. Contracture of the muscles was a prominent feature of one case. A third case with onset at about the age of 4 years also showed a progressive course (138). Other substances were also present within the reducing bodies (RNA and glycogen), but the presence of sulfhydryl groups was striking enough to make the histochemical reaction a useful screening technique (Fig. 9.38). A few structures resembling reducing bodies were also seen in a boy of 14 with a benign congenital myopathy, although there were differences in the ultrastructure of these bodies compared to the ones described above (50). Additionally, this latter case showed marked Type 1 fiber predominance and was quite similar to the congenital hypotonia with Type 1 predominance.

Reducing bodies were so numerous in the muscle of a 7-year-old girl with progressive asymmetrical weakness that a partial biochemical characterization of the structures was possible (140). Two abnormal proteins of molecular weight 62,000 and 53,000 were identified. When sucrose density gradient fractionation was used to isolate the 53,000 Dalton protein, conglomerates of reducing bodies were noted in the solution. Electron microscopy in the same case has confirmed the presence of filaments with a diameter of 17 nm and a 4-nm lumen. The reducing bodies were not reproduced in tissue culture nor was there any evidence of a viral etiology as judged by negative results in following injection of muscle homogenate into rats and primate kidney culture.

Myopathy with Tubular Aggregates

The tubular aggregate is a pathological change in which compact collections of tubules replace part of the muscle fiber. They are visible as tubules only

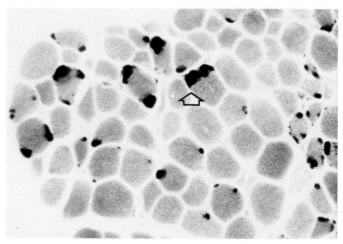

Figure 9.38. Reducing body myopathy. With this stain for reducing substances the abnormal structures are intensely staining (*arrow*) (direct nitro blue tetrazolium (NBT) stain).

under the electron microscope since they have a diameter of 500–600 Å. With the histochemical reaction at the light microscopic level they are easily recognized as intensely blue staining areas with some of the oxidative enzyme reactions (Fig. 9.39). They have been seen in many different diseases, such as the periodic paralyses, and it has also been suggested that the change may be associated with toxins or medications (141). Morgan-Hughes and associates (142) described this change as the characteristic finding in a 60-year-old man who experienced pain and stiffness in the muscles, particularly in the leg, after exercise. Over a 6-year period his exercise tolerance had decreased until he was able to walk only half a mile on level ground or 2–3 minutes uphill. The pain and stiffness would then become severe and could persist for 24 hours or more following the exercise. He had been treated previously for depression and was taking diazepam and nialamide. There were no abnormal laboratory tests other than the muscle biopsy and the ischemic exercise test was normal (142). Four women and one man were affected in three generations of a family whose members experienced aching, stiffness, and leg cramps with mild activity (143). Some degree of proximal weakness was noted. CK levels were mildly to moderately elevated in all the patients. EMG was either normal or showed some myopathic changes. The tubular aggregates were analyzed by immunofluorescent staining with antibodies to sarcoplasic reticular calcium protein and calsequestrin. Both of these proteins are sarcoplasmic reticular components and the tubular aggregates were reactive to both (144). The studies also suggested that the aggregates markedly increased the calcium loading capacity of the affected fibers.

The biopsy of another patient with identical symptoms but no family history is illustrated (Fig.9.39). He had been taking aspirin on an average of twice daily but had not taken any medication for 5 weeks prior to the biopsy.

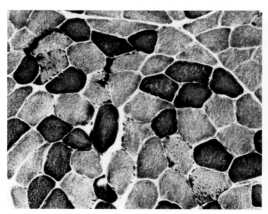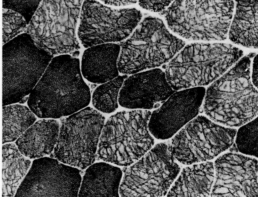

Figure 9.39 (*left*). Myopathy with tubular aggregates. A 45-year-old man had a history of muscle pains for 3 years prior to the biopsy. He had taken aspirin to relieve his discomfort but had not been taking any other mediations. The tubular aggregates can be seen as dark staining areas scattered throughout the muscle biopsy (NADH-tetrazolium reductase).
Figure 9.40 (*right*). In a patient whose only complaint was "toe walking," the oxidative enzyme reaction revealed an abnormal "stranded" appearance to the muscle fibers particularly of the Type 2 fibers. The electron microscopy did not reveal any marked abnormality (NADH tetrazolium reductase).

Toe Walkers

A child who walks with the ball of the foot hitting the ground first rather than the heel may have some serious illness such as Duchenne dystrophy, or "Stick Man" dystrophy, in which case the toe walking is no more than part of a spectrum of signs and symptoms. Occasionally children present with this as the only complaint. In the majority no diagnosis is ever made, passive stretching exercises are prescribed, and the child seems to recover, either because of, or in spite of, the physical therapy.

Sometimes the condition is familial as illustrated by the following example. A 3-year-old girl was referred to the clinic because she was "stiff." Apart from a very slight hip waddle she usually walked in a normal fashion, but on occasion, and particularly when excited, she would walk on her toes. She tired rather easily but she was able to run and keep up with the other children in a normal fashion. There was no other neuromuscular symptom in her history and her motor development had been quite normal. Eleven relatives in four generations had the same symptom including her father. The disease was inherited as an autosomal dominant. On examination, she had mild weakness of the hips so that she stepped up onto a stool with transient unilateral hand support and used bilateral hand support to stand from a squatting position. The deep tendon reflexes were slightly decreased. The strength in the arms appeared normal. The heel cords were tight and dorsiflexion of the foot was possible only to 90°.

Her father was also examined at the age of 31. His only complaint had been that he felt some stiffness of his joints, particularly of the knees and ankles. He also tired more easily than most people. When arising from a very low chair, he occasionally had to use his hands for support but he was able to take part in athletics at high school without any problem. On examination, there was no detectable weakness but the heel cords were tight and dorsiflexion of the foot was not possible beyond 90°. Deep tendon reflexes were normal. The laboratory studies were all normal with the exception of the muscle biopsy which is illustrated (Fig. 9.40). Both father and daughter had identical changes. The oxidative enzyme reaction showed a lacy distortion of the intermyofibrillar network pattern which is, in my experience, unique. Electron microscopic examination of the tissue revealed no abnormality that we could detect, thereby compounding the mystery. The significance of these "lace fibers" remains in doubt.

REFERENCES

1. Dubowitz, V. *The Floppy Infant.* Spastics International Medical Publications, London, 1969.
2. Walton, J. N. Amyotonia congenita. A follow-up study. Lancet *1:* 1023–1028, 1956.
3. Walton, J. N. The limp child. J. Neurol. Neurosurg. Psychiatry *20:* 144–154, 1957.
4. Zellweger, H., and Schneider, H. J. The syndrome of hypotonia, hypomentia, hypogonadism, obesity (HHHO) or Prader-Willi syndrome. Am. J. Dis. Child. *115:* 588, 1958.
5. Bray, G. A., Dahms, W. T., Swerdloff R. S., Fiser R. H., Atkinson R. L., and Carrel, R. E. The Prader-Willi syndrome: a study of 40 patients and a review of the literature. Medicine *62:* 59–80, 1983.
6. Theodoridis, C. H., Brown, C. A., Chance, G. W., and Rudd, B. T. Plasma growth hormone levels in children with Prader-Willi syndrome. Aust. Paediatr. J. *7:* 24, 1971.
7. Afifi, A. K., and Zellweger, H. Pathology of muscular hypotonia in the Prader-Willi syndrome. Light and electron microscopic study. J. Neurol *9:* 49–61, 1969.

8. Windsor, E. J., and Welch J. P., Prader-Willi syndrome associated with inversion of chromosome 15. Clin. Genet. *24:* 456–461, 1983.
9. Hasegawa, T., Hara, M., Ando, M., Osawa, M., Fukuyama, Y., Takahashi, M., and Yamada, K. Cytogenetic studies of familial Prader-Willi syndrome. Hum. Genet. *65:* 325–330, 1984.
10. Mattei, J. F., Mattei, M. G., and Giraud, F. Prader-Willi syndrome and chromosome 15. A clinical discussion of 20 cases. Hum. Genet. 64: 356–362, 1983.
11. Koussett, B. G. The cytogenetic controversy in the Prader-Labhart-Willi syndrome. Am. J. Med. Genet. *13:* 431–439, 1982.
12. Wharton, B. S. An unusual variety of muscular dystrophy. Lancet *1:* 248–249, 1965.
13. Banker B. W., Victor, M., and Adams, R. Arthrogryposis multiplex due to congenital muscular dystrophy. Brain *80:* 319–333, 1957.
14. Short, J. K., Congenital muscular dystrophy. Neurology *13:* 526–530, 1963.
15. Gubbay, S. S., Walton, J. N., and Pearce, G. W. Clinical and pathological study of a case of congenital muscular dystrophy. J. Neurol. Neurosurg. Psychiatry *29:* 500–508, 1966.
16. Pearson, C. M., and Fowler, W. G. Hereditary nonprogressive muscular atrophy inducing arthrogryposis syndrome. Brain *86:* 75–88, 1963.
17. Zellweger, H., Afifi, A., McCormick, W. F., and Mergner, W. Severe congenital muscular dystrophy. Am. J. Dis. Child. *114:* 591–602, 1967.
18. Fukuyama, Y., Haruna, H., and Kawazura, M. A peculiar form of congenital progressive muscular dystrophy. Pediatr. Univ. Tokyo *4:* 4–5, 1960.
19. Fowler, M. C., and Manson, J. L. Congenital muscular dystrophy with malformation of the central nervous system. In: *Clinical Studies in Myology*, edited by B. A. Kakulas. Amsterdam, Elsevier, 1973, pp. 192–197.
20. Fukuyama, Y., Osaw, M., and Suzuki, H. Congenital muscular dystrophy of the fukuyama type—clinical, genetic and pathological considerations. Brain Dev. *3:* 1–29, 1981.
21. Nonaka, I., Sugita, H., Takada, K., and Kumagai, K. Muscle histochemistry in congenital muscular dystrophy with central nervous system involvement. Muscle Nerve *5:* 102–106, 1982.
22. Yoshioka, M., Okuno, T., Honda, Y., and Nakano, Y. Central nervous system involvement in progressive muscular dystrophy. Arch. Dis. Child, *55:* 589–594, 1980.
23. Yoshioka, M., Okuno, T., Ito, M., Konishi, Y., Itagaki, Y., and Sakamoto, Y. Congenital muscular dystrophy (Fukuyama type); repeated CT studies in 19 children. Comput. Tomogr. *5:* 81–88, 1981.
24. Misugi, N. Light and electron microscopic studies of congenital muscular dystrophy. Brain Dev. *2:* 191–199, 1980.
25. Chijiiwa, T., Mishimura, M., Inomata, H., Yamana, T., Narazaki, O., and Kurokawa, T. Ocular manifestations of congenital muscular dystrophy (Fukuyama type). Ann. Ophthalmol. *15:* 921–928, 1983.
26. Kamoshita, S., Konishi, Y., Segawa, M., and Fukuyama, Y. Congenital muscular dystrophy as a disease of the nervous system. Arch. Neurol *33:* 513–516, 1976.
27. Bernier, J. P., Brooke, M. H., Naidich, T. P., and Carroll, J. E. Myoencephalopathy cerebral hypomyelination revealed by CT scan of the head in a muscle disease. Trans. Am. Neurol. Assoc. *104:* 244–246, 1979.
28. Segawa, M., Nomoura, Y., Ogiso, M., et al. Steroid therapy on Fukuyama type congenital muscular dystrophy is effective on the CNS pathology. Brain Dev. *4:* 301, 1982.
29. Ullrich, O. Kongenitale, atonisch-sklerotische Muskel Dystrophie. Z. Gesamte Neurol. Psychiatrie *126:* 171–201, 1930.
30. Furukawa, T., and Toyokura, Y. Congenital hypotonic-sclerotic muscular dystrophy. J. Med. Genet. *14:* 426–429, 1977.
31. Goebel, H. H., Lenard, H. G., Langenbeck, U., and Mehl, B. A form of congenital muscular dystrophy. Brain Dev. *2:* 387–400, 1980.
32. Dubowitz, V. Rigid spine syndrome: a muscle syndrome in search of a name. Proc. R. Soc. Med. *66:* 219, 1973.
33. Jones, R., Khan, R., Hughes, S., and Dubowitz, V. Congenital muscular dystrophy: the importance of early diagnosis and orthopaedic management in the long-term prognosis. J. Bone Joint Surg. *61B:* 13–17, 1979.
34. Brooke, M. H., and Engel, W. K. The histographic analysis of human muscle biopsies with regard to fiber types. 4. Children's biopsies. Neurology *19:* 591–599, 1969.
35. Brooke, M. H. Congenital fiber type disproportion. In: *Clinical Studies in Myology*, edited by B. A. Kakulas. Excerpta Medica, Amsterdam, 1973.
36. Curless, R. G., and Nelson, M. B. Congenital fiber type disproportion in identical twins. Ann. Neurol. *2:* 455–459, 1977.
37. Kinoshita, M., Satoyoshi, E., and Kumagai, M. Familial type 1 fiber atrophy. J. Neurol. Sci. *25:* 11–17, 1975.

38. Lenard, H. G., and Goebel, H. H. Congenital fiber type disproportion. Neuropaediatrie *6:* 220–231, 1975.

39. Fardeau, M., Harpey, J. P., and Caille, B. Disproportion congénitale des différents types de fibre musculaire, avec petitesse relative des fibres de type I. Rev. Neurol. *131:* 745–766, 1975.

40. Martin, J. J., Clara, R., Centerick, C., and Joris, C. Is congenital fiber type disproportion a true myopathy? Acta Neurol. Belg. *76:* 335–344, 1976.

41. Cavanagh, N. P. C., Lake, B. D., and McMeniman, P. Congenital fiber type disproportion myopathy. Arch. Dis. Child. *54:* 735–743, 1979.

42. Argov, Z., Gardner-Medwin, D., Johnson, M. A., and Mastaglia, F. L. Patterns of muscle fiber type disproportion in hypotonic infants. Arch. Neurol. *41:* 53–57, 1984.

43. Goebel, H. H., Lenard, H. G., Goerke, W., and Kunze, K. Fibre type disproportion in the rigid spine syndrome. Neuropaediatrie *8:* 467–477, 1977.

44. Seay, A. R., Ziter, F. A., and Petajan, J. H. Rigid spine syndrome. A type 1 myopathy. Arch. Neurol. *34:* 119–122, 1977.

45. Shy, G. and Magee, K. R. A new congenital nonprogressive myopathy. Brain *79:* 610–621, 1956.

46. Telerman-Toppet, N., Gerard, J. M., and Coers, C. Central core disease; a study of clinically unaffected muscle. J. Neurol. Sci. *19:* 207–223, 1973.

47. Morgan-Hughes, J. A., Brett, E. M., Lake, B. D., and Tome, F. M. S. Central core disease or not? Observations on a family with a nonprogressive myopathy. Brain *96:* 527–536, 1973.

48. Neville, H. E., and Brooke, M. H. Central core fibers; structured and unstructured. In: *Basic Research in Myology,* edited by B. A. Kakulas. Excerpta Medica, Amsterdam, 1973.

49. Engel, W. K., Foster, J. B., Hughes, B. P., Huxley, H. D., and Mahler, R. Central core disease; an investigation of a rare muscle cell abnormality. Brain *84:* 167–185, 1961.

50. Afifi, A. K., Smith, J. W., and Zellweger, H. Congenital nonprogressive myopathy. Central core disease and nemaline myopathy in one family. Neurology *15:* 371–381, 1965.

51. Armstrong, R. M., Koenigsberger, R., Mellinger, J., and Lovelace, R. E. Central core disease with congenital hip dislocation. Neurology *21:* 369–376, 1971.

52. Bethlem, J., van Wijngaarden, G. K., Meijer, A. E. F. H., and Fleury, P. Observations on central core disease. J. Neurol. Sci. *14:* 293–299, 1971.

53. Cohen, M. E., Duffner, P. K., and Heffner, R. Central core disease in one of identical twins. J. Neurol. Neurosurg. Psychiatry *41:* 659–663, 1978.

54. Dubowitz, V., and Roy, S. Central core disease of muscle, clinical, histochemical, and electron microscopic studies of an affected mother and child. Brain *93:* 133–146, 1970.

55. Dubowitz, V., and Sharrard, J. Congenital clubfoot with (?) central core disease. Proc. R. Soc. Med. *61:* 1258–1260, 1968.

56. Gonatas, N. K., Perez, M. C., Shy, G. M., and Evangelist, I. Central "core" disease of skeletal muscle. Am. J. Pathol. *47:* 503–513, 1965.

57. Mrozek, K., Strugalska, M., and Fidzianska, A. A sporadic case of central core disease. J. Neurol. Sci. *10:* 339–348, 1970.

58. Saper, J. R., and Itabashi, H. H. Central core disease. A congenital myopathy. Dis. Nerv. Syst. *37:* 649–653, 1976.

59. Shy, G. M., Engel, W. K., and Wanko, T. Central core disease: a myofibrillary and mitochondrial abnormality of muscle. Ann. Intern. Med. *56:* 511–520, 1962.

60. Byrne, E., Blumbery, P. C., and Hallpike, J. F. Central core disease. Study of a family with five affected generations. J. Neurol. Sci. *53:* 77–83, 1982.

61. Engel, W. K., Brooke, M. H., and Nelson, P. G. Histochemical studies of denervated or tenotomized cat muscle. Ann. N.Y. Acad. Sci. *138:* 160–185, 1966.

62. Frank, J. P., Harat, Y., Butler, I. J., Nelson, T. E., and Scott C. I. Central core disease and malignant hyperthermia syndrome. Ann. Neurol. *7:* 11–17, 1980.

63. Eng, G. D., Epstein, B. S., Engel, W. K., McKay, D. W., and McKay, R. Malignant hyperthermia and central core disease in a child with congenital dislocating hips. Arch. Neurol. *35:* 189–197, 1978.

64. Karpati, G., Carpenter, S., and Eisen, A. A. Experimental corelike lesions and nemaline rods. Arch. Neurol. *27:* 237–251, 1972.

65. Isaacs, H., Heffron, J. J. A., and Badenhorst, M. Central core disease. J. Neurol. Neurosurg. Psychiatry *38:* 1177–1186, 1976.

66. Radu, H., Rosu Servu, A. M., Ionescu, V., and Radu, A. Focal abnormalities in mitochondrial distribution in muscle. Acta Neuropathol. *39:* 25–31, 1977.

67. Ringel, S. P., Bender, A. N., and Engel, W. K. Extrajunctional acetylcholine receptors. Alterations in human and experimental neuromuscular diseases. Arch. Neurol. *33:* 751–758, 1976.

68. Coers, C., Telerman-Toppet, N., Gerard, J. M., Szliwowski, H., Bethlem, J., and van Wijngaarden, G. K. Changes in motor innervation and histochemical pattern of muscle fibers in some congenital myopathies. Neurology *26:* 1046–1053, 1976.

69. Kar, N. C., Pearson, C. M., and Verity, M. A. Muscle fructose-1:6-diphosphatase deficiency associated with an atypical central core disease. J. Neurol. Sci. *48:* 243–256, 1980.

70. Shy, G. M., Engel, W. K., and Wanko, T.: Central core disease: a myofibrillary and mitochondrial abnormality of muscle. Ann. Intern. Med. *56:* 511–520, 1962.

71. Shy, G. M., Engel, W. K., Somers, J. E., and Wanko, T. Nemaline myopathy; a new congenital myopathy. Brain *86:* 793–810, 1963.

72. Conen, P. E., Murphy, G. E., and Donohue, W. L. Light and electron microscopic studies of "myogranules" in a child with hypotonia and muscle weakness. Can. Med. Assoc. J. *89:* 983–986, 1963.

73. Engel, A. G. Late onset rod myopathy (a new syndrome?). Light and electron microscopic observations in two cases. Mayo Clin. Proc. *41:* 713–741, 1966.

74. Kulakowski, S., Flament-Durand, J., Malaisse-Lagae, F., Chevallay, M., and Fardeau, M. Myopathie a batonnets. Arch. Franc. Pediatr. *30:* 505–526, 1973.

75. Feigenbaum, J. A., and Munsat, T. L. A neuromuscular syndrome of scapuloperoneal distribution. Bull. Los Angeles Neurol. Soc. *35:* 47–57, 1970.

76. Kuitunen, P., Rapola, J. Noponen, A.-L., and Donner, M. Nemaline myopathy. Acta Paediatr. Scand. *61:* 353–361, 1972.

77. Kinoshita, M. and Satoyoshi, E. Type I fiber atrophy and nemaline bodies. Arch. Neurol. *31:* 423–425, 1974.

78. Arts, W. F., Bethlem, J., Dingemans, K. P., and Eriksson, A. W. Investigations on the inheritance of nemaline myopathy. Arch. Neurol. *35:* 72–77, 1978.

79. Badurska, B., Fidzianska, A., and Jedrzejowska, H. Nemaline myopathy. Neuropatol. Pol. *8:* 390–397, 1970.

80. Bender, A. N., and Willner, J. P. Nemaline (rod) myopathy. The need for histochemical evaluation of affected families. Ann. Neurol. *4:* 37–42, 1978.

81. Dahl, D. S., and Klutzow, F. W. Congenital rod disease; further evidence of innervational abnormalities as the basis for the clinico-pathological features. J. Neurol. Sci. *23:* 371–385, 1974.

82. Engel, W. K., Wanko, T., and Fenichel, G. M. Nemaline myopathy. Arch. Neurol. *11:* 23–39, 1964.

83. Fukuhara, N., Yuasa, T., Tusubaki, T., Kushiro, S., and Takasawa, N. Nemaline myopathy—histological, histochemical and ultrastructural studies. Acta Neuropathol. *42:* 33–41, 1978.

84. Fulthorpe, J. J., Gardner-Medwin, D., Hudgson, P., and Walton, J. N. Nemaline myopathy. Neurology *19:* 735–748, 1969.

85. Gonatas, N. K. The fine structure of the rod-like bodies in nemaline myopathy and their relation to the Z-discs. J. Neuropathol. Exp. Neurol. *25:* 409–420, 1966.

86. Heffernan, L. P., Rewcastle, N. B., and Humphrey, J. G. The spectrum of the rod myopathies. Arch. Neurol. *18:* 529–542, 1968.

87. Hopkins, I. J., Lindsey, J. R., and Ford, F. F. Nemaline myopathy. A long-term clinico-pathologic study of affected mother and daughter. Brain *89:* 299–310, 1966.

88. Hudgson, P., Gardner-Medwin, D., Fulthorpe, J. J., and Walton, J. N. Nemaline myopathy. Neurology *17:* 1125–1142, 1967.

89. Karpati, G., Carpenter, S., and Andermann, F. A new concept of childhood nemaline myopathy. Arch. Neurol. *24:* 291–303, 1971.

90. Price, H. M., Gordon, G. B., Pearson, C. M., Munsat, T. L., and Blumberg, J. M. New evidence for excessive accumulation of Z-band material in nemaline myopathy. Proc. Natl. Acad. Sci. U.S.A. *54:* 1398–1406, 1965.

91. Radu, H., and Ionescu, V. Nemaline (neuro)myopathy. J. Neurol. Sci. *17:* 53–60, 1972.

92. Sreter, F. A., Astrom, K. E., Romanul, F. C. A., Young, R. R., and Royden-Jones, H. Characteristics of myosin in nemaline myopathy. J. Neurol. Sci. *27:* 99–116, 1976.

93. Shafiq, S. A., Dubowitz, V., Peterson, H. deC., and Milhorat, A. T. Nemaline myopathy. Report of a fatal case with histochemical and electron microscopic studies. Brain *90:* 817–828, 1967.

94. Tsujihata, M., Shimomura, C., Yoshimura, T., Sato, A., Ogawa, T., Tsuji, Y., Nagataki, S., and Matsuo, T. Fatal neonatal nemaline myopathy: a case report. J. Neurol. Neurosurg. Psychiatry *46:* 856–859, 1983.

95. Norton, P., Ellison, P., Sulaiman A. R., and Harb, J. Nemaline and myopathy in the neonate. Neurology *33:* 351–356, 1983.

96. Kondo, K., and Yuasa, T., Genetics of congenital nemaline and myopathy. Muscle Nerve *3:* 308–315, 1980.

97. Engel, W. K., and Warmolts, J. R. The motor unit. Diseases affecting it in toto or in portio. In: *New Developments in Electromyography and Clinical Neurophysiology,* edited by J. E. Desmedt. Karger, Basel, 1973, pp. 141–177.

98. Robertson, W. C., Kawamura, Y., and Dyck, P J. Morphometric study of motoneurons in congenital nemaline myopathy and Werdnig-Hoffman disease. Neurology *28:* 1057–1061, 1978.

99. Karpati, G., Carpenter, S., and Andermann, F. A new concept of childhood nemaline myopathy. Arch. Neurol. *24:* 291–303, 1971.

100. Martinez, A. J., Hay, S., and McNeer, K. W. Extraocular muscles. Light microscopic and ultrastructural features. Acta Neuropathol. *34:* 237–253, 1976.

101. Stromer, M. H., Tabatabai, L. B., Robson, R. M. Goll, D. E., and Zeece, M.G. Nemaline myopathy, an integrated study; selective extraction. Exp. Neurol. *50:* 402–421, 1976.

102. Jennekens, F. G., Roord, J. J., Veldman, H., Willemse, J., and Jockusch, B. M.: Congenital nemaline myopathy; I. Defective organization of alpha actinin is restricted to muscle. Muscle Nerve *6:* 61–68, 1983.

103. Stuhlfauth, I., Jennekens, F. G., Willemse, J., and Jockusch, B. M. Congenital nemaline myopathy; II. Quantitative changes in alpha actinin and myosin in skeletal muscle. Muscle Nerve *6:* 69–74, 1983.

104. Rewcastle, N. B., and Humphrey, J. G. Vacuolar myopathy; clinical, histochemical and microscopic study. Arch. Neurol *12:* 570–582, 1965.

105. Sato, T., Walker, D. L., Peters, H. A., Reese, H. H., and Chou S. M. Chronic polymyositis and myxovirus-like inclusions. Arch. Neurol. *24:* 409–418, 1971.

106. Meltzer, H. Y., McBride, E., and Poppei, R. W. Rod bodies in the skeletal muscle of an acute schizophrenic patient. Neurology *23:* 769–780, 1973.

107. Spiro, A. J., Shy, G. M., and Gonatas, N. K. Myotubular myopathy. Arch.Neurol. *14:* 1–14, 1966.

108. Munsat, T. L., Thompson, L. R., and Coleman, R. F. Centronuclear (myotubular) myopathy. Arch. Neurol. *20:* 120–131, 1969.

109. Badurska, B., Fidzianska, A., Kamieniecka, Z., Prot, J., and Strugalska, H. Myotubular myopathy. J. Neurol. Sci. *8:* 563–571, 1969.

110. Bethlem, J., Meijer, A. E. F. H., Schellens, J. P. M., and Vroom, J. J., Centronuclear myopathy. Eur. Neurol. *1:* 325–333, 1968.

111. Coleman, R. F., Thompson, L. R., Neihuis, A. W., Munsat, T. L., and Pearson, C. M. Histochemical investigation of myotubular myopathy. Arch. Pathol. *86:* 365–376, 1968.

112. Headington, J. T., McNamara, J. D., and Brownell, A. K. Centronuclear myopathy. Histochemistry and electron microscopy. Arch. Pathol. *99:* 16–24, 1975.

113. PeBenito, R., Sher, J. H., and Cracco, J. B. Centronuclear myopathy: clinical and pathologic features. Clin. Pediatr. *17:* 259–265, 1978.

114. Sher, J. H., Rimalovski, A. B., Athanassiades, T. J., and Aronson, S. M. Familial centronuclear myopathy. Neurology *17:* 727–742, 1967.

115. Bethlem, J., Van Wijngaarden, G. K., Meijer, A. E. F. H., and Hulamann, W. C. Neuromuscular disease with Type 1 fiber atrophy; central nuclei and myotube-like structures. Neurology *19:* 705–710, 1969.

116. Goulon, M., Fardeau, M., Got, C., Babinet, P., and Manko, E. Myopathie centronucleaire d'expression clinique tardive. Rev. Neurol. *132:* 275–290, 1976.

117. Harriman, D. G. F., and Haleem, M. R. Centronuclear myopathy in old age. J. Pathol. *108:* 237–248, 1972.

118. Inokuchi, T., Umezaki, H., and Santa, T. A case of type 1 muscle fiber hypotrophy and internal nuclei. J. Neurol. Neurosurg. Psychiatry *38:* 475–482, 1975.

119. Van Wijngaarden, G. K., Fleury, T. Bethlem, J., and Meijer, A. E. F. H. Familial myotubular myopathy. Neurology *19:* 901–908, 1969.

120. McLeod, J. G., Baker, W. De C., Lethlean, A. K., and Shorey, C. D. Centronuclear myopathy with autosomal dominant inheritance. J. Neurol. Sci. *15:* 375–387, 1972.

121. Schochet, S. S., Zellweger, H., Ionasescu, V., and McCormick, W. F. Centronuclear myopathy; disease entity or syndrome. J. Neurol. Sci. *16:* 215–228, 1972.

122. Vital, C. Vallat, J.-M., Martin, F., Le Blanc, M., and Bergouignan, M. Étude clinique et ultrastructurale d'un cas de myopathie centronucléaire (myotubular myopathy) de l'adulte. Rev. Neurol. *123:* 117–130, 1970.

123. Karpati, G., Carpenter, S., and Nelson, R. F. Type 1 muscle fiber atrophy and central nuclei; a rare familial neuromuscular disease. J. Neurol. Sci. *10:* 489–500, 1970.

124. Pepin, B., Mikol, J., Goldstein, B., Haguenau, M., and Godlewski, S. Forme familiale de myopathie centronucleaire de l'adulte. Rev. Neurol. *132:* 845–857, 1976.

125. Barth, P. G., Van Wijngaarden, G. K., and Bethlem, J. X-linked myotubular myopathy with fatal neonatal asphyxia. Neurology *25:* 531–536, 1975.

126. Engel, W. K., Gold, G. N., and Karpati, G. Type 1 fiber hypotrophy and central nuclei. Arch. Neurol. *18:* 435–444, 1968.

127. Meyers, K. R., Gollomb, H. M., Hansen, J. L., and McKusick, V. A. Familial neuromuscular disease with "myotubes." Clin. Genet. *5:* 327–337, 1974.

128. Engel, A. G., Gomez, M. R., and Groover, R. V. Multicore disease; a recently recognized congenital myopathy associated with multifocal degeneration of muscle fibers. Mayo Clin. Proc. *46:* 666–681, 1971.

129. Heffner, R., Cohen, M., Duffner, and P., Diagler, G. Multicore disease in twins. J. Neurol. Neurosurg. Psychiatry *39:* 602–606, 1976.

130. Bonnette, H., Roelofs, R., and Olson, W. H. Multicore disease: report of a case with onset in middle age. Neurology *24:/* 1039–1044, 1974.

131. van Wijngaarden, G. K., Bethlem, J., Dingemans, K. P., Coers, C., Telerman-Toppet, N., and Gerard J. M. Familial focal loss of cross striations. J. Neurol. *216:* 163–172, 1977.

132. Jerusalem, F., Engel, A. G., and Gomez, M. R. Sarcotubular myopathy. Neurology *23:* 897–906, 1973.

133. Engel, A. G., Angelini, C., and Gomez, M. R. Fingerprint body myopathy; a newly recognized congenital muscle disease. Mayo Clin. Proc. *47:* 377–388. 1972.

134. Tomé, F. H. S. and Fardeau, M. Fingerprint inclusions in muscle fibers in dystrophia myotonica. Acta Neuropathol. *24:* 62–67, 1973.

135. Carpenter, S., Karpati, G., Eisen, A, Andermann, F., and Watters, G. Childhood dermatomyositis and familial collagen disease. Neurology *22:* 425, 1972.

136. Sengel, A. and Stoebner, P. Une inclusion musculaire atypique rare: les "corps en empreintes digitales" ou "fingerprint bodies." Acta Neuropathol *27:* 61–68, 1974.

137. Brooke, M. H., and Neville, H. E. Reducing body myopathy. Neurology *22:* 829–840, 1972.

138. Dubowitz, V., and Brooke, M. H. *Muscle Biopsy: A Modern Approach.* W. B. Saunders, London, 1973, p. 351.

139. Tomé, F. H. S. and Fardeau, M. Congenital myopathy with "reducing bodies" in muscle fibers. Acta Neuropathol. *31:* 207–217, 1975.

140. Carpenter, S., Karpati, G., and Holland, P. New observations in reducing body myopathy. Neurology *35:* 818–827, 1985.

141. Engel, W. K., Bishop, D.W., and Cunningham, G. G. Tubular aggregates in type II muscle fibers; ultrastructural and histochemical correlation. J. Ultrastruc. Res. *31:* 507–525, 1970.

142. Morgan-Hughes, J. A., Mair, W. G. P., and Lascelles, P. T. A disorder of skeletal muscle associated with tubular aggregates. Brain *93:* 873–880, 1970.

143. Pierobon-Bormioli, S., Armani, M., Ringel, S. P., Angelini, C., Vergani, L., Betto, R., and Salviati, G. Familial neuromuscular disease with tubular aggregates. Muscle Nerve *8:* 291–198, 1985.

144. Salviati, G., Pierobon-Bormioli, S., Betto, R., Damiani, E., Angelini, C., Ringel, S. P., Salvatori, S., and Margreth, A. Tubular aggregates: sarcoplasmic reticulum origin, calcium storage ability and functional implications. Muscle Nerve *8:* 299–306, 1985.

Index